Clinical Manual of Psychiatric Diagnosis and Treatment: A Biopsychosocial Approach

Clinical Manual of Psychiatric Diagnosis and Treatment: A Biopsychosocial Approach

Ronald W. Pies, M.D.
Associate Clinical Professor of Psychiatry
Tufts University School of Medicine
Boston, Massachusetts;
Lecturer on Psychiatry
Harvard University School of Medicine
Boston, Massachusetts;
Director, Psychopharmacology Service
Dr. Harry C. Solomon Mental Health Center
Lowell, Massachusetts

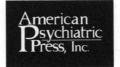

Washington, DC
London, England

Copyright © 1994 American Psychiatric Press, Inc.

ALL RIGHTS RESERVED
Manufactured in the United States of America on acid-free paper

First Edition 97 96 95 94   4 3 2 1

American Psychiatric Press, Inc.
1400 K Street, N.W., Washington, DC 20005

Library of Congress Cataloging-in-Publication Data
Pies, Ronald W., 1952–
    Clinical manual of psychiatric diagnosis and treatment : a biopsychosocial approach / Ronald W. Pies. — 1st ed.
        p.   cm.
    Includes bibliographical references and index.
    ISBN 0-88048-534-5 (alk. paper)
        1. Psychology, Pathological. 2. Mental illness—Diagnosis.
    3. Mental illness—Treatment. I. Title.
        [DNLM: 1. Mental Disorders—diagnosis. 2. Mental Disorders—therapy. WM 100 P624c 1994.
    RC454.P524 1994
    616.89—dc20
DNLM/DLC   93-48517
for Library of Congress   CIP

British Library Cataloguing in Publication Data
A CIP record is available from the British Library.

Contents

List of
Tables and Figures

Tables

Figures

Foreword

It is more than three decades since George Engel defined an approach for the understanding of human diversity. His model encompassed the conceptually separable disciplines of biology, psychology, and social science and became a touchstone for psychiatric education. The model challenged us to be inclusive and, with that, to extend our depth of understanding. Much has been written about the virtue of Engel's model and relatively little within the framework he erected.

Psychiatry, however, has recently traveled a road away from that position. The direction has been toward objectivity as the ideal, and there has been a narrowing of psychiatric inquiry in favor of the first part only of Engel's trinity. One can see this direction in the publishing trends in psychiatric journals and the emphasis on reductionism in the training of clinicians. Funding in research is directed more and more toward less and less. Board examiners also often find that candidates cannot obtain a comprehensive history and are then unable to articulate a clinically useful picture of a human in distress. There is a growing avoidance of the patient's unique perception of his or her world. The aim of psychiatry is now locked onto a restricted scientific target, in deference to a scientific paradigm borrowed from classical physics and misapplied. Psychiatry bears the risk (as Leon Eisenberg, among others, suggests) of becoming "mindless."

In a manner of speaking, all psychiatry is "biological psychiatry," and the rest is the province of theology. We are *in* nature and a part of it, and, at least since we entered the Holocene, we have shaped nature so profoundly that we speak, for good reasons, of another form of nature, that is, human nature. We connect with each other and change each other, and the environment we create changes us. Neuronal tissue grows in response to its environment at least as much as it is obedient to any lockstep process choreographed immutably by the "gene machine." We are creatures in nature, but we create our own nature and select each other on the basis of the fitness to that human environment, so that civilization is enfolded into genetic mechanism, and genetic mechanism into civilization. If we are to understand patients and, as doctors, to help them, we require the broadest base. Yes, biopsychosocial—and that includes civilization—ours and others'. We certainly need reductionistic research, but we should also pursue greater understanding of the psychological and social environment. That task is further informed by literature—poetry, philosophy, theater. That is our "biology" also.

Now Dr. Ronald Pies has taken on the major task of writing a book *within* the biopsychosocial model, not writing about it, as I am doing far more easily in this foreword. He comes to this task prepared. He is a highly respected psychopharmacologist with a strong background in neurology and neuroscience. He has now put into print his years as a clinician and teacher. Yet his enthusiastic and eloquent pursuit of understanding human complaints has always been accompanied by widest acquaintance with world literature. He writes poetry when he is not doing psychiatry. Although his own work as a poet is not seen in this volume, his way of understanding the range of human diversity is found here in the poetry and philosophy of others.

Dr. Pies' initial disclaimer about not presenting a "comprehensive text" is written in sincere humility by the author; there is, however, in this volume a broad base for general information. Dr. Pies presents the psychiatric disorders by means of interspersed clinical vignettes and sections on treatment and management. His references are always current and relevant. The conclusion at the end of every chapter tells you where you have been and points the direction back to where you might find something you missed.

The biopsychosocial model is a large envelope to fill. Dr Pies stays focused on the clinical picture. He makes use of theoretical constructions and much of the empirical data of the separate disciplines within the model, and, with the empathy of the teacher, he is aware that he is taking the reader on a long journey. What helps, of course, is his easy manner. The book you will read is authentic and assiduously researched, but the tone is relaxed, as in conversation with somebody who has thought long and deeply on extremely complex issues.

The author says that he has written the book for third- and fourth-year residents in psychiatry. Indeed this could be a most helpful volume for The Board examinations. But all will find it textured yet readable, and very user friendly.

Theodore Nadelson, M.D.

Introduction

It is probably unusual to introduce a book by describing what the work is not; yet in this instance I think such a negative description will help orient and guide the reader.

First, this is not a "comprehensive textbook" of psychiatry. I did not include chapters on eating disorders or impulse control disorders, for example. These are important topics, but they did not fit into the overarching purpose of this book, which is to familiarize the reader with the most common, pervasive, and incapacitating disorders he or she is likely to encounter in adult clinical psychiatry. Second, this is neither a manual of psychopharmacology nor a book on "how to do psychotherapy." Rather, in the "Treatment Directions and Goals" section of each major topic, I have tried to point out the most important issues in the pharmacological and psychotherapeutic treatment of the patient. I believe I have included enough basic information to guide the reader in the fundamental concepts of pharmaco- and psychotherapy. In some instances—particularly in reference to some psychotropics—I have made rather specific comments as to dosage, blood levels, etc. Appropriate references are always given for more detailed information.

This book, finally, is not a variant or alternative "DSM." It was both frustrating and liberating to write most of the book during the transitional period from DSM-III-R to DSM-IV; frustrating, because of the long "wait" to see what the new manual would say, and liberating, because I was induced to capture the "essence" of the various disorders without recourse to DSM-type lists of criteria. Instead, each major topic has a "Central Concept" section that depicts the principal features of the illness by means of a clinical vignette. Indeed, such vignettes abound throughout the book, based on my conviction that nothing teaches so well as a clinical example. That these anecdotes may omit one or another of the "official" criteria is of less concern to me than that the reader remember the clinical example. To this end, I have sometimes employed humorous fictitious names or bilingual puns, which, I am sure, will not amuse everyone—but then, good teaching often flourishes atop a bad joke.

All of us, of course, are indebted to the authors of both DSM-III-R and its recent offspring, DSM-IV, for their commitment to clear and rigorous diagnostic thinking. I have included material from DSM-IV in instances when it differs significantly from DSM-III-R, or when it contributes to an important "teaching point."

I have consistently provided a "historical perspective" for each of the major syndromes discussed. I don't assume that this material will be of interest to everyone, but I do maintain that it is of importance to the beginning clinician—particularly the resident in psychiatry, who sometimes gets the message that our current nosology sprang full-blown from the brow of some official committee. I have tried to show how the various DSM categories have evolved from many earlier concepts of mental illness, sometimes dating from classical times. I have also included a good deal of material on psychological testing, on the premise that we psychiatrists need to be able to communicate with our colleagues in clinical psychology. To be sure, the psychiatric resident is unlikely to do psychological testing, but he or she will constantly be exposed to data from the MMPI, WAIS-R, Bender-Gestalt, and even the Rorschach.

By now, it should be evident that my intended readership is primarily the third- or fourth-year resident in psychiatry who is eager to go beyond the cookbook approach to diagnosis, and who wishes to gain a broad understanding of the "biopsychosocial" model. Indeed, the latter is the cornerstone of the entire book. The central assumption throughout the text is that the clinican must be able to integrate the complex biological, psychological, and sociocultural data of the case at hand. I believe this text will also be helpful to the more experienced clinician who wishes to review the biopsychosocial aspects of diagnosis and treatment—either in preparation for board examinations or in pursuit of enriched understanding.

Many individuals deserve credit for whatever merits this book possesses. I wish first to thank Carol Nadelson for her encouragement over the 6 years in which the book took shape. Claire Reinburg and

Pam Harley provided expert editorial assistance. My students over the years—particularly those at Tufts—have been an important source of inspiration and instruction. My teachers and colleagues in Syracuse and Boston were important influences on my "biopsychosocial" orientation. Finally, I want to thank Nancy Butters, L.I.C.S.W., for her unflagging support during many a despairing hour, and her invaluable editorial suggestions. The book would not have reached "parturition" without her help.

1

The Diagnostic Formulation

I never know what I think until I read what I write.
—attributed to E. M. Forster

What is a diagnostic formulation? It is as close an approximation to understanding the "whole person" as a psychiatrist initially can achieve. It is a comprehensive attempt to utilize the "biopsychosocial" model (Engel 1977) in a practical clinical manner. Most important, perhaps, the diagnostic formulation embodies all that is unique about psychiatry—for no other discipline strives so rigorously to uncover and integrate biological, psychological, and social components of mental illness.

In DSM-III-R (American Psychiatric Association 1987), some attempt was made to delineate the "psychosocial stressors" in the patient's life and the "global functioning" of the patient. Axis IV, for example, instructed the clinician to code "the overall severity of a psychosocial stressor or multiple psychosocial stressors that have occurred in the year preceding the current evaluation" (p. 18) and that may have contributed to the patient's psychopathology (e.g., death of a spouse, becoming a parent, etc.). DSM-IV (American Psychiatric Association 1994) drops this quantitative approach and instead uses a more descriptive approach to "psychosocial and environmental problems" (p. 29). The categories now include "occupational problems," "problems related to the social environment," "economic problems," and so on. Even "good" stressors may be listed when they are psychologically disruptive (e.g., a job promotion that imposes new burdens on the patient). (If the social problem is the main focus of treatment, it should be coded on Axis I.)

Axis V indicates the clinician's judgment of the individual's overall level of psychosocial functioning. It utilizes the semiquantitative Global Assessment of Functioning (GAF) Scale, which assesses such dimensions as ability to maintain personal hygiene, "test reality," and function on the job.

Although important in itself, the use of these DSM-IV axes does not yield an integrated understanding of the whole person—to the extent that one's limited knowledge may permit. This *gestalt* is the aim of the diagnostic formulation. The diagnostic formulation incorporates the classical "psychodynamic formulation" of the patient, but goes well beyond it. The diagnostic formulation attempts to show how a variety of biomedical and sociocultural factors impinge on and transmute the patient's "psychodynamics." Indeed, sometimes our psychodynamic "understanding" of a patient proves illusory, in light of overwhelming biomedical or social factors. Witness the futility of understanding the dynamics of "hysterical conversion symptoms" when these prove to be secondary to multiple sclerosis (MS). But, of course, even in MS the patient can go on to develop conversion symptoms, just as pseudoseizures are often "installed" on an underlying organic disorder. It is this complex interplay of the organic and functional, which we explore in Chapter 3, that makes the diagnostic formulation so critical. So, too, with the role of sociocultural factors. A lower-social-class rural black woman from Haiti who speaks of a "hex" upon her, or a Mexican-American who speaks of *mal ojo* ("the evil eye"), is not to be understood solely in "psychodynamic" terms, which are essentially the product of Euro-American psychiatric theory.

With these complexities in mind, let's examine the keystone of our diagnostic formulation: the biopsychosocial model.

The Biopsychosocial Model

In 1960, George Engel, M.D., began to elaborate "a unified concept of health and disease"—a concept that evolved the *biopsychosocial model.* This model posits that whether a cell or a person, every system is influenced by the continuation of the systems of which each is a part (e.g., one's family, community, culture, and nation). It is not my intention to elaborate on Engel's concept, but to provide the specific clinical underpinnings of his model. How, in other words, can the psychiatrist utilize the biopsychosocial model in understanding the patient? What are the "bio-," "psycho-," and "social" parts of this model? What are the practical instances in which this model is useful?

Biomedical Factors in Psychiatric Illness

From birth to death, the human being is both the product and the target of biochemical forces. What we are is limited, primordially, by our genetic endowment. What we become is further shaped by neo-natal traumata, childhood illnesses, hormonal and neurological disorders, a plethora of other physical ailments, and the substances we put into our bodies. All these factors are of relevance to the psychiatrist and may be directly implicated in the patient's psychopathology.

Vignette

Lenny was a reclusive and shy 16-year-old who did poorly in school and was often teased by his classmates for being overweight and "an airhead." Occasionally, Lenny would get in trouble for breaking windows or stealing from other students. Psychological testing revealed an IQ of 70 (subnormal). Physical examination revealed underdeveloped secondary sexual characteristics and small, firm testes. Chromosomal analyses showed the XXY karyotype of Klinefelter's syndrome.

A host of chromosomal abnormalities may be associated with psychiatric symptoms. Down's syndrome, marked by mental deficiency but no specific behavioral disturbance, is quite well known. Less recognized, and still poorly understood, is the 47-chromosome XYY genotype. Some evidence—though controversial—points to an unexpectedly high incidence of aggressive, impulsive behavior in these XYY individuals.

The genetic contribution to psychopathology, of course, goes beyond gross chromosomal aberrations. A variety of neuropsychiatric syndromes have well-defined genetic inheritance patterns.

Vignette

A 14-year-old girl showed "neurotic" traits sufficient to warrant psychotherapy. Over the ensuing 5 months she became psychotically depressed and manifested a peculiar combination of tremor and choreoathetoid movements. Her liver functions were elevated and her ceruloplasmin level was low. The diagnosis of Wilson's disease was made.

Wilson's disease is inherited in an autosomal recessive fashion. Huntington's chorea, which may manifest with *psychiatric* symptoms before neurological ones, is inherited as an autosomal dominant condition. These are but a few of the genetically based conditions that may have psychiatric complications (see Table 1–1).

If we are fortunate enough to find ourselves in the womb with all our chromosomes in good shape, we must still square off against a

Table 1–1. Genetically based conditions with neuropsychiatric complications

---

Chromosomal aberrations

Down's syndrome: trisomy (chromosome) 21

Cri du chat (cat-cry) syndrome: deletion of short arm, chromosome 5

Edwards syndrome: trisomy (chromosome) 18

Autosomal recessive conditions

Phenylketonuria

Wilson's disease

Lesch-Nyhan syndrome

Autosomal dominant conditions

Huntington's disease

Tuberous sclerosis

Source. Extensively modified from Jervis 1975.

host of pre-, peri-, and postnatal assailants. Toxemia of pregnancy, uncontrolled maternal diabetes, maternal malnutrition, and placenta previa may all threaten the developing brain. Complications of labor or delivery—such as "breech birth" or prolonged labor—can lead to fetal hypoxia and attendant brain damage. Postnatal factors, such as meningoencephalitis, lead poisoning, or malnutrition, can permanently damage the infant's central nervous system (CNS) and produce neuropsychiatric complications in later life. (This is why a "developmental" history and "prenatal" history are critical parts of the complete psychiatric history.)

A variety of neuropsychiatric disorders that have their onset in childhood have profound effects on adult psychopathology. Consider the following vignette.

Vignette

A 21-year-old male carried the diagnosis of "borderline personality disorder." His behavior was impulsive, labile, and often violent. He had several arrests for shoplifting and disorderly conduct. He complained of frequent bouts of anxiety and depression and of "feeling hyper all my life." A school history revealed an inability to sit still in class, difficulty with attention, and "rowdy" behavior on the playground. His parents related the patient's inability as a child to watch television "for more than 5 minutes at a stretch." A diagnosis of "adult attention-deficit disorder" was made. The patient was treated with methylphenidate, 20 mg/day, and showed marked improvement in behavior and mood.

There is good evidence that attention-deficit disorder has a strong biological component, as is also the case with Tourette's disorder. However, both conditions are affected by—and, in turn, affect—the psychosocial milieu in which the child or adolescent develops.

The biological part of the biopsychosocial model is heavily influenced by a variety of neuroendocrine disorders (Table 1–2). The organs most often implicated are the thyroid, parathyroid, and adrenal glands. However, we are just beginning to appreciate the role of more subtle neuroendocrine factors, such as neuropeptides. Thus, there is evidence that adrenocorticotropic hormone (ACTH), β-endorphin, vasopressin, and related peptides affect motivation, attention, and memory. Abnormalities in levels of some neuropeptides have been found in the brains of patients with Alzheimer's disease and Huntington's disease; for example, there may be reduced levels of somatostatin in the brains of Alzheimer's disease patients (Ferrier et al. 1983).

Vignette

A 34-year-old businessman complained of easy fatigability, generalized weakness, insomnia, and weight loss. He said his appetite was "fine." Three months later, he seemed agitated, hyperactive, and disoriented, stating that he was "King of the Jews." On physical examination, the patient showed hyperreflexia, tachycardia, and moist, warm skin. Laboratory studies revealed marked hyperthyroidism.

While endocrine disorders may directly affect the CNS, a variety of nonendocrine organic conditions are associated with psychiatric symptoms. Some clinicians refer to these as "somatopsychic" disorders, implying that the "direction" of cause and effect is from soma to psyche. (The time-honored *psychosomatic disorders* are incorporated in DSM-IV under the heading "Psychological Factors Affecting Medical Condition." Examples include migraine headache, asthma, duodenal ulcer, and ulcerative colitis.) We do not generally know the mecha-

Table 1–2. Neuroendocrine disorders with psychiatric complications

Hyper-, hypothyroidism

Hyper-, hypoparathyroidism

Adrenocortical insufficiency (Addison's disease)

Adrenocortical excess (Cushing's syndrome)

Pheochromocytoma

Diabetes mellitus

Insulinoma

nisms by which such somatic factors act on the psyche. Thus, pancreatic carcinoma is associated with an unexpectedly high incidence of depression, long before the patient is aware of the diagnosis, and in excess of the depression associated with other abdominal malignancies. (Could some as yet undetected neuropeptide be involved?) Pernicious anemia, systemic lupus erythematosus (SLE), and parkinsonism are also associated with depression. A multitude of prescription drugs can affect the psyche, especially antihypertensive and steroid medications.

Vignette

A 40-year-old female had boarded up all the windows of her house because "the neighbors are spying on me." The patient was fully oriented, and recent and remote memory were intact. The physical examination was normal, but laboratory testing showed normocytic anemia, leukopenia, and red cell casts in the urine. Antinuclear antibody (ANA) testing was strongly positive. A diagnosis of "SLE, r/o lupus cerebritis" was made. Treatment with prednisone led to reduction in the patient's psychosis.

An important component of the "bio-" part of our model is the *intercurrent physical illness* that may be affecting the patient's psyche. This influence is probably not via neuropeptides or specific chemical factors, but through effects on the patient's coping mechanisms, self-esteem, and body image. For example, a patient who becomes aware that he or she has a chronic, unremitting illness may undergo a period of marked depression or regression. This has become poignantly evident in patients with acquired immune deficiency syndrome (AIDS), but it may also be true for patients with emphysema, parkinsonism, or cerebrovascular disease. (There may also be neurochemical or neuroendocrine mechanisms involved in the depression associated with parkinsonism or stroke.) Frequently, patients with chronic illness become angry with their family or physician. They may become overly dependent on the physician for attention, medication, or both. Hospitalization may promote severe, "childlike" regression, and discharge may provoke further psychological deterioration. The patient's family may also experience anger and frustration in having to care for their chronically ill relative. All these facts become relevant in the diagnostic formulation of the psychiatric patient with intercurrent physical illness.

Vignette

A 78-year-old female was admitted to the psychogeriatric service for treatment of depression. She had suffered from severe chronic obstructive pulmonary disease (COPD) for many years, but had been cared for at home, with the aid of "home oxygen," by her son and daughter-in-law. Recently, the patient's COPD had worsened, and the patient expressed suicidal ideation. She ate poorly and lost 18 pounds over a 2-month period. Her son and daughter-in-law expressed anger that the patient "is damn ungrateful for all the care we've given her." On physical examination, old and new burn marks were discovered on the patient's back and buttocks. "Elder abuse" was confirmed after a social service investigation.

Another area of critical concern to the psychiatrist is that of *substance abuse, dependence,* and *withdrawal.* The drug-abusing patient often poses a diagnostic dilemma, because it is virtually impossible to make a "psychiatric" diagnosis in the presence of severe drug abuse or withdrawal. Thus, many seemingly "depressed" alcoholic persons—once "detoxed" in an inpatient setting—lose their depressive features quite rapidly. Similarly, patients with drug-induced psychoses may remit in a matter of days, having been admitted with a diagnosis of "r/o schizophrenia." As we shall see in Chapter 10, treatment decisions are often adversely affected by the failure to recognize a primary substance abuse problem.

Vignette

A 43-year-old divorced male was admitted for treatment of "severe depression." He gave a history of recent weight loss, poor concentration, and insomnia, which he attributed to his divorce, some 6 weeks prior to admission. However, the resident in charge of Joe's care uncovered a history of severe alcohol abuse for the past

4 months. Although the patient had an abnormal dexamethasone suppression test (DST: see Chapter 2) and a high score on the Beck Depression Inventory (BDI), he was not treated with an antidepressant. After 3 weeks on the unit, the patient's DST normalized and his score on the BDI dropped into the "mildly depressed" range. Group therapy and regular Alcoholics Anonymous attendance resulted in dramatic improvement.

Let us summarize the biological component of our biopsychosocial model. The diagnostic formulation must consider a host of biomedical factors related to the patient's psychiatric symptoms. These include genetic endowment; pre-, post-, and neonatal traumata; neurological illness; neuroendocrine disorders; intercurrent medical illness; and substance abuse or withdrawal.

Psychological Factors in Psychiatric Illness

When we are confronted with a psychiatric patient in distress, there are two basic "psychological" questions we must answer: how is this person psychically "put together," and how is the individual's "core conflict" to be understood? But what do we mean by "put together" and "core conflict"? There are many answers to these questions, but among the most useful are those given by Roger A. MacKinnon (1980) and—in the area of the "core conflict"—by Perry, Cooper, and Michels (1987).

The Ego and Its Defenses

MacKinnon (1980) has outlined what he calls the "organization of ego functions." The ego, of course, is the "executive apparatus" of the mind. As MacKinnon notes, "All ego functions serve the basic task of the organism's adaptation to the environment to ensure survival while allowing for the gratification of needs" (pp. 913–914). MacKinnon points out that the "biological substrate of the ego lies within the basic physiological processes of perception, concentration, motor behavior, memory, cognition" (p. 914), and other cognitive processes. In short, the "ego" is not some monolithic structure in the mind, but rather the integrated product of many adaptive functions. By assessing these functions, we can gauge the individual's "ego strength." This, in turn, has profound implications for treatment. For example, one would not treat a schizophrenic patient with classical psychoanalysis; the patient usually lacks the "ego strength" to withstand such an intense psychic exploration. Even most "borderline" patients (see Chapter 9) would not be suitable for unmodified psychoanalysis, and, indeed, they were described historically as patients who "fall apart on the couch." Thus, MacKinnon's framework is of more than theoretical importance.

MacKinnon lists eight general types of ego functions (Table 1–3; see below). A complete psychological understanding of the patient would include an appraisal of these functions, as well as the "psychodynamic formulation"—that is, the understanding of the core conflict. Of course, one doesn't necessarily (or even commonly) include all such material in a "case write-up"; but one must keep these issues in mind in order to provide good therapy.

Vignette

A 19-year-old male schizophrenic patient regularly received fluphenazine decanoate injections every 2 weeks, following a brief meeting with his outpatient psychiatric resident. At one such meeting, the patient commented that "they must get these needles from

Table 1–3.   Organization of ego functions

Defense formation

Regulation and control of drives, affects, and impulses

Relationship to others

Self-representation/self-esteem

Synthetic-integrative functioning

Stimulus regulation

Adaptive regression in the service of the ego

Reality testing and sense of reality

Source.   Extensively modified from MacKinnon 1980.

the horse doctors." He appeared quite anxious, and the resident felt that "an interpretation" was necessary. The resident commented that "sometimes long needles can be sexually threatening to men." The patient seemed to ignore this comment and changed the subject. He received his injection but never again appeared for his treatment.

MacKinnon has described these eight functions in considerable detail. But the clinician can compress an assessment of these functions into 16 basic questions, as follows:

Defense formation

1. Do the patient's defense mechanisms successfully mediate between id and superego demands?
2. Are the patient's defenses mainly primitive or mature?

Regulation and control of drives, affects, and impulses

1. Can the patient tolerate delay, tension, and frustration?
2. Can the patient sublimate—that is, channel drives into acceptable substitute behaviors?

Relationship to others

1. Can the patient experience others as "whole" persons with both good and bad traits?
2. Can the patient form emotionally rich and enduring relationships?

Self-representation/self-esteem

1. Does the patient have a reasonable degree of self-confidence and self-esteem?
2. Does the patient possess a balanced, "holistic" sense of self, incorporating both good and bad traits?

Synthetic-integrative functioning

1. Can the patient reconcile inconsistent or contradictory aspects of

self and others, and act appropriately in the face of such contradictions?
2. Can the patient integrate knowledge gained from new experiences
in a constructive way?

Stimulus regulation

1. Can the patient "screen out" extraneous or excessive stimuli in
order to pursue constructive goals (e.g., reading, job task, etc.)?
2. Can the patient provide himself or herself with sufficient stimulation to maintain intrapsychic and interpersonal stability?

Adaptive regression in the service of the ego

1. Can the patient "relax" enough to enjoy sex, music, hobbies, and
so forth?
2. Is the patient open to new experiences in these areas?

Reality testing and sense of reality

1. Can the patient maintain adequate boundaries between "self" and
"other"?
2. Can the patient reason objectively to distinguish wish or imagina-
tion from external reality?

Admittedly, the ego functions described by MacKinnon cover
a lot of ground. How can we understand their practical and clinical
importance? Let us consider the case of Saul R., with MacKinnon's
ego functions clearly in mind:

Saul was a 23-year-old single male who presented in the emergency
room after slashing his wrists. He stated that this occurred "after my
girlfriend bummed me out." It emerged that Saul had witnessed his
girlfriend coming out of a convenience store with a young man, who
appeared to be joking with her. Saul concluded, "She's gotta be
fooling around behind my back." He described the girlfriend as

"a total dirtball . . . a real bitch." When the ER resident, a young male, suggested that Saul might be overreacting to the incident, Saul became enraged, shouting, "What are you, queer or something?" Saul had to be physically restrained. At that point, he began to sob, stating, "I knew she'd leave me. I'm just garbage, anyway."

It should be evident that Saul has deficits in a number of the ego functions we have delineated. His totally negative view of his girlfriend suggests the use of "splitting." His ability to regulate affect is clearly impaired, as exemplified in his wrist cutting. He appears to have rather shallow and unstable interpersonal relationships, though we do not have sufficient history to state this with confidence. Saul's self-representation and self-image appear to be quite distorted ("I'm just garbage anyway"), though, again, we need more longitudinal information to decide whether this is a "state" or "trait." (By the way, one might speculate that Saul's extremely negative description of his girlfriend is actually a *projection* of his own split-off representation of "bad me.") Clearly, Saul's capacity to integrate new experience and to test reality is quite limited, if his current response is typical for him. We might reach quite different conclusions, of course, if it turned out that Saul was intoxicated on amphetamines. Again, the distinction between "state" and "trait" is crucial.

Understanding the Core Conflict: The Psychodynamic Formulation

Having arrived at some idea of how the patient is "put together," we must now understand how he or she has come "unglued." Perry, Cooper, and Michels (1987) approach this question by means of the *psychodynamic formulation,* which, in essence, explains the patient's central or "core" conflicts, their role in the current (dysfunctional) situation, and their developmental origins. The psychodynamic formulation relies on psychoanalytic principles, such as the interpretation of unconscious fantasies, but goes beyond "Freudian" formulations. Indeed, Perry and colleagues incorporate *ego-psychological, self-psychological,* and *object-relations* models into their schema. A detailed exploration of these models would itself require several chapters. Instead, we shall briefly describe them and then quickly move on to their practical application. We shall also add a "fourth dimension" to the psychodynamic formulation: the *cognitive-behavioral model*. Although "cognitive-behavioral" factors are usually contrasted with "psychodynamic" ones, we shall see that this distinction is largely illusory. Indeed, a richer understanding of the patient's conflict is gained when the cognitive-behavioral dimension is integrated with the other three models.

The ego-psychological model emphasizes the "defensive compromises" mediated by the ego. For example, such compromises may occur in mediating among primitive wishes, superego constraints, and the demands of reality. This model is directly linked to MacKinnon's description of the ego functions. After all, the "compromises" we make depend on how strong a "hand" we hold. Thus the symptoms we develop are determined by the characteristic ego defenses at our disposal. The ego-psychological model explores these defenses in relation to the individual's unconscious wishes and fears.

Vignette

A 19-year-old female developed a functionally "paralyzed" right arm. In the course of psychotherapy, it emerged that the patient had been fondled inappropriately by her father when she was 3 years old. She also recalled that on the day prior to her paralysis, her father had approached her in her bedroom and remarked, "You look really hot tonight, baby." The patient felt "a mixture of hating him and being turned on." She slapped her father's face but awakened the next morning unable to move the arm she had used to slap him.

The ego-psychological model would explain the patient's symptom as a *defensive compromise* between her (illicit) attraction and her rage. Developmentally, the patient was "set up" for such a reaction by her father's sexual abuse. (Recalling MacKinnon's ego functions, we would conclude that *conversion,* a relatively primitive defense, was employed by the patient's ego.)

The self-psychological model emphasizes the empathic failures in the child's development that distort and inhibit the self. For example, extremely cold, withholding parents may foster the development of an insecure, approval-hungry child. The defensive compensations of such a child form the basis of some narcissistic disorders, and the self-psychological model is quite useful in understanding such patients.

The object-relations model emphasizes the "internal representation" of self and others. (Recall that two of the ego functions described by MacKinnon involved the ability to construct a balanced sense of self and others.) To the extent that the child develops a stable, coherent, and "holistic" view of self and others, he or she is able to achieve self-esteem, trust, and—in later life—intimacy. To the extent that self and others are represented internally as fragmented—"all good" or "all bad"—the individual will be hindered in achieving these goals. A child who maintains such an internal representation might well see himself or herself as "all good" one day and "all bad" the next. One often sees such "splitting" in patients with borderline personality disorder. These split-off parts of the self may be *projected* onto others so that they, too, are experienced as all good or all bad—a common development in the psychotherapy of borderline patients.

Vignette

Allen was a 24-year-old single male who had an extremely disturbed childhood. His mother was extraordinarily "cold" at times and at other times inappropriately sexual with Allen. In psychotherapy, Allen would sometimes present with a kind of swaggering, euphoric mood, wondering "why the hell I even need all this therapy." At other times, Allen would describe himself as "garbage" and barely communicate with his therapist. On some such days, however, he would have angry outbursts, shouting at his therapist, "You must be the most incompetent jerk in the whole damn field."

The object-relations model helps us understand how Allen's pathology developed—that is, how his split-off "good me" and "bad me" are analogues of the all-good or all-bad internal representation of his mother, fostered, it appears, by the mother's own pathology.

Finally, there is the cognitive-behavioral model. At first, this model may seem like a strange bedfellow among the three "psychodynamic" partners. Indeed, the cognitive-behavioral model has little use for constructs like the unconscious, the ego, or the internal object. Instead, it emphasizes the *irrational cognitions* and *maladaptive behaviors* we learn and practice. The cognitive-behavioral model views psychopathology as primarily the outcome of such irrational or self-destructive cognitions. Thus, the depressed patient may be "propagandizing" himself or herself with ideas such as "I must have everyone's love, or I am worthless," "I must do well at everything I attempt, or I am an incompetent jerk," and so on. By helping the patient alter these cognitions we can help him or her get better.

Perhaps an analogy can be made between the object-relations term "splitting" and the cognitive-behavioral term "irrational cognition." Both involve an "all-or-none" approach to the self or others. The patient who is in touch only with "bad me" is very likely to ignore any of his or her positive accomplishments and, indeed, to discredit them. This may take the form of the irrational cognition "I'm no good unless I do everything perfectly." Thus, the cognitive-behavioral model complements the object-relations model and has affinities with the other psychodynamic models as well. Nevertheless, these models may dictate different interventions in the course of psychotherapy.

Before moving on to the "social" part of our biopsychosocial approach, let us attempt to integrate the four models discussed above. Can we understand a patient's central conflict by means of the ego-psychological, self-psychological, object-relations, and cognitive-behavioral perspectives? Let us consider the following clinical history:

Karen is a single 24-year-old who seeks help for her chronic "binge-purge" pattern (bulimia nervosa). For the past 7 years, Karen has been inducing vomiting and abusing laxatives in order, as she puts it, "to make sure I don't explode." Her weight at interview is actually well within normal limits. Karen gives a history of a very disturbed family system. "My house was like a cross between Grand Central Station and Hiroshima," the patient stated, adding, "There was never any time to solve problems . . . the fur was always flying, and everyone was trying to grab the scraps of meat." Karen had three siblings: two older sisters and a younger brother. She described her sisters as "real sharks . . . very competitive for Mom and

Dad's attention, boys, clothes, you name it." Karen described her mother as "kind of a phony . . . I mean, always saying how smart I was but then discouraging me every time I wanted to strike out on my own, take piano lessons, or whatever. But "little brother . . . well, he was always gonna win the Nobel Prize." Karen described her father as "the iceman . . . no matter what I did, even stand on my head, I couldn't get dad to like me."

Karen felt extremely guilty about her binging and purging, stating, "I really feel like a piece of crap . . . sometimes I think that's all I really am . . . just that piece of crap floating in the toilet bowl after I upchuck." Nevertheless, Karen acknowledged a certain pleasure at the distress her behavior caused in her family, stating with a grin, "Yeah, the Iceman and the Bitch Queen [her father and mother] really go bananas when I tell them what I do." Despite her obvious anger with her parents, Karen felt unable to express this openly, saying, "They'd never talk to me again . . . besides, why should I waste my time with them?"

We have given an extremely condensed clinical history of Karen; nevertheless, it will serve to demonstrate the fourfold approach to the psychodynamic formulation. The ego-psychological model would tell us that Karen's binge-purge behavior is a defensive compromise between unconscious wishes and fears (e.g., between the wish to strike back at her parents and the fear of losing their interest). This model might also hypothesize that Karen's vomiting represents forbidden sexual and aggressive impulses directed at her father. In an almost literal sense, Karen is still "standing on her head" in order to get her father's attention—but what she "throws up" at him is scarcely to his liking. She also effectively punishes her mother—"the Bitch Queen"— while at the same time identifying with her mother's punitive stance ("discouraging me every time I wanted to strike out on my own").

The self-psychological model would point to the empathic failures in Karen's early family environment and view Karen's personality as having become "distorted." As a consequence, she manifests a strong need for the approval of others and correspondingly low self-esteem. Paradoxically, Karen shows some narcissistic traits (e.g., she would be "wasting her time" by talking with her parents, whom she derisively dismisses as the Iceman and the Bitch Queen). The self-psychological model would see this haughtiness as Karen's unconscious attempt to compensate for her low self-esteem.

The object-relations model would focus on Karen's failures to form well-balanced internal representations of herself and others. Rather, Karen views herself as "a piece of crap" and is equally negative about her parents. The object-relations model might hypothesize that Karen's description of her parents is actually a projection of her own, internalized "bad me," which has been split off from her "good me." This bad, angry self is strongly repressed but "breaks through" in the form of Karen's binging and purging.

Finally, the cognitive-behavioral model would focus on Karen's irrational, "all-or-none" cognitions and her dire need for approval. What is the evidence, for example, that one is a "piece of crap" simply because one's behavior is sometimes inappropriate? And what would be so horrible if Karen's parents *didn't* love her—would it be the end of the world? Where is the evidence that Karen's parents "would never talk to her again" if she expressed anger? And if they didn't speak to her again, would her life be over?

Clearly, there are many ways to formulate Karen's case. The four models we have examined complement each other, and each contributes a bit of truth.

By the way, one study of "bulimic" versus "control" families suggests that Karen's case is not unique. Johnson and Flach (1985) found that the families of persons with bulimia set high expectations but discouraged their daughters from pursuing these lofty goals. The "bulimic" families were also more disorganized ("like a cross between Grand Central Station and Hiroshima") than control families, showing little ability to solve individual problems. These considerations lead us directly into the final portion of our "biopsychosocial" triad.

Sociocultural Factors in Psychiatric Illness

A poor, Mexican-American woman tells a psychiatry resident that "my heart problem is God's will . . . it is perhaps a punishment for my sins." An elderly immigrant from Czechoslovakia, recently diagnosed as having fractured his hip, refuses to seek medical care, stating, "I'll call the doctor when I really need to." A 19-year-old Puerto Rican woman is brought to the emergency room after disrobing in public, screaming, and falling to the sidewalk in a convulsive stupor. All of her actions occurred minutes after a sexual assault.

Is the Mexican-American woman psychotically depressed? Is the Czechoslovakian immigrant demonstrating "denial"? Is the Puerto Rican woman "hysterical"? Perhaps your answers to these questions would change if you were aware that, for many Mexican-Americans, illness is subject to "God's will" and a consequence of having sinned (Martinez 1978); that Slovaks often view illness as a form of weakness and defer medical care as long as possible (Stein 1976); or that in Puerto Rico, severe stress is often "handled" by means of the *ataque*— a culturally recognized and legitimate cry for help (Abad and Boyce 1979).

Ethnicity, of course, is merely one dimension of "social psychiatry." The social part of our biopsychosocial approach also deals with the family unit, educational and socioeconomic status, peer group relations, life stresses, and social role. The consequences of these factors may be considerable. For example, Hollingshead and Redlich (1958), in their classic study, showed an association between low socioeconomic status and the incidence of mental illness. Durkheim's (1897/1951) seminal investigation showed an inverse relationship between suicide and the individual's degree of integration into a network of enduring ties. More recently—and perhaps, more unexpectedly—Waitzkin (1984) has shown that "doctor-patient communication" is influenced by socioeconomic factors. Specifically, doctors from upper-class and upper-middle-class backgrounds tend to give out more information to patients than do doctors from lower socioeconomic backgrounds. Moreover, patients from upper-class or upper-middle-class backgrounds receive more "doctor time" and more information than do patients from lower-socioeconomic-class backgrounds.

But do such socioeconomic or ethnic factors actually influence *psychiatric diagnosis*? Some research suggests that blacks and other minorities are more often misdiagnosed than whites (Adebimpe 1981; Mukherjee et al. 1983). Specifically, the increased likelihood of hallucinations in black and Hispanic patients with bipolar disorder may contribute to the misdiagnosis of schizophrenia in these groups (Lawson 1986). Even "objective" evidence may lead us into diagnostic error. For example, because the Minnesota Multiphasic Personality Inventory (MMPI) was not standardized on a black population, blacks tend to score higher on the paranoia and schizophrenia scales than do whites (Gyunther 1981).

There are some interesting connections between the social and the biological parts of our model. For example, some data indicate that Asians require lower doses of psychotropics than do non-Hispanic whites—including lithium, antidepressants, and antipsychotics (Lawson 1986; Lin and Finder 1983). Hispanic patients also seem to require less antidepressant medication than do whites and report more side effects (Marcos and Cancro 1982). Blacks reportedly have significantly higher plasma tricyclic levels for a given oral dose than do whites (Ziegler and Biggs 1977).

On a more theoretical level, racial differences may have implications for the so-called biological markers of mental illness. For example, serum creatinine phosphokinase (CPK) may be elevated in some acutely psychotic patients (Meltzer 1969), but serum CPK is significantly higher in healthy blacks than in whites (Meltzer and Hoy 1974).

Lefley (1990) has elegantly summarized the many ways in which "culture" may affect chronic mental illness. For example, in its nine-culture study, the International Pilot Study of Schizophrenia found a better prognosis for this illness in developing countries than in the industrialized West (Sartorius et al. 1986); other studies have supported this finding. What factors have contributed to this somewhat surprising outcome? Various workers have posited greater familial support, reduced emphasis on the "sick role," and differing concepts of the "self" in nonindustrialized societies (Lefley 1990). Lefley pointed out the ways in which ethnicity or culture can shape the individual's "receptivity" to particular models of disease and treatment; for example, a physiological or medical model of mental illness "fits" the belief system of many Hispanic families. Similarly, Haitian patients often prefer injections to pills, believing the former to be powerful weapons against some external invasion of mind or body (Lefley 1990).

Let us now try to bring together a number of ethnic, social, and socioeconomic factors in a clinical vignette.

Vignette

A 37-year-old Puerto Rican–born male presented to the ER after a suicide attempt. The patient's brother accompanied him and provided some information. Both the patient and his brother had come to the United States 2 years earlier and settled in Boston. Whereas the patient's brother had become quite successful as a computer programmer, the patient had grown increasingly despondent and dysfunctional over the past year. He recently "broke up" with a Puerto Rican woman he had met in Boston, and had also lost his job as a grocery store clerk. In the ER the patient appeared quite agitated and anxious, alluding to a *mala influencia* ("evil influence") that was possessing him. His brother—who spoke better English than the patient—explained that the patient believed himself possessed by an "evil spirit," and that he had been to a local Puerto Rican "spiritist" (healer-medium) for *despojo* ("exorcism"). When the ritual of *dando la luz spiritu* ("giving the spirit light") failed to help him, the patient took an overdose of sleeping pills. A family history revealed that the patient's father had died when the patient was 7 years old and that afterward the patient seemingly became more withdrawn.

What can we conclude from this admittedly sketchy history? Is our patient "psychotically depressed"? How do cultural factors impinge on the diagnosis? First of all, this patient has several sociocultural risk factors that predispose him to depressive illness—for example, his status as an immigrant, recent loss of job, and breakup with his girlfriend. The loss of one or both parents during childhood is also correlated with adult-onset depression. On a more "interactional" level, we may speculate that the patient views himself as inadequate in comparison to his more successful brother.

Is the patient psychotic? The answer is not readily apparent. Normally, we view ideas such as possession by "evil influences" as delusions. But what should we think when such ideas are culturally tolerated, if not encouraged? In a study of 79 Puerto Rican households in New York City, Harwood (1977) found that 47% of all adults identified themselves as "spiritists," performed rituals at home to cleanse the premises of harmful spiritual influences, or reported some other involvement with spiritism. In some Moslem cultures, demonic spirits (*jinn* or *zar*) are thought to be one cause of mental illness, especially in women (Racy 1970). When such beliefs are clearly syntonic with the patient's culture, it is inappropriate to speak of "psychosis." (The patient's family may provide critical information in such cases.) Nonetheless, the patient in our last vignette was clearly depressed and in need of treatment, regardless of the cultural nuances in his belief system.

Summing Up the Biopsychosocial Perspective: The Diagnostic Formulation

Let us now draw together the three strands of our biopsychosocial model and construct a diagnostic formulation of the following case history.

Vignette

Sylvia is a 26-year-old married white female who presented with a chief complaint of "severe panic . . . like I'm crawling out of my skin . . . my heart feels like it's about to stop." As a consequence of these attacks, the patient had become virtually housebound. The patient states that the onset of the attacks followed the smoking of a single "joint" at a friend's party, approximately 2 years ago. The attack began that evening, and the patient had to leave the party, accompanied by her husband of 6 months. Reportedly, he was "really pissed" at her for "being such a wimp." Over the subsequent year, the patient developed panic episodes, lasting around 20 to 40 minutes, two or three times per week. These episodes were characterized by tachycardia, dyspnea, dizziness, tingling in the fingers, and "a feeling that I am going to lose my mind." The attacks often occurred without any obvious precipitant, although their frequency and intensity increased when the patient left home or when she was "thinking of something upsetting, like having a heart attack."

Sylvia regarded her marriage as "O.K." but acknowledged that "my husband definitely likes to wear the pants in the family." At the same time, the patient acknowledged her gratefulness that "he's there to help me . . . he helps me get out to shop and so forth . . . I'd be in real trouble without him." Her husband, Jim, revealed to the interviewer that "I kind of enjoy taking care of Sylvia, but lately, its gotten to be a pain." He recently admitted his attraction to a female co-worker and had warned Sylvia, "I don't know if I can resist much longer." Both the patient and her husband acknowledged that their sexual life had deteriorated over the past year.

The patient's past psychiatric history was essentially negative, though she acknowledged, "I've always been a little bit depressed." She also recalled a period of "school phobia" at age 5, which lasted for 2 months.

Sylvia's biological mother died when Sylvia was 2 years old, and the patient had only fragmentary recollections of a "pretty, smiling face." Sylvia acknowledged feeling "always a little hurt and angry" that her mother had "left" her. Her father—a businessman who was often out of town—remarried when Sylvia was 3. Sylvia recalled him as being "a real strict fundamentalist type." Her stepmother was "kind of schizo . . . like sometimes she'd hardly talk to me or hold me, and at other times it was like she folded herself right around me." The patient's biological mother, Sylvia had learned, had had a history of panic attacks "a lot like mine."

Sylvia had done well academically and had obtained a master's degree in business administration. She described herself as "real sharp at work . . . on top of everything. I've always been the one who solves everyone's problems at work—the troubleshooter." In the past month, however, Sylvia had "gotten into some hassles" with her boss. Two weeks prior to evaluation, Sylvia received word that she was facing an imminent layoff because of her company's "problems with the stock market." Since that time, Sylvia's panic attacks increased to around two or three per day. Other than making the trip to and from work—accompanied by her husband, who drove her both ways—Sylvia had been virtually housebound over the past month. Sylvia described herself as "strongly religious" and "felt really bad" that she could not get to church anymore.

A medical exam 1 year ago had been completely normal except for a "midsystolic click and late systolic murmur" noted by the patient's internist. An echocardiogram revealed mitral valve prolapse. The patient was given a small dose (10 mg tid) of propranolol (Inderal), which reduced some of her anxiety symptoms but left her depressed. She discontinued it and did not return to her internist.

Drug history was negative for current alcohol abuse, cocaine, amphetamines, or other "street drugs." The patient acknowledged a "bad coffee habit," usually in excess of six cups per day.

This patient begins with a number of biological factors that may predispose her to panic attacks and, secondarily, to agoraphobia. Mitral valve prolapse has been associated with panic disorder, although the meaning of this finding remains controversial. That Sylvia's biological mother also had panic-like symptoms suggests a familial vulnerability to the disorder. In a recent study by Torgersen (1983), monozygotic twins were found to have significantly higher rates of panic disorder and agoraphobia than did dizygotic twins, suggesting a true genetic component. Sylvia's consumption of caffeine may also play a role in her panic attacks. Caffeine may be "panicogenic," and persons with panic disorder may be more sensitive than normal control subjects to the anxiety-inducing effects of caffeine (Boulenger et al. 1984; Shear and Fyer 1988). Finally, it is not uncommon, in the author's experience, for panic attacks to *begin* after the first use of marijuana or other "street drugs," even though subsequently the attacks occur quite spontaneously. Both cocaine and marijuana have been implicated in the onset of panic attacks (Aronson and Craig 1986; Beaconsfield et al. 1972; Katon 1986). Primary alcohol abuse and recurrent withdrawal may lead to a "kindling" effect on the CNS that facilitates the onset of panic disorder (Katon 1986; Stockwell et al. 1984).

Sylvia's history points to a number of contributing psychological factors, and her disorder may be conceptualized using several of the models we have examined. Naturally, these psychological factors do not vitiate the biochemical mechanisms we have just discussed; rather, the two components complement and reinforce each other.

First, it is interesting that although Sylvia recalls her biological mother in positive terms ("a pretty, smiling face"), she also felt hurt and angry that her mother had "left" her. De Moor (1985) and others (Buglass et al. 1977) have suggested that agoraphobic women, in comparison with normal control subjects, harbor ambivalent feelings toward their mothers. In Sylvia's case, we might speculate that her panic attacks represent a defensive compromise between expressing *anger* on the one hand and *dependence* on the other. The ego-psychological model might apply this analysis to Sylvia's relationships with her biological and adoptive mothers and—more recently—with her husband.

The self-psychological and object-relations models allow us to focus on Sylvia's loss of "mothering" during the critical separation-individuation stage of development. Kohut (1971) has speculated that adult panic states are related to failures of empathic self-selfobject (child-mother) merger in childhood. Tolpin (1971) has argued that such "empathic failures" lead to poor internalization of anxiety-reduction mechanisms and that this, in turn, predisposes the individual to self-fragmentation. Diamond (1985, p. 121) contends that agoraphobia "is an attempt to avoid . . . environments that will provoke or worsen disruption in the already endangered state of self-cohesiveness" resulting from panic attacks; thus, staying home "will bandage the wound to the self opened by the panic state" (p. 121). Again, using the ego-psychological and self-psychological models, it is interesting to recall Sylvia's comment that sometimes her stepmother was extremely aloof and that sometimes she "folded herself right around me." Friedman (1985) has noted two patterns of maternal-child interactions in adult agoraphobic patients: 1) the mother may distance herself excessively, or 2) the mother may "shadow" the child excessively, thus discouraging independent striving.

With respect to Sylvia's "school phobia," we should recall the hypothesis that panic attacks represent a biological alarm mechanism that is evoked when the individual is threatened with separation from a significant other (Gittelman and Klein 1984). For example, there is demonstrated an abnormally high rate of "school phobia" in panic disorder patients. In Sylvia's case, the threat of losing her husband to another woman may well have recapitulated her earlier separation anxiety ("school phobia").

More recently, clinicians have begun applying the cognitive model to the understanding of panic-agoraphobic symptoms (Craske 1988). De Moor (1985) notes that in panic attack sufferers, "the intensity of the anxiety experience is proportional to the subjectively estimated degree of probability that the hypothetical danger will occur" (p. 381–382)—for example, that one will die or "go crazy" during a panic attack. This is interesting, in light of Sylvia's remark that the attacks increased when she would think of "something upsetting, like having a heart attack." Roberts (1984) has presented an integrated therapeutic approach to panic disorder, in which patients are educated as to the *actual* dangers of their attacks (i.e., that they will not "go crazy," "drop dead," etc.).

The sociocultural perspective on Sylvia's case might begin with the observation that Sylvia's marriage is in deep trouble. Her husband's flirtation with his co-worker is not merely a threat to Sylvia's self-esteem and security; it also represents the possible loss of a "phobic partner"—the person who takes Sylvia to work, to the grocery, and so forth. Yet Sylvia's culture of origin might make it difficult for her to express anger toward her husband; after all, her "strict fundamentalist" father might have disapproved of such assertiveness. (At the same time, his fundamentalist values, internalized by Sylvia, would make it virtually impossible to accept marital infidelity.) The sociocultural perspective, finally, would point to Sylvia's imminent "layoff" as a source of great stress; indeed, on the Holmes and Rahe Scale of Psychosocial Stressors, "fired at work" rates a 47 on a scale from 1 to 100, and "trouble with boss" rates a 23.

Conclusion

The "biopsychosocial approach" is not a cliché. When taken seriously, it is the very heart of the diagnostic formulation. It may be summed up in "the three M's": *molecules, mentation,* and *milieu.* Although DSM-IV emphasizes the objective and observable correlates of mental illness, the psychiatrist must probe more deeply and search more broadly if genuine diagnosis is to occur.

References

Abad V, Boyce E: Issues in psychiatric evaluations of Puerto Ricans: a sociocultural perspective. Journal of Operational Psychiatry 10:28–39, 1979

Adebimpe VR: Overview: white norms and psychiatric diagnosis of black patients. Am J Psychiatry 138:279–285, 1981

American Psychiatric Association: Diagnostic and Statistical Manual of Mental Disorders, 3rd Edition, Revised. Washington, DC, American Psychiatric Association, 1987

American Psychiatric Association: Diagnostic and Statistical Manual of Mental Disorders, 4th Edition. Washington, DC, American Psychiatric Association, 1994

Aronson TA, Craig TJ: Cocaine precipitation of panic disorder. Am J Psychiatry 143:643–645, 1986

Beaconsfield P, Ginsburg J, Rainsbury R: Marijuana smoking: cardiovascular effects in man and possible mechanisms. N Engl J Med 287:209–212, 1972

Boulenger J-P, Uhde TW, Wolff EA, et al: Increased sensitivity to caffeine in patients with panic disorders: preliminary evidence. Arch Gen Psychiatry 41:1067–1071, 1984

Buglass P, Clarke J, Henderson AS, et al: A study of agoraphobic housewives. Psychol Med 7:73–86, 1977

Craske MG: Cognitive-behavioral treatment of panic, in American Psychiatric Association Review of Psychiatry, Vol 7. Edited by Frances AJ, Hales RE. Washington, DC, American Psychiatric Press, 1988, pp 121–137

De Moor W: The topography of agoraphobia. Am J Psychother 39:371–388, 1985

Diamond DB: Panic attacks, hypochondriasis, and agoraphobia: a self psychology formulation. Am J Psychother 39:114–125, 1985

Durkheim E: Suicide: A Study in Sociology (1897). Translated by Spaulding JA. Edited with and introduction by Simpson G. New York, Free Press, 1951

Engel G: The need for a new medical model: a challenge for biomedicine. Science 196:129–133, 1977

Ferrier IN, Cross AJ, Johnson JA, et al: Neuropeptides in Alzheimer-type dementia. J Neurol Sci 62:159–170, 1983

Friedman S: Implications of object-relations theory for the behavioral treatment of agoraphobia. Am J Psychother 39:525–540, 1985

Gittelman R, Klein DF: Relationship between separation anxiety and panic and agoraphobic disorders. Psychopathology 17 (suppl 1):56–65, 1984

Gyunther MD: Is the MMPI an appropriate assessment device for blacks? Journal of Black Psychology 7:67–75, 1981

Harwood A: Rx: Spiritist as Needed: A Study of Puerto Rican Community Mental Health Resource. New York, Wiley, 1977

Hollingshead AB, Redlich FC: Social Class and Mental Illness. New York, Wiley, 1958

Jervis GA: Biomedical types of mental deficiency, in American Handbook of Psychiatry, 2nd Edition, Vol 4. Edited by Arieti S. New York, Basic

Books, 1975, pp 463–473

Johnson C, Flach A: Family characteristics of 105 patients with bulimia. Am J Psychiatry 142:1321–1324, 1985

Katon W: Panic disorder: epidemiology, diagnosis, and treatment in primary care. J Clin Psychiatry 47(No 10, Suppl):21–27, 1986

Kohut H: The Analysis of the Self: A Systematic Approach to the Psychoanalytic Treatment of Narcissistic Personality Disorders. New York, International Universities Press, 1971

Lawson WB: Racial and ethnic factors in psychiatric research. Hosp Community Psychiatry 37:50–54, 1986

Lefley HP: Culture and chronic mental illness. Hosp Community Psychiatry 41:277–286, 1990

Lin K-M, Finder E: Neuroleptic dosage for Asians. Am J Psychiatry 140:490–491, 1983

MacKinnon RA: Psychiatric history and mental status examination, in Comprehensive Textbook of Psychiatry/III, 3rd Edition. Edited by Kaplan HI, Freedman AM, Sadock BJ. Baltimore, MD, Williams & Wilkins, 1980, pp 906–920

Marcos LR, Cancro R: Pharmacotherapy of Hispanic depressed patients: clinical observations. Am J Psychother 36:505–512, 1982

Martinez RA (ed): Hispanic Culture and Health Care: Fact, Fiction, Folklore. St Louis, MO, CV Mosby, 1978

Meltzer H: Muscle enzyme release in the acute psychoses. Arch Gen Psychiatry 21:102–112, 1969

Meltzer HY, Hoy PA: Black-white differences in serum creatinine phosphokinase (CPK) activity. Clinica Chimica Acta 54:215–224, 1974

Mukherjee S, Shukla S, Woodle J, et al: Misdiagnosis of schizophrenia in bipolar patients: a multiethnic comparison. Am J Psychiatry 140:1571–1574, 1983

Perry S, Cooper AM, Michels R: The psychodynamic formulation: its purpose, structure, and clinical application. Am J Psychiatry 144:543–550, 1987

Racy J: Folk psychiatry, in Psychiatry in the Arab east. Acta Psychiatr Scand Suppl 211:62–67, 1970

Roberts R: An integrated approach to the treatment of panic disorder. Am J Psychother 38:413–430, 1984

Sartorius N, Jablensky A, Korten A, et al: Early manifestations and first-contact incidence of schizophrenia in different cultures. Psychol Med 16:909–928, 1986

Shear MK, Fyer MR: Biological and psychopathologic findings in panic disorder, in American Psychiatric Press Review of Psychiatry, Vol 7. Edited by Frances AJ, Hales RE. Washington, DC, American Psychiatric Press, 1988, pp 29–53

Stein HF: A dialectical model of health and illness attitudes and behavior among Slovak-Americans. Int J Ment Health 5:325–330, 1976

Stockwell T, Smail P, Hodgson R, et al: Alcohol dependence and phobic anxiety states, II: a retrospective study. Br J Psychiatry 144:58–63, 1984

Tolpin M: On the beginnings of a cohesive self: an application of the concept of transmuting internalization to the study of transitional object and signal anxiety. Psychoanal Study Child 26:316–352, 1971

Torgersen S: Genetic factors in anxiety disorders. Arch Gen Psychiatry 40:1085–1089, 1983

Waitzkin H: Doctor-patient communication: clinical implications of social scientific research. JAMA 252:2441–2446, 1984

Ziegler VE, Biggs J: Tricyclic plasma levels: effect of age, race, sex, and smoking. JAMA 238:2167–2169, 1977

2

Adjunctive Testing in Psychiatry

In the course of treating psychiatric patients, you will find that clinical observation and careful history taking are the most important tools you possess. Nevertheless, as psychiatry continues to expand its biopsychosocial mode, you will often find it helpful to involve allied disciplines and their unique testing procedures in your overall approach to the patient. The fields of clinical psychology and neuropsychology, neuroradiology, and neuroendocrinology have made important contributions to the adjunctive testing procedures available to psychiatrists. In this chapter I cannot hope to explore each of these areas in detail; rather, I give you an overview of the tests at your disposal, their indications, and a basic understanding of their "mechanics."

Psychological Testing

Although psychological and neuropsychological testing is usually delegated to psychologists in most clinical settings, you should be at least conversant with the more commonly used tests and scales. To that end, we summarize the basics of some "classic" tests and then describe a few commonly used rating scales.

Tests are usually classified as either "objective" or "projective." The former are usually "paper and pencil" tests based on specific items and questions with right or wrong answers; the latter are generally ambiguous arrays of stimuli designed to elicit the patient's unique feelings, conflicts, and perceptions. Tests may be further described as intelligence, personality, or neuropsychiatric testing (Kaplan and Sadock 1988).

Intelligence Testing

The Weschsler Adult Intelligence Scale (WAIS) and its revised counterpart, the WAIS-R, are the most widely used IQ tests in clinical psychiatry. The WAIS consists of six verbal and five performance subtests, yielding a "verbal" IQ, a "performance" IQ, and a combined "full scale" score. Each subtest is influenced by a variety of educational, cultural, and affective factors. (For example, an uneducated, anxious patient from a Southeast Asian background may perform poorly on the WAIS, despite normal or above-average intelligence.) Psychotropic medication may also affect results on the WAIS (House and Lewis 1985). A disparity of greater than 15 points between the verbal and performance IQs may indicate psychopathology or organic brain damage, although the interpretation of such discrepancies is somewhat controversial (House and Lewis 1985). The various subtests of the WAIS and a very brief description of each are listed in Table 2–1.

Let's now see how the WAIS-R might turn out for a particular patient, whose diagnosis you may wish to formulate as you read the (qualitative) test results:

> Mr. Fretter, a 35-year-old engineer, showed a high full-scale score, with the verbal score exceeding the performance score. He displayed a meticulous approach to the block design and object assembly subtests. He also did very well on the vocabulary, similarities, and comprehension subtests. However, in a few instances, Mr. Fretter showed difficulties in "changing set" on the similarities test, and his overall score on this subtest was lower than his intelligence suggested. He did well on the arithmetic and digit span tests.

As you may have deduced, Mr. Fretter shows a pattern consistent with obsessive-compulsive traits. We would have seen quite a different pattern if we had looked at a patient with, say, conversion disorder;

such patients usually do poorly on comprehension, similarities, and picture arrangement, and seldom show overall high IQs (Meyer 1983).

The classification of intelligence by IQ range is summarized in Table 2–2.

Personality Testing

Rorschach Test

The Rorschach has so infiltrated our culture that we use the term to describe almost any situation in which an idiosyncratic response is evoked by some particular (usually ambiguous) stimulus. The test was pioneered by the Swiss psychiatrist Hermann Rorschach around 1910 and has been the subject of many volumes of commentary. What follows is merely a "sketch" of a very complex picture (see Carr 1985 for a good synopsis).

Essentially, the Rorschach consists of a standard set of 10 inkblots: 5 black and white, and 5 including colors. The cards are shown to the patient in a specified order, and his or her reactions are carefully

Table 2–1. Weschsler Adult Intelligence Scale (WAIS) subtests

Verbal subtests

Information: tests general knowledge.

Comprehension: assesses social judgment.

Arithmetic: tests simple calculations.

Similarities: tests abstraction (sensitive indicator of IQ).

Digit span: tests immediate retention.

Vocabulary: highly correlated with IQ but also education.

Performance subtests

Picture completion: detects visuoperceptive defects.

Block design: assesses left-right brain function.

Object assembly: tests visuoperception and manual dexterity.

Digit symbol: tests concentration and rapidity of learning.

Source. Extensively modified from Kaplan and Sadock 1988.

logged. Scoring of responses is based on a symbol system related to four qualities: location, determinants, content, and popularity. *Location* refers to what portion of the blot the patient used as a basis for responding—for example, the whole blot (coded as W) or only an odd detail (Dd). The quality *Determinants* refers to the form, shading, color, or movement (human vs. animal) that prompted the patient's response. *Content* refers to whether the patient's responses reflect interest in human, animal, anatomic, or sexual themes. *Popularity* reflects the fact that certain responses are more common than others.

Each of these response patterns is said to have psychological significance. For example, the use of the whole inkblot (W) is associated with the ability to "interact actively and efficiently with the environment" (Erdberg 1985, p. 68). In contrast, when uncommon details (Dd) are utilized, this may suggest "significant difficulties with operation in society" (Erdberg 1985, p. 69). The relative balance between form (F) and color (C) may give us a sense, respectively, of how much "internal control" versus "responsiveness" the patient shows. The best indicator of "reality-testing ability" is the accuracy of form perception, coded F+%. A high percentage of C responses may indicate emotional lability or suggestibility. "Animal movement" responses (FM) may give clues as to "some sort of drive state experience that has the ability to intrude into consciousness [and] disrupt concentration" (Erdberg 1985). In contrast, human movement responses

Table 2–2.   Classification of intelligence based on range of intelligence quotient (IQ)

Classification	IQ range
Mental retardation	< 20–70
Borderline	70–79
Dull normal	80–90
Normal	90–110
Bright normal	110–120
Superior	120 and higher

Source. Extensively modified from Kaplan and Sadock 1988.

(M) signify abstract thinking and thoughtfulness.

Knowing these bare-bones facts about the Rorschach, what would you guess about the following patient? He shows a long reaction time to the cards and makes only 20 responses total. He shows very few C responses and a high percentage of F responses; he shows few M and W responses. We might conclude that this patient displays little tendency to "react" to the environment, has a high degree of internal control or restraint, and has difficulty with abstract thinking. This is the Rorschach pattern we would expect in a patient with major depression (Meyer 1983). In similar fashion, other diagnoses tend to show characteristic Rorschach patterns. Thus, schizophrenic patients tend to show poor form responses (low F+%), a paucity of popular responses, and overgeneralization (e.g., "This card is a cat, because I see a whisker right here"). We will say more about the Rorschach in our discussion of the individual disorders in later chapters.

Thematic Apperception Test (TAT)

The TAT consists of a series of 30 pictures and one blank card, the former generally depicting human relationships of an ambiguous nature. For example, picture No. 2 shows a country scene of a young woman with books in her hand, a man working in the fields, and an older woman looking on. The patient is shown these pictures and asked to "make up a story" about them. Interpretation of the patient's stories relies, in part, on knowledge of how the pictures are usually interpreted (Carr 1985). For example, the card just described (No. 2) usually elicits a story about a schoolgirl, her mother, and her father. We might expect a patient with poor communication in his or her family to describe no interaction among the three figures. Alternatively, a story involving competition between the young and the old women may reveal oedipal-level struggles in the patient's family (Carr 1985).

Minnesota Multiphasic Personality Inventory (MMPI)

The MMPI is a self-report inventory consisting of 550 statements requiring a response of "True," "False," or "Cannot say." It is the most widely used of the "objective" personality tests and may be scored by computer. The MMPI gives scores on 10 empirically derived scales, each designed to detect various forms of psychopathology (e.g., hypochondriasis, paranoia, hypomania). Three additional scales (L, F, and K) are designed to increase the validity of the test by "exposing" individuals who try to manipulate the outcome of the test in various ways—for example, by casting themselves in a bad light ("faking bad") or by minimizing psychopathology ("faking good"). The scales and their symbols are listed in Table 2–3.

Experts in the interpretation of the MMPI caution against literal interpretations of the clinical scales and instead emphasize the relationships between the scales (Newmark 1985). Thus, "two-point codes" have been devised that show the relationship between the two highest scales above a T (true) score of 70—what we might call the "twin peaks" effect. The higher of the two scales is coded first; thus, a "4-8" pattern might be seen in a patient who scored 85 on scale 4 (psychopathy) and 81 on scale 8 (schizophrenia). This 4-8 pattern is often seen in patients demonstrating irritability, suspiciousness, and "acting out in asocial ways" (Newmark 1985). A synopsis of some important two-point codes is given in Table 2–4. Note that these codes do not point to a specific diagnosis, but rather to characteristic tendencies or attributes.

Neuropsychological Testing

These tests are generally designed to assess "brain function," with the aim of detecting disease or injury in the central nervous system.

Table 2–3. Minnesota Multiphasic Personality Inventory (MMPI) scales

? Cannot say scale	4 Psychopathic deviant (Pd)
L Lie scale	5 Masculinity-femininity (Mf)
F Faking bad	6 Paranoia (Pa)
K Faking good	7 Psychasthenia (Pt)
1 Hypochondriasis (Hs)	8 Schizophrenia (Sc)
2 Depression (D)	9 Hypomania (Ma)
3 Hysteria (Hy)	0 Social introversion (Si)

Note. See Newmark 1985 for further details.

Specific functions such as visual memory, psychomotor skill, and perceptuomotor performance are assessed; in some cases, cerebral lesions may be localized with considerable precision.

Halstead-Reitan Battery

One of the most commonly used tests of brain function, the Halstead-Reitan Battery, is composed of 10 subtests, summarized in Table 2–5. A detailed discusion is provided by Barth and Macciocchi (1985). The following vignette, adapted from Barth and Macciocchi, is an example of how the Halstead-Reitan Battery works in practice.

Vignette

Mr. Zetz is a 32-year-old attorney who suffered a head injury after falling from a ladder. A computed tomography (CT) scan of the brain and an electroencephalogram (EEG) obtained shortly after the accident had been normal, and the patient had been released. However, on follow-up examination 6 weeks later, Mr. Zetz complained of headaches, dizziness, difficulties in word finding, memory problems, and mild anxiety and depression. On the WAIS, Mr. Zetz showed disruption of the performance subtest. On the Halstead-Reitan Battery, he showed difficulties in abstract reasoning and concept formation on the category test, and reduced attention on the trail making test. He showed no major motor or sensory deficits

Table 2–4. MMPI two-point scales

1-2/2-1	Depression, worry, pessimism
1-8/8-1	Anger, alienation, somatic delusions
2-6/6-2	Hostility, resentment, early psychosis
3-8/8-3	Immature, vulnerable, schizoid
4-6/6-4	Impulsive, narcissistic, hostile
6-8/8-6	Paranoid, irritable, grandiose
7-8/8-7	Introspective, ruminative, insecure

Source. Extensively modified from Newmark 1985.

on the tactual performance, finger oscillation, or sensory-perceptual tests. Taken together, these findings were strongly suggestive of the typical response to head trauma. The patient was told that his symptoms were normal and that he should see significant recovery over the next 6 months.

Bender-Gestalt Test

The Bender-Gestalt was originally designed to assess maturational levels in children; however, it is now used most commonly as a screening device for organic brain dysfunction in adults (Kaplan and Sadock 1988). It consists of nine designs, each printed on a separate card against a white background. The patient is asked to copy each design with the particular card in view and without time limit.

The designs include, for example, a circle whose edge touches the corner of a square; a series of dots; and so forth. Many clinicians include a subsequent recall phase in which the patient must reproduce from memory as many of the designs as possible. (Psychiatrists often administer a truncated version of the Bender-Gestalt when they ask a patient, for example, to copy a drawing of a cube.)

Table 2–5.   Halstead-Reitan Battery subtests and what each measures

---

Category test: abstract thinking

Tactual performance test: dexterity, spatial memory

Rhythm test: auditory perception, attention, concentration

Finger-oscillation test: dexterity, motor speed

Speech-sounds perception test: auditory discrimination

Trail making test: visuomotor perception, motor speed, attention

Critical flicker frequency: visual perception

Time sense test: memory and spatial perception

Aphasia screening test: verbal and nonverbal brain functions

Sensory-perceptual test: stereognosis, tactile perception

Source. Extensively modified from Kaplan and Sadock 1988.

Psychological Rating Scales

There are dozens of rating scales used in clinical psychiatry, of which we will mention only a few. The main features of some of these scales are summarized in Table 2–6.

You should be aware of two major formats for structured or semistructured interviews: the Diagnostic Interview for Borderlines (DIB), developed by Gunderson and colleagues, and the Schedule for Affective Disorders and Schizophrenia (SADS), developed by Spitzer, Endicott, and associates. Both formats have been used widely for clinical and research purposes. Of special interest in the DIB is its inclusion of "psychosis" as one of five (equally weighted) areas of dysfunction (the others being social adaptation, impulse control, affect, and interpersonal relations). Recent editions of the *Diagnostic and Statistical Manual* have placed less emphasis on the presence of psychotic features in defining borderline personality disorder; DSM-IV, however, now includes brief psychotic symptoms among the criteria for borderline personality disorder (see Chapter 9).

The SADS is a highly detailed (78-page) protocol that assesses both present and "historical" functioning. Eight summary scales relate to current psychopathology: depressive mood and ideation, endogenous features, depressive-associated features, suicidal ideation and behavior, anxiety, manic symptoms, delusions-hallucinations, and formal thought disorder. The SADS-C contains only those items pertaining to the preceding week and may be used to measure change during treatment (Carr 1985).

Neuroimaging Techniques

For much of the 19th century, attempts to discern the pathoanatomic basis of schizophrenia and manic-depressive illness ended mainly in disappointment or contradiction. Although today these matters are hardly resolved, several neuroimaging techniques have yielded substantial information about these conditions (Jaskiw et al. 1987; Morihisa 1987). We are beginning to turn up intriguing findings in the area of anxiety disorders as well. Neuroimaging techniques can be

Table 2–6.   Psychiatric rating scales

Scale	Type	Description	Comments
Zung Depression Scale	Self-report	20 items rated on a 4-point scale of severity.	Assesses affective, psychic, and somatic features of depression.
Beck Depression Inventory	Self-report	21 symptom and attitude categories rated on a 4-point scale.	Results depend greatly on motivation of both patient and examiner; may measure "asthenia" > depression in some populations. May be good "screening" test.
Hamilton Rating Scale for Depression	Other-rated	17 items rated on a 3- or 5-point scale.	Includes items for somatic and hypochondriacal symptoms. Most useful in assessing severity in patient already diagnosed as depressed.
Brief Psychiatric Rating Scale	Other-rated	18 items rated on a 7-point scale.	Helpful for following response to treatment.
Global Assessment Scale	Other-rated	Scale of 1 to 100, from very sick to very healthy.	Modified version used for DSM-III-R Axis V; reflects present state based on chart, interview, family informants.
Andreasen Scale for Assessment of Negative Symptoms	Other-rated	6-point scales for 5 symptom complexes.	Differentiates positive from negative symptoms of schizophrenia.

Source. Adapted from Carr 1985.

divided into "structural" and "dynamic" types, although this distinction is rapidly beginning to blur. The former includes X-ray computed tomography (CT) and magnetic resonance imaging (MRI); the latter includes positron-emission tomography (PET), single-photon emission computed tomography (SPECT), and various types of computerizd electroencephalographic "brain mapping" techniques. These techniques and some of their clinical applications to date are summarized in Table 2–7.

When should you consider utilizing one or more of these imaging techniques? The clearest answers can be given with respect to the structural imaging techniques (e.g., CT, MRI); at this point, use of the dynamic techniques (e.g., PET, SPECT), with the exception of electroencephalography and polysomnography, is largely confined to research investigations. Weinberger (1984) has proposed that a CT scan of the brain be obtained in patients with any one of seven conditions accompanying or accounting for their psychiatric presentation: 1) the presence of confusion, dementia, or delirium; 2) first episode of psychosis; 3) movement disorder; 4) anorexia nervosa; 5) prolonged catatonia; 6) first affective episode after age 50; and 7) personality change after age 50. All of these conditions may reflect structural brain pathology.

The indications for obtaining an MRI are similar, and some authorities assert that MRI is virtually always preferable to CT, even though the former is considerably more expensive—and, I might add, extremely uncomfortable for some patients, owing to the high noise level and confined space. Actually, each technique—CT and MRI—has its own advantages and disadvantages, as summarized in Table 2–8. This list will undoubtedly change as we learn more about MRI and as the technique is refined in various ways (e.g., use with contrast agents, use of ultrarapid serial "cuts," etc.).

Various types of electroencephalographic studies can be extremely helpful in certain neuropsychiatric conditions. When you suspect temporal lobe epilepsy, disordered brain metabolism causing delirium, or a specific sleep disorder such as nocturnal myoclonus, you should generally obtain an EEG. With respect to temporal lobe epilepsy, the most sensitive study (though often difficult to arrange) is probably a sleep-deprived EEG using either nasopharyngeal or sphenoidal

Table 2–7.   Neuroimaging techniques

Technique	Methodology	Demonstrable pathology	Clinical relevance
Structural techniques			
CT	X rays from different angles are displayed in single reconstructed image, reflecting cross section or "slice" of subject.	May reveal ventricular enlargement, cerebellar atrophy, widening of cortical sulci, reversed asymmetries, brain density abnormalities. May excel (vs. MRI) for intracranial calcification, tumor margins, old vs. new hemorrhage.	Has revealed high VBRs in chronic schizophrenic and bipolar patients; cerebellar atrophy and third ventricle enlargement in schizophrenic patients; high % reversal of asymmetry in schizophrenic patients.
MRI	Tissues are placed in strong magnetic field causing alignment of hydrogen protons; radio waves excite protons, and subsequent "decay" in excitation can be measured and assigned various shades depending on intensity. Tissues have varying proton density and decay rates (T_1, T_2).	As above for CT, but has better resolution; is superior for demyelinating diseases and posterior fossa, temporal lobe, and brain stem lesions.	Has revealed smaller frontal and temporal lobes in schizophrenic patients; cortical and subcortical atrophy, basal ganglia lesions in depressed elderly patients; T_1 values in Alzheimer's disease patients correlate with cognitive deficits.
Dynamic techniques			
PET	Subject is injected with positron-emitting isotope (FDG), yielding estimate of glucose metabolism in brain regions; color map depicts regional 3-D glucose utilization.	May reveal abnormalities in regional cerebral blood flow; abnormal anterior/posterior gradient; correlations with abnormal brain functional activity/metabolism.	Abnormal glucose metabolism in prefrontal cortex, caudate in OCD patients; "hypofrontality" in subcortical dementia and schizophrenic (?) patients

Table 2–7. Neuroimaging techniques (*continued*)

Technique	Methodology	Demonstrable pathology	Clinical relevance
Dynamic techniques (*continued*)			
SPECT	Is based on detection of gamma rays from a single-photon–emitting radionuclide such as ^{123}I, which is administered to subject. Gamma detector system creates 3-D image of radionuclide distribution, yielding measure of blood flow.	Can show abnormalities in cerebral blood flow; physiologically specific radionuclides can show abnormalities in receptor binding.	Has shown focal perfusion deficits and abnormal muscarinic receptor distribution in Alzheimer's patients (^{123}I-labeled ligand was used).
BEAM and other EEG	Electrical activity in upper layers of cortex measured using scalp, NP, or sphenoidal electrodes; latent abnormalities may be unmasked using photic stimulation, hyperventilation; response (evoked potential) to various stimuli is measured; computed topographic mapping (BEAM).	Can aid detection of frank seizure activity; abnormal perception of novel stimulus (evoked potential); abnormal sleep-related events; abnormal pattern of electrical activity (regional EEG frequencies).	Has shown left-hemisphere dysfunction in schizophrenic patients (BEAM); decreased P300 response in schizophrenic and borderline patients.

Note. CT = computed tomography; MRI = magnetic resonance imaging; VBR = ventricular-brain ratio; PET = positron-emission tomography; FDG = fluorodeoxyglucose; SPECT = single-photon emission computed tomography; BEAM = brain electrical activity mapping; EEG = electroencephalography.
Source. Casanova et al. 1990; Gilman 1992a, 1992b; Guenther and Breitling 1985; Hendren and Hodde-Vargas 1992; Rabins et al. 1991.

leads, although the value (not to mention the comfort) of nasopharyngeal leads has been questioned.

The polysomnogram (PSG) is essentially a "sleep" EEG, with additional monitoring of eye movement, muscle activity, cardiac rhythm, and sometimes respiratory function (Rosse et al. 1989). The sleep EEG may also be helpful in atypical cases of depression, because a shortened rapid eye movement (REM) latency (among other abnormalities) is often seen in patients with major depression (Ballenger 1988). A number of primary sleep disorders may also present with "atypical depression," and a PSG may be helpful in diagnosis (Pies et al. 1989).

A particularly interesting adaptation of the EEG entails the use of specific sensory stimuli to "evoke" brain responses—so-called evoked potential studies. The stimuli may be auditory, visual, or "somatosensory" (usually involving a brief electrical stimulus to an extremity). Visual evoked potentials can assist in distinguishing "organic" from hysterical blindness; they are also used to confirm the presence of demyelinating diseases such as multiple sclerosis. One evoked potential—the P300—may be abnormal in some patients with schizophrenia or borderline personality disorder (Kutcher et al. 1987).

Although PET and SPECT are still largely research techniques, they may prove to be increasingly important in confirming the presence of various types of dementing illness. In one study of patients with Alzheimer's disease, cortical perfusion as measured by SPECT showed focal deficits that correlated closely with cognitive impairment (Besson et al. 1990). Alzheimer's disease patients may also show significant reductions in metabolic rate when studied by PET scanning, particularly in the parietal lobes (Cutler et al. 1985).

Let us close this section with a clinical vignette (adapted from Weller and Weller 1982).

Vignette

A 15-year-old girl presented with classic symptoms of anorexia nervosa, including food hoarding, distorted body image, self-induced vomiting, and amenorrhea. Her family history strongly suggested the "typical anorexic" dynamics. (For example, the patient was described as quiet and obedient in her childhood, but recently had developed a need to gain attention and control family members through her eating habits.) A routine neurological examination at the time of hospitalization revealed mild right-arm weakness and abnormal gait. A CT scan showed a left frontal tumor in

Table 2–8. Computed tomography (CT) and magnetic resonance imaging (MRI): a comparison

Indications/advantages	Contraindications/disadvantages
Computed tomography	
Preferable in acute trauma with much medical equipment.	Without contrast, insensitive to detection of acute brain infarction and meningiomas.
Preferable in uncooperative, claustrophobic patients or in those who cannot remain immobile for MRI.	Limited detection of posterier fossa and inferior temporal lesions because of bony structure artifacts.
Indicated in patients with cardiac pacemaker, mechanical heart valves, intracranial clips.	Patient subjected to ionizing radiation.
Procedure of choice after acute injury to head or spine, because of rapidity.	Contrast cannot be used in patients with iodine allergy.
Probably better than MRI in visualizing intracranial blood and calcified lesions.	
Less expensive than MRI.	
Magnetic resonance imaging	
Especially helpful in viewing posterior fossa lesions.	Contraindicated if aneurysm clip, ferromagnetic foreign body, pacemaker present.
Useful in detecting heavy metal deposits (e.g., in Hallervorden-Spatz disease).	Possibly traumatic for patients with claustrophobia.
Superior to CT scan for detecting most cerebral lesions, especially in white matter.	Not widely available, and costlier than CT.

Source. Adapted from Gilman 1992a; Rosse et al. 1989.

the thalamic-hypothalamic region, later diagnosed as an astrocytoma. Radiation therapy resulted in remission of both the patient's neurological signs and her "anorexia nervosa."

Neuroendocrine Techniques

In the past 15 years, a variety of neuroendocrine stimulation and "challenge" tests have been developed. Most have involved some measure of thyroid, adrenocortical, or hypothalamic-pituitary function. The most popular and widely used of these has been the dexamethasone suppression test (DST). In the 1980s this test appeared quite promising as a rather sensitive and specific test for major depression. Since then, both the sensitivity and the specificity of the DST have been impugned. We will discuss this test in more detail in Chapter 4. More recently, the thyrotropin-releasing hormone (TRH) stimulation test (TRHST) and various tests measuring growth hormone have received much attention, mainly as indicators of affective illness. Various "challenge" tests using amphetamine, sodium lactate, m-CPP (*m*-chloropenylpiperazine, a serotonin agonist), and other agents are finding increasing use in research settings; a few of these may have clinical utility in selected cases. These diverse neuroendocrine tests are summarized in Table 2–9.

Miscellaneous Tests

Many other physiological tests and procedures are being investigated in clinical psychiatry, some of which we will discuss in more detail in the chapters that follow. For example, the Amytal interview will be described in the chapters on somatoform and dissociative disorders (see Chapters 7 and 8, respectively).

Keep in mind that none of the tests we have discussed is 100% reliable for the condition tested and that diagnosis ultimately rests on clinical judgment. A good illustration is the diagnosis of temporal lobe epilepsy. A patient may have two or more "negative" EEGs before someone—perhaps a member of the nursing staff—notices the patient

Table 2–9. Neuroendocrine tests

Test	Physiology and technique	Indications and utility	Limitations
DST	Synthetic cortico-steroid normally suppresses secretion of cortisol; non-suppression may indicate HPA axis pathology or depression. Dexamethasone 1 mg given at 11 P.M.; serum cortisols checked next morning, 4 P.M., 11 P.M. Levels > 5 μg/dl = abnormal.	May be useful in ambiguous cases (e.g., psychotic affective illness vs. acute schizophrenia); persistent elevation after apparent recovery warrants scrutiny.	"Negative" test (normal should not impede vigorous treatment of depression; many false positive and false negative outcomes.
TRH stimulation test	Normally, release of hypothalamic TRH leads to surge of pituitary TSH. Patients with primary hypothyroidism have exaggerated surge; hyperthyroid patients have "flat" TSH response. Some depressed patients may have subclinical thyroid disease.	Some treatment-resistant depressed patients may show augmented TSH response with other TFTs normal; a blunted TSH response is seen in approx. 25% of patients with major depression; a blunted TSH response may be correlated with severity/suicidality.	Blunted TSH also seen in alcoholism, bulimia, and BPD. Results confounded by age (decreased response to TRH in elderly persons), weight loss, and steroid or cocaine use.
GH response	GH response may be index of limbic system dopamine activity; GH response to the dopamine agonist apomorphine may reflect status of hypothalamic dopamine receptor	There is blunting of GH release in some manic patients, in response to desipramine (suggests α_2 down-regulation); GH responses to to clonidine	Both blunted and excessive GH responses to apomorphine are seen in schizophrenic patients—may reflect subtype of patient?

Table 2–9.   Neuroendocrine tests (*continued*)

Test	Physiology and technique	Indications and utility	Limitations
GH response (*cont'd*)	sensitivity. GH also released via α_2-adrenergic mechanism in hypothalamus (e.g., clonidine and desipramine lead to GH surge).	and desipramine are blunted in unipolar and bipolar depressive patients. GH response may be blunted in process schizophrenic patients given apomorphine.	
Lactate challenge test	Sodium lactate causes many changes in normal subjects and panic patients (e.g., increased heart rate, blood pressure, HCO_3, prolactin; decreased pCO_2, serum cortisol, calcium). Panic disorder patients show further drop in pCO_2, abrupt increase in heart rate, and exaggerated autonomic response.	About 70% of panic disorder patients show lactate-induced panic; panic may be blocked by tricyclics or benzodiazepines. Panic with lactate infusion is not usually seen in patients with social phobia, generalized anxiety, or OCD.	Specificity is not clear; panic may depend on rate and concentration of infusion.

Note. DST = dexamethasone suppression test; HPA = hypothalamic-pituitary-adrenal; TRH = thyroid-releasing hormone; TSH = thyroid-stimulating hormone; TFT = thyroid function test; GH = growth hormone; OCD = obsessive-compulsive disorder.
Source. Liebowitz et al. 1985; Malas et al. 1987; Rosse et al. 1989.

carrying out stereotypic movements in an altered state of consciousness. You may or may not manage to get a "stat" EEG revealing seizure activity in such circumstances; you would, however, be justified in making the diagnosis on clinical grounds if the patient showed other classic symptoms of temporal lobe epilepsy. Despite some very impressive new technology, psychiatry remains fundamentally a clinical science.

References

Ballenger JC: Biological aspects of depression: implications for clinical practice, in American Psychiatric Press Review of Psychiatry, Vol 7. Edited by Frances AJ, Hales RE. Washington, DC, American Psychiatric Press, 1988, pp 169–187

Barth JT, Macciocchi SN: The Halstead-Reitan Neuropsychological Test Battery, in Major Psychological Assessment Instruments. Edited by Newmark CS. Boston, MA, Allyn & Bacon, 1985, pp 381–413

Besson JAO, Crawford JR, Parker DM, et al: Multimodal imaging in Alzheimer's disease: the relationship between MRI, SPECT, cognitive and pathological changes. Br J Psychiatry 157:216–220, 1990

Carr AC: Psychological testing of personality, in Comprehensive Textbook of Psychiatry/IV, 4th Edition, Vol 1. Edited by Kaplan HI, Sadock BJ. Baltimore, MD, Williams & Wilkins, 1985, pp 514–535

Casanova MF, Goldberg TE, Suddath RL, et al: Quantitative shape analysis of the temporal and prefrontal lobes of schizophrenic patients: a magnetic resonance image study. J Neuropsychiatry Clin Neurosci 2:363–372, 1990

Cutler NR, Hazby JV, Duara R, et al: Clinical history, brain metabolism, and neuropsychological function in Alzheimer's disease. Ann Neurol 18:298–309, 1985

Erdberg P: The Rorschach, in Major Psychological Assessment Instruments. Edited by Newmark CS. Boston, MA, Allyn & Bacon, 1985, pp 65–88

Gilman S: Advances in neurology, Part 1. N Engl J Med 326:1608–1616, 1992a

Gilman S: Advances in neurology, Part 2. N Engl J Med 326:1671–1676, 1992b

Guenther W, Breitling D: Predominant sensorimotor area left hemisphere dysfunction in schizophrenia measured by brain electrical activity mapping. Biol Psychiatry 20:515–532, 1985

Hendren RL, Hodde-Vargas J: Neuroimaging in schizophrenia. Psychiatric Times 9(9):17–21, 1992

House AE, Lewis ML: Wechsler Adult Intelligence Scale—Revised, in Major Psychological Assessment Instruments. Edited by Newmark CS. Boston, MA, Allyn & Bacon, 1985, pp 323–380

Jaskiw GE, Andreasen NC, Weinberger DR: X-ray computed tomography and magnetic resonance imaging in psychiatry, in Psychiatry Update: American Psychiatric Association Annual Review, Vol 6. Edited by Hales RE, Frances AJ. Washington, DC, American Psychiatric Press, 1987, pp 260–299

Kaplan HI, Sadock BJ: Synopsis of Psychiatry, 5th Edition. Baltimore, MD, Williams & Wilkins, 1988

Kutcher SP, Blackwood DHR, St Clair D, et al: Auditory P-300 in borderline personality disorder and schizophrenia. Arch Gen Psychiatry 44:645–650, 1987

Liebowitz MR, Gorman JM, Fyer AJ, et al: Lactate provocation of panic attacks, II: biochemical and physiological findings. Arch Gen Psychiatry 42:709–719, 1985

Malas KL, van Dammen DP, de Fraites EA, et al: Reduced growth hormone response to apomorphine in schizophrenic patients with poor premorbid social functioning. J Neural Transm 69:319–324, 1987

Meyer RG: The Clinician's Handbook. Boston, MA, Allyn & Bacon, 1983

Morihisa JM: Functional brain imaging techniques, in Psychiatry Update: American Psychiatric Association Annual Review, Vol 6. Edited by Hales RE, Frances AJ. Washington, DC, American Psychiatric Press, 1987, pp 300–325

Newmark CS: The MMPI, in Major Psychological Assessment Instruments. Edited by Newmark CS. Boston, MA, Allyn & Bacon, 1985, pp 1–64

Pies R[W], Adler DA, Ehrenberg BL: Sleep disorders and depression with atypical features: response to valproate. J Clin Psychopharmacol 9:352–357, 1989

Rabins PV, Pearlson GD, Aylward E, et al: Cortical magnetic resonance imaging changes in elderly inpatients with major depression. Am J Psychiatry 148:617–620, 1991

Rosse RB, Grese AA, Deutsch SI, et al: Laboratory and Diagnostic Testing in Psychiatry. Washington, DC, American Psychiatric Press, 1989

Weinberger DR; Brain disease and psychiatric illness: when should a psychiatrist order a CAT scan? Am J Psychiatry 141:1521–1527, 1984

Weller RA, Weller EB: Anorexia nervosa in a patient with an infiltrating tumor of the hypothalamus. Am J Psychiatry 139:824–825, 1982

3

Medical Disorders Presenting With Psychiatric Symptoms

In an important sense, we should place quotation marks around the two key words in the title of this chapter: "medical" and "psychiatric." Clearly, there is no simple definition of these terms that permits us to dichotomize all disorders into one or the other category. Many psychiatrists have also been dissatisfied with the term "organic," as in, "distinguishing organic from functional mental disorders"—a point the authors of DSM-IV have been at pains to emphasize, and one with which I have expressed some disagreement (Tucker et al. 1990; Pies 1991). Whether one places delirium, dementia, and the amnestic disorders under the general heading "Organic Mental Disorders" (as in DSM-III-R) or under the heading "Cognitive Disorders" (as in DSM-IV) is of little concern to the clinician; it is a matter of import mainly to nosologists and third-party payers. What matters critically to clinicians is the ability to diagnose an apparently "psychiatric" symptom as an essentially "medical" problem. Before defining these terms and subdividing our topic into convenient categories, let us launch into an illustrative vignette, adapted from Weissberg (1979).

Vignette

A 56-year-old woman with chronic alcohol and intravenous drug abuse was brought to the emergency room by family members,

51

because of her increasing agitation since the death of her husband 2 days earlier. The previous night, the patient had misidentified her brother as her dead husband, and she had defecated in her own living room. On admission to the ER, the patient denied recent alcohol abuse. Pulse and blood pressure were normal but temperature was not taken. A mental status examination was not performed. The patient was "medically cleared," with a referral to the psychiatry service; her diagnosis was "grief reaction." On admission to the psychiatric unit, the patient was noted to be disoriented to day and place ("This is a hotel . . ."). The psychiatrist noted slight scleral icterus and ordered liver function tests, which came back markedly elevated. The patient's temperature was 100.4 degrees. Subsequent labs suggested acute hepatitis A and B, and hepatic encephalopathy was suspected.

This vignette illustrates two important points: 1) the label "medically clear" should never be accepted without critically evaluating the medical workup (or lack thereof); and 2) the presence of an "obvious" psychosocial stressor (e.g., the death of a spouse) does not rule out the presence of medical illness—the body can have as many diseases as it pleases! In a recent study by Koran et al. (1989), medical illness was assessed in 529 patients in the California public mental health system. Of these patients, 12% had newly detected medical illness, and 6% had physical illness causally related to their "psychiatric" symptoms. The most common illnesses detected were (from highest to lowest frequency) neurologic, endocrine/nutritional, cardiovascular, gastrointestinal, and respiratory. Many other studies have confirmed the high prevalence of undetected medical illness in psychiatric populations.

When we refer to "medical" disorders in this chapter, we are not implying some special etiology different in kind from that of "psychiatric" disorders. We are simply using a convenient short-hand term for the range of neurologic, metabolic, infectious, hematological, and endocrinological disorders that make up the traditional curriculum of clinical medicine. Similarly, we use the term "psychiatric" to encompass the range of symptoms commonly seen in disorders such as schizophrenia, major depression, and various anxiety disorders. We surely do not wish to imply that one category involves "biological" factors and the other does not. As DSM-IV points out, "There is much 'physical' in 'mental' disorders and much 'mental' in 'physical' disorders" (American Psychiatric Association 1994, p. xxi). Indeed, the thrust of this chapter is to demonstrate how "psychiatric" symptoms may be reflections of common, biologically based ("organic") diseases.

I have divided the discussion into two main categories: medical illness resulting primarily in cognitive loss or an abnormal level of consciousness; and medical illness leading to disturbed reality testing, sensory perception, mood, or behavior. The first category encompasses the classical terms delirium and dementia, as well as the so-called amnestic disorders. The second category embraces the "old" (DSM-III-R) terms organic delusional disorder, organic hallucinosis, organic mood (and anxiety) disorders, and organic personality disorders. In DSM-IV, a different scheme is used, as we will see in later chapters. (For example, a mood disorder due to hypothyroidism would be classified under the category "Mood Disorder Due to a General Medical Condition.")

Of course, in clinical practice, patients rarely fit neatly into one or another of these categories. For example, a patient who presents with a medically based disturbance in reality testing (i.e., psychosis) frequently has an accompanying disorder of perception (i.e., hallucinations). An excellent review of the category "Physical Disorders Presenting as Psychiatric Illness" has been provided by Drooker and Byck (1992).

Cognitive Loss or Abnormal Level of Consciousness

Delirium and Dementia

Delirium and dementia are the most common conditions in this general category; pure amnestic disorders are less frequently encountered. Delirium and dementia have also been termed, respectively, "acute" and "chronic" organic brain syndrome. The differences between these categories are summarized in Table 3–1.

Clinical Presentation and Diagnosis

The hallmark of delirium is a fluctuating level of consciousness, a condition that is not usually seen in dementia until quite late in the disease process. The delirious patient, for example, may "nod off" every few minutes or show a marked inability to attend to your questions for more than a few minutes. In contrast, the demented patient shows primarily an impairment in memory (especially for recent events), calculation, and abstract thinking. Of course, patients may have superimposed delirium and dementia—but you cannot diagnose dementia until the delirium "clears."

As you might expect, there are dozens of medical conditions that cause delirium (Table 3–2). You should always keep in mind the most urgent and life-threatening causes of delirium: acute cerebrovascular accident, hypertensive encephalopathy, hypoglycemia, hypoxia, meningoencephalitis, poisoning, and severe thiamine deficiency, among others.

Given the myriad of conditions that can cause delirium, is there any way of making a "first cut" diagnosis? La Bruzza (1981) points out that many cases of delirium can be categorized as either anticholinergic or hyperadrenergic in nature. The former type may be due to toxicity from atropine-like compounds, tricyclics, antipsychotics, over-

Table 3–1.   Acute and chronic brain dysfunction: a comparison

	Delirium	Dementia
Onset	Acute	Usually insidious
Duration	Usually < 1 month	Usually months to years
Awareness/attention	Reduced, fluctuating	Often intact, stable
Perception	Often distorted	Often normal except at dusk
Thinking	Disorganized	Impoverished, concrete
Sleep/wake	Disrupted, reversed	Often normal for age

Source. Extensively modified from Lipowski 1980.

the-counter sleeping pills, and so forth. The latter type may be due to stimulant toxicity, sedative withdrawal, hypoglycemia, delirium tremens, thyrotoxicosis, and other conditions leading to hyperfunction of the sympathetic nervous system. The patient with anticholinergic-type delirium usually shows a rapid, weak pulse; large, nonreactive pupils; and dry, flushed skin. In contrast, the patient with hyperadrenergic delirium typically shows a rapid pulse; large, reactive pupils; and profuse sweating associated with pale (vasoconstricted) skin. Of course, patients often "overdose" on a mixture of medications and may present with a puzzling array of physical and psychological features.

Dementia, like delirium, may arise from a plethora of causes (Table 3–3). However, around 90% of patients with dementing illness have either Alzheimer's disease (approximately 65%) or multi-infarct dementia (approximately 25%).

The principal clinical differences between Alzheimer's disease and multi-infarct dementia lie in the course and complications of the two conditions. Alzheimer's disease usually presents as a chronic, insidious decline in cognitive function; multi-infarct dementia usually takes a stepwise or "stuttering" course marked by fairly sudden decrements in cognitive function. Alzheimer's disease usually does not present with focal neurological findings (e.g., hemiparesis), whereas multi-infarct dementia often does.

Table 3–2. Causes of delirium

Hypoxemia	Hyperparathyroidism
Electrolyte disturbance	Addison's disease
Acid-base disturbance	Corticosteroids
Uremia	Thiamine deficiency
Hypoglycemia	Thyroid dysfunction
Hypoparathyroidism	Porphyria
Pellagra	Hepatic failure
Acute cerebrovascular accident	Meningoencephalitis
Drug intoxication	Drug withdrawal

Dementia is not always an insidious illness, as the following vignette demonstrates.

Vignette

A 60-year-old male was brought into the ER by his wife because, according to his wife, he had been "acting very strangely over the last month." She elaborated, "Doctor, he doesn't seem to care about anything anymore, and his memory is terrible. And his behavior—why, he can't even control his urine anymore." She explained that the problem had begun fairly suddenly, about 2 months ago, after the patient had received a mild blow on the head. Since then, he had become apathetic, forgetful, incontinent of urine, and unable to walk without assistance. The ER physician suspected a chronic subdural hematoma. However, a computed tomography (CT) scan of the brain revealed enlarged ventricles and periventricular edema, without a focal lesion.

A provisional diagnosis of normal-pressure (i.e., communicating)

Table 3–3.   Causes of dementia

Progressive degenerative brain disease

Alzheimer's disease

Pick's disease

Subcortical dementias (e.g., parkinsonism, Huntington's disease)

Arrestable or reversible causes

Intoxications (e.g., heavy metals)

Infections (e.g., cryptococcal meningitis)

Metabolic disorders (e.g., hypocalcemia)

Nutritional disorders (e.g., B_{12} deficiency)

Vascular disorders (e.g., multi-infarct dementia)

Space-occupying lesions (e.g., subdural hematoma)

Normal-pressure hydrocephalus

Endocrine (e.g., myxedema)

Source. Adapted from Pies and Weinberg 1990; based on Consensus Conference 1987.

hydrocephalus was made; subsequent ventricular-peritoneal shunting alleviated the patient's gait disturbance and, to a moderate extent, his cognitive difficulties.

A good deal of attention in recent years has been focused on dementia related to acquired immune deficiency syndrome (AIDS) or human immunodeficiency virus (HIV). Such dementia may appear even in the absence of opportunistic infections associated with AIDS, such as toxoplasmic encephalitis. Early signs of HIV-related dementia may show up on complex tests of spatial and motor coordination, or as clinically evident impairment of memory, loss of concentration, or confusion (Westreich 1990). The symptoms and signs of the so-called AIDS dementia complex (ADC) are summarized in Table 3–4.

Keep in mind that patients with advanced HIV disease may present with a variety of opportunistic infections affecting the central nervous system (CNS). Consider the following case (extensively modified from Chaisson and Griffin 1992):

A 43-year-old homosexual male presented with progressive memory loss, confusion, and difficulty speaking for the past week. He had been diagnosed with AIDS 1 year earlier and had recently been treated for Pneumocystis pneumonia. On admission, he denied fever, sweats, headache, or stiff neck. His speech showed incomplete

Table 3–4.   AIDS dementia complex

Cognitive	Mood/Behavior	Motor
Impaired memory	Apathy	Ataxia
Poor concentration	Withdrawal	Leg weakness
Confusion	Personality change	Tremor
Slowed mentation	Psychosis	Impaired fine motor skills
Impaired attention	Decreased spontaneity	Dysarthria
	Anxiety	Dysgraphia
	Depression	

Source.   Extensively modified from Westreich 1990.

sentences with missing articles, poor syntax, and some perseveration. Cranial nerve examination showed right-lateral gaze nystagmus and mild right-facial weakness. He also showed decreased vibratory and pinprick sensation in the lower extremities. Magnetic resonance imaging of the brain showed a left frontal lobe lesion and an area of hyperintensity involving the right parieto-occipital region. Stereotactic biopsy of the brain revealed inclusions that reacted with antibody against polyoma virus antigen. The presumptive diagnosis was progressive multifocal leukoencephalopathy.

Drooker and Byck (1992) point out that the "Great Imitator" of 19th-century neuropsychiatry—tertiary syphilis—is increasingly common in persons with AIDS, often presenting with a disturbance of memory or mood.

Finally, dementia is sometimes difficult to distinguish from what was once called "depressive pseudodementia," which is now termed "the dementia of depression." (The change in terminology reflects the growing sense that depression may actually change the brain's ability to function in a very "real" way.) The differences between these conditions are summarized in Table 3–5.

Table 3–5. Differential diagnosis of dementia and dementia of depression

	Dementia	Dementia of depression
Duration	Months, years	Days, weeks
Past history	Systemic illness	Affective illness
Neurological features	Dysphasia, dyspraxia, incontinence	Usually absent
Answers to questions	Erroneous, confabulated perseverative	Often, "I don't know"
CT, EEG	Often abnormal	Usually normal
Response to antidepressant	Usually modest	Positive

Note. CT = computed tomography; EEG = electroencephalogram.
Source. Extensively modified from Binder 1988.

Management

Treatment of delirium and dementia, whenever possible, is directed at the underlying cause. In delirious patients with no known etiology for their condition, you will virtually never go wrong by administering glucose and thiamine—and you may avert brain damage from severe hypoglycemia or Wernicke-Korsakoff syndrome. Correction of electrolyte abnormalities, hypoxia, and so forth must occur before the patient is likely to improve very much. However, the agitated delirious patient may benefit temporarily from haloperidol, orally or parenterally, in doses ranging from 0.5 mg to 10 mg iv (or higher) every 20 or 30 minutes (Murray 1991). Surprisingly, this regimen does not appear to provoke significant extrapyramidal side effects. Murray (1991) emphasizes, in addition to haloperidol, the use of psychosocial and behavioral interventions in delirium (e.g., orientation of the patient, "human contact" with staff and and relatives). Benzodiazepines such as lorazepam (0.5 to 2 mg up to tid) are sometimes used to manage agitated delirium, but these medications are more likely to result in further confusion or paradoxical agitation than is haloperidol.

We have no specific "treatments" for the most common type of dementia, Alzheimer's disease. As of this writing, studies are under way with the agent tetrahydroaminoacridine (THA), but the preliminary results have not been spectacular. Other agents sometimes used to treat Alzheimer's disease include acetylcholine-enhancing agents such as physostigmine or arecoline, and the dihydrogenated ergot alkaloids (Spar and LaRue 1990). The latter—originally thought to act as cerebral vasodilators—may have a beneficial effect on brain glucose metabolism in early Alzheimer's disease. The day-by-day "management" of Alzheimer's disease usually focuses on various forms of behavioral agitation and disinhibition (e.g., screaming, head banging, aggressive behavior toward nursing home staff or family, etc.). In general, behavioral approaches are worth trying, although the Alzheimer's patient has a limited ability (in the middle to late stages of the illness) to learn and retain new material. Education and support of family members are important at all stages of the illness. Pharmacological approaches to behavioral agitation and disinhibition include use of low-dose, high-potency antipsychotics (e.g., haloperidol or pimozide); serotonergic agents such as trazodone; beta-blockers; anticonvulsants; lithium carbonate; and benzodiazepines (Jenike 1985; Spar and LaRue 1990). Each type of agent has advantages and disadvantages; for example, antipsychotics pose a high risk of tardive dyskinesia in elderly persons (Pies 1992), and benzodiazepines can lead to cognitive confusion and further behavioral disinhibition (Greenblatt et al. 1991). I have had good results using trazodone 50 to 200 mg/day in demented patients with markedly aggressive and agitated behavior. This agent may also be helpful in Alzheimer's patients with concomitant depression. Highly anticholinergic agents (e.g., thioridazine, amitriptyline) are best avoided in patients with Alzheimer's disease because they promote further cognitive dysfunction. Haloperidol 0.5 to 2.0 mg/day or pimozide in similar doses may be of help in the behaviorally disinhibited Alzheimer's patient.

Other types of dementia are managed in similar fashion. We should note that in multi-infarct dementia, control of hypertension and cardiac arrhythmias is particularly important in reducing long-term morbidity. Finally, the demented patient should be carefully assessed for the presence of concurrent mood disorder; "poststroke depression" and depression in the context of subcortical dementias (e.g., Parkinson's disease or Huntington's disease) may respond dramatically to antidepressant treatment.

Amnestic Syndromes

Among the most common "medically based" amnestic disorders is so-called Wernicke-Korsakoff syndrome, which we will discuss presently. Other causes of amnesia include head trauma, hippocampal infarction, herpes simplex encephalitis, neoplasms, and anoxic injury (Cummings 1985).

Vignette

A 52-year-old male was seen by the psychiatric resident on call for the ER because, according to the ER physician, the patient "seems confused and irrational. . . . He told me I'm his brother." The ER physician, noting the patient's somewhat ataxic gait, suspected alcohol intoxication; however, a blood alcohol level was read as "unde-tectable," and electrolytes and CBC were within normal limits. No neurological examination was performed. On interview by the psy-chiatric resident, the patient appeared apathetic and somewhat drowsy. He was disoriented to day and date and could recall none of three items after 2 minutes. The patient misidentified the resident as an old friend named Charlie, and stated, "I saw you yesterday outside the post office." The patient showed mild nystagmus and difficulty with heel-to-toe walking. A diagnosis of Wernicke-Korsa-koff syndrome was made, and the patient improved markedly after administration of thiamine hydrochloride intravenously.

Another amnestic syndrome sometimes seen by psychiatrists is that of transient global amnesia. This syndrome presents as an acute period of memory loss consisting of two components: an ongoing anterograde amnesia that persists for several hours, and a retrograde amnesia that lasts a few weeks (Cummings 1985). Its etiology is probably some alteration in cerebrovascular flow. We will discuss the differential diagnosis of transient global amnesia from various "func-tional" types of amnesia in our chapter on dissociative disorders (see Chapter 8).

Medical Illness Leading to Disturbed Reality Testing, Perception, Mood, or Behavior

Disturbances of Reality Testing

A large number of "medical" conditions can present with psychotic features. Cummings (1985) notes that Schneiderian first-rank fea-tures of schizophrenia may result from several medical conditions (Table 3–6). (As we will see in our chapter on schizophrenia [Chap-ter 5], Kurt Schneider believed that several symptoms, which he termed "first-rank," were especially useful in making the diagnosis of schizophrenia [e.g., auditory hallucinations that comment on one's behavior, the experience of having one's thoughts controlled].)

Are there any generalizations we can make about so-called organic psychoses? Typically, they are characterized by paranoid delusions, persecutory thoughts, and ideas of reference. Frequently, the temporal lobes are involved, as is suggested in the following vignette (extensively modified from Lishman 1987).

Vignette

A 53-year-old female with no psychiatric history was admitted to the hospital after attacking her husband with a knife. She accused her family of trying to poison her and of spraying the house with poison gas. She believed that her son was "turning her into a dog." The patient also complained of severe headache. On physical examination, there were no abnormal neurological signs. The patient showed bizarre facial mannerisms and unexpected movements from time to time. After 3 weeks in the hospital, the patient became stuporous and died. On autopsy, a glioblastoma of the right temporal lobe was discovered.

Table 3–6.   Medical conditions associated with first-rank Schneiderian symptoms

Central nervous system disorders

Temporal lobe malignancy

Viral encephalitis

Cerebrovascular disease

Temporal lobe epilepsy

Hydrocephalus

Basal ganglia disease

Metabolic/systemic conditions

Hypothyroidism

Addison's disease

Amphetamines, LSD, toxins, alcohol

Source.   Extensively modified from Cummings 1985.

Although not noted in this case, the presence of visual, tactile, or olfactory hallucinations in a "psychotic" patient ought to tip the clinician off to the presence of an organic process—particularly involving the temporal lobes.

McAllister (1992) gives us several other pointers, as summarized in Table 3–7. We might add the observation (presaged in the 1960s by Sir Martin Roth) that many patients with late-life delusional disorders ("paraphrenia") turn out to have either organic delusional syndromes or some neurological impairment, such as hearing loss, contributing to their psychosis.

The clinician should be especially alert to medications, drugs, and substances of abuse that may be associated with psychotic symptoms. Dopamine agonists (such as bromocriptine) and anticholinergic agents (including benztropine) are but two examples. A variety of alcohol-related paranoid states may be difficult to distinguish from paranoid schizophrenia (Lishman 1987). For example, prolonged excessive alcohol use is often associated with delusions of jealousy, infidelity, or other sexual themes. (Alcohol hallucinosis is discussed later in this chapter.) Finally, many psychotropic medications—including antidepressants and lithium—may induce psychotic symptoms in predisposed individuals or in patients with toxic levels of these agents.

Table 3–7.   Central nervous system disorders and associated delusions

Condition	Comment
Cerebrovascular disorders	More common with right posterior infarcts; subcortical atrophy may predispose.
Degenerative disorders	In around 40% of the cases, delusions, usually of the simple persecutory type, will occur at some point.
Extrapyramidal disorders	Delusions are often complex and "tightly held."
Epilepsy	Delusions are more common with temporal lobe foci; left temporal lobe foci are associated with first-rank schizophrenic symptoms

Source.   Extensively modified from McAllister 1992.

The management of organically based psychosis is, of course, directed at the underlying cause. Antipsychotics may be palliative, but they also run the risk of worsening the patient's mental status; highly anticholinergic agents are especially to be avoided. In some cases of psychosis secondary to substance abuse (e.g., phencyclidine or LSD), benzodiazepines may be helpful (Anderson and Tesar 1991) but also run the risk of "disinhibiting" some agitated patients.

Medical Causes of Perceptual Disturbance

Let us consider the following case. A 42-year-old male presents in the ER with the chief complaint that "they're driving me nuts . . . the voices . . . I can't stand it anymore." He described the acute onset of "bad voices" in his head, which he did not identify as his own voice or thoughts. Typically, the voices would say, "Let's get him," or other threatening statements. The patient was fully oriented and denied any illicit substance or amphetamine use. There was no history of head trauma or seizures. The patient had a surprising degree of reality testing surrounding the voices. For example, he was able to say, "I guess there's something wrong with me . . . I don't really think any-one could be out to get me . . . but sometimes it feels real." On close questioning, the patient acknowledged "drinking quite a bit" for the week prior to onset of the voices and as recently as 2 days before the voices began. He denied visual hallucinations, and his vital signs were essentially normal, with a slightly elevated pulse. A diagnosis of alco-hol hallucinosis was made. The patient responded to lorazepam 1 mg po tid and two "prn" doses of thiothixene, 2 mg po. He was dis-charged from the emergency service 36 hours after presenting. [Of course, one is never sure that two doses of an antipsychotic truly had a specific "psychotolytic" effect—as opposed to acting as a nonspecific sedative. Remember also that most antipsychotic agents can lower the seizure threshold in patients withdrawing from alcohol or other CNS depressants.]

Alcohol hallucinosis in "pure culture" is not always seen; often, the "voices" may be accompanied or supplanted by visual hallucina-tions (as you would expect in delirium tremens [DTs]), and the patient may show significant loss of reality testing (American Psychiatric Association 1987; Lishman 1987). In chronic cases, the differential between alcohol hallucinosis and paranoid schizophrenia may be difficult. Other medical conditions that may produce isolated disturbances of sensation (auditory, visual, tactile, or olfactory distortions and hallucinations) are listed in Table 3–8. Note, by the way, that the classic DTs present with visual or tactile hallucinations in the presence of clouded sensorium. We will say more about this and other psychiatric symptoms secondary to substance abuse in Chapter 10.

A good clinical rule of thumb is that visual or olfactory hallucinations are "organic" in origin, until proved otherwise. When reality testing is preserved, the clinician should be especially skeptical of a "psychiatric" diagnosis such as schizophrenia. In temporal arteritis, for example, the patient may complain of seeing "rainbows" or "faces," usually in the context of persistent headaches. Migraine headache may present with vivid visual distortions or hallucinations with intact reality testing. For example, in addition to the classic symptoms of teichopsia, the patient may report micropsia, macropsia, or even the "autoscopic" experience of seeing himself or herself crossing the street (Lishman 1987). Temporal lobe epilepsy—particularly when originating in the uncinate process—may present with olfactory or gustatory hallucinations. When the seizure focus is nearer the occipital lobe, visual hallucinations may be reported. In such cases, the accompanying features of déjà vu, stereotypies, amnesic periods, and postictal confusion should help the clinician make the diagnosis. (The electroencephalogram is sometimes helpful but not always sensitive enough, even with sphenoidal or nasopharyngeal leads [see Soreff 1987].) Although many writers have emphasized temporal lobe pathology as a source of

Table 3–8. Medical conditions associated with perceptual abnormalities

Alcohol hallucinosis	Posterior occipital lesions
Temporal lobe epilepsy	Narcolepsy
Migraine headaches	Anticholinergic drugs
Temporal arteritis	Amphetamines, barbiturates, cocaine

Source. Extensively modified from Soreff 1987.

perceptual disturbances, Fornazzari et al. (1992) recently reported three cases of frontal lobe seizures associated with "violent" visual imagery but without motor disturbance or loss of consciousness.

As with organic psychoses, treatment of organically based perceptual dysfunction is directed at the underlying cause. For example, temporal arteritis may respond dramatically to a course of steroids; migraine, to beta-blockers; and so forth. Alcohol hallucinosis is a somewhat controversial condition (see Lishman 1987) that may respond to either benzodiazepines, antipsychotics, or both; keep in mind, however, that antipsychotics may lower the seizure threshold and thus pose an additional risk in patients with various withdrawal syndromes. In the three cases of frontal lobe seizures reported by Fornazzari et al. (1992), two patients responded well to carbamazepine.

Medical Causes of Disturbed Mood

For purposes of exposition, I am "lumping" together so-called organic anxiety syndromes with the more narrowly defined organic "mood" disorders (i.e., disorders leading to depressive or manic symptoms). (In clinical practice, it is often difficult to separate anxiety from depressive or manic conditions.) We will expand on this brief overview in Chapters 4 and 6. Some of the medical conditions that may be associated with significant mood disturbance (depression, mania, anxiety) are listed in Table 3–9.

Let us now consider the following case:

A 65-year-old married male without prior psychiatric history presented to his family doctor with a chief complaint of "feeling down" for about 2 months. He gave a 2-week history of vague gastrointestinal distress, poor appetite, and a 5-pound weight loss. After very sensitive questioning by his doctor, the patient revealed that 1 month earlier, a close friend had died. The patient attributed his depression to this loss and said that he had come for the appointment "to please my wife." The physical examination was remarkable for a slightly enlarged, nontender gallbladder, and very slight jaundice. Urinary amylase was increased. A provisional diagnosis of pancreatic carcinoma with secondary depression was made.

Besides demonstrating the diagnostic utility of Couvoisier's sign—jaundice in the presence of an enlarged, nontender gallbladder—this case demonstrates an important principle in differential diagnosis: Beware the ready-made psychodynamic explanation. It may be true, of course, that the patient's loss contributed to his depression, but that did not provide him with immunity to pancreatic cancer.

Given the multitude of organic causes of depression, how, upon hearing those hoofbeats, can you sort out the "horses" from the "zebras"? Rundell and Wise (1989) reviewed 755 cases seen by the psychiatric consultation-liaison service in a general hospital. The study found that 38% of depressed patients had a diagnosis of organic mood disorder. The most frequent causes or precipitants were as follows: stroke (18.5%); Parkinson's disease (11.1%); lupus cerebritis (11.1%); and HIV infection (also 11.1 %). Hypothyroidism and multiple sclerosis both accounted for about 7% of cases. Somewhat surprisingly, medications accounted for only about 7% of cases; in the two cases noted, propranolol and corticosteroids were implicated. Because "stroke" was the number one cause of depression in this study, it is worth noting that depression following cerebrovascular accident is often correlated with left frontal lesions or with lesions in the basal ganglia. The degree of "poststroke depression" is not correlated with the degree of functional impairment following the stroke. (Presumably, it is the destruction of various neurotransmitter tracts that underlies the phenomenon.) The second most common organic cause of depression in the Rundell and Wise study—Parkinson's disease—was recently reviewed by Cummings (1992), whose findings are summarized in Table 3–10.

What should "clue" the clinician to the presence of an organic basis for depression? Although major depression can occur at any age, onset after age 45 should start yellow lights flashing—particularly if the patient's family psychiatric history is negative, there has been considerable weight loss, and no psychosocial precipitant can be found. (But to repeat: The presence of a precipitant does **not** imply the absence of organic factors!)

Finally, we consider an often-neglected diagnosis, primary sleep disorder, as a cause of depression (Pies et al. 1989). A variety of conditions, including nocturnal myoclonus, sleep apnea, and the so-

Table 3–9.   Medical conditions associated with mood disturbance

Medical condition	Mania	Depression	Anxiety
Infectious	Viral encephalitis Tertiary syphilis	Mononucleosis Encephalitis Hepatitis Tertiary syphilis	Septicemia Meningitis Encephalitis Neurosyphilis
Neoplastic	Brain tumor	Pancreatic cancer Bronchogenic cancer Brain tumor Lymphoma	
Cardio-vascular/respiratory		Hypoxia Sleep apnea CHF	Angina CHF Pulmonary embolus Pneumothorax Acute asthma COPD
Endocrine	Hyperthyroidism Cushing's disease Addison's disease Carcinoid syndrome	Hypo-/hyper-thyroidism Cushing's syndrome Addison's disease Parathyroid disease Diabetes mellitus	Hypo-/hyper-thyroidism Hypopara-thyroidism Hypoglycemia Pheochromocytoma Carcinoid
Metabolic	Uremia Dialysis	Uremia Hyponatremia Hypokalemia	Uremia Hypokalemia Hypocalcemia Low magnesium Acute intermittent porphyria Liver failure
Nutritional	Pellagra B_{12} deficiency	Pellagra Thiamine deficiency B_{12} deficiency Folate deficiency B_6 deficiency	B_{12} deficiency Thiamine deficiency Nicotinic acid deficiency

Table 3–9.   Medical conditions associated with mood disturbance (*continued*)

Medical condition	Mania	Depression	Anxiety
GI	Carcinoid tumor	Cirrhosis Crohn's disease Pancreatitis Celiac disease	Peptic ulcer Esophageal reflux Gallbladder disease Ulcerative colitis
Collagen-vascular		SLE (lupus) Rheumatoid arthritis Giant cell arteritis	

CNS disease	Multiple sclerosis
	Tumor
	Epilepsy
	Post-CVA
	Posttrauma
	Huntington's disease
	Wilson's disease
	Pick's disease
		Multiple sclerosis
		Parkinson's disease
		Alzheimer's disease
		Huntington's
		  disease
		Stroke
		Brain tumor
			Multiple sclerosis
			Alzheimer's disease
			Huntington's
			  disease
			Subarachnoid
			  hemorrhage
			CNS tumor
			Ménière's disease

Drugs/toxins	Steroids
	L-Dopa
	Bromocriptine
	Isoniazid
	Tricyclics
	Anticholinergics
	Cocaine
	Amphetamines
	Cyclobenzaprine
	Disulfiram
		Steroids
		Reserpine
		Propranolol
		Alpha-methyldopa
		Clonidine
		Digitalis
		Isoniazid
		Disulfiram
		Cimetidine
		Physostigmine
		Benzodiazepines
			Sympathomimetics
			Sedative
			  (withdrawal)
			Neuroleptics
			  (akathisia)
			Lead, mercury
			Organophosphates

Miscella-neous	Thalamotomy Postpartum	Amyloidosis Psoriasis Wilson's disease Postpartum	

Note. CHF = Congestive heart failure; COPD = chronic obstructive pulmonary disease; GI = gastrointestinal; SLE = systemic lupus erythematosus; CNS = central nervous system; CVA = cerebrovascular accident.
Source. Extensively modified from Cummings 1985, McNeil 1987.

called alpha-delta anomaly associated with fibrositis (Moldofsky 1986), may present as "atypical depression." A history of daytime somnolence, headaches, and musculoskeletal pain may help point the clinician toward the diagnosis of fibrositis (rheumatic pain modulation disorder). Depression, hypersomnolence, and a history of "very loud snoring" in a moderately obese, hypertensive male should prompt an investigation for obstructive sleep apnea. (Incidentally, benzo-diazepines for "insomnia" will only worsen sleep apnea.) In short, remember that while depression can cause disordered sleep, the con-verse is also true.

Management of Organic Mood Disorders

It will probably come as no surprise to you that the management of organic mood disorders generally rests on treatment of the underlying condition: correct the patient's hypo- or hyper- whatever and the patient will tend to improve. However, depressed patients with certain chronic and incurable conditions such as parkinsonism, or irreversible conditions such as severe cerebrovascular accident, may require on-going antidepressant therapy. Depression secondary to subcortical dementing illness (e.g., Huntington's disease or Parkinson's disease)

Table 3–10.   Depression and Parkinson's disease

Depression is present in about 40% of Parkinson's patients.

Depression in Parkinson's disease is characterized by high anxiety and low self-punitive ideation compared with other depressive disorders.

Risk factors for depression in Parkinson's disease are low CSF 5-HIAA and past depression history.

Depression in Parkinson's disease is associated with bradykinesia and gait impairment more than tremor.

Depressed Parkinson's disease patients have greater frontal lobe dysfunction than do nondepressed Parkinson's patients.

Depressed Parkinson's disease patients respond to tricyclics, bupropion, or ECT.

Note.   5-HIAA = 5-hydroxyindoleacetic acid.
Source.   Extensively modified from Cummings 1992.

may respond quite well to antidepressants (Cassem 1991). (Huntington's patients tend to be sensitive to highly anticholinergic agents, so the clinician might consider desipramine or fluoxetine.) "Poststroke depression" may respond well to nortriptyline, trazodone, psychostimulants, or electroconvulsive therapy (ECT) (Cassem 1991). Cassem (1991) states that "early and aggressive treatment of poststroke depression is required . . . to minimize the cognitive and performance deficits which this mood disorder inflicts on the patient in the recovery period" (p. 243). Prescribing antidepressants in medically ill patients demands close attention to such side effects as orthostatic hypotension, anticholinergic effects, and cardiac conduction problems (Cassem 1991; Harnett 1989). In general, nortriptyline, desipramine, psychostimulants, and bupropion have a better side-effect profile in medically ill patients than do the first-generation tertiary tricyclics such as amitriptyline or imipramine. The selective serotonin reuptake inhibitors (SSRIs) such as fluoxetine and sertraline may prove safe and effective in medically ill depressed patients, based on their side-effect profiles, but more research is needed to confirm this.

Medical Conditions Leading to Alteration in Personality

It is rare to find a "pure" alteration in someone's personality without any trace of cognitive impairment, anxiety, depression, altered perception, and so forth. Indeed, DSM-III-R noted as one of the chief features of organic personality syndrome, "affective instability, e.g., marked shifts from normal mood to depression, irritability, or anxiety" (American Psychiatric Association 1987, p. 115). The line between this condition and organic mood or anxiety syndromes is sometimes hard to discern. With these caveats in mind, let us look at a case of classic organic alteration in personality.

Vignette

Mr. D'Argent, a 62-year-old bank vice president, was brought to the ER by his very distressed wife. "I don't know what's happening to him," she said. "We went to the theater, and in the middle of the performance, he started swearing at the actors. Then we left, and he . . . he urinated right in the lobby!" This sort of disinhibited behavior had been going on for approximately 3 months but had worsened in the past few weeks. The patient had no psychiatric history or family history of depression or psychosis. On mental status examination, he was alert and fully oriented. Neurological examination was notable for positive "grasp" reflex but was otherwise normal. A CT scan of the brain with contrast revealed a probable meningioma in the prefrontal cortex.

Some of the more common organic causes of disturbed personality are listed in Table 3–11. Of course, many individuals with such a disturbance will go on to develop full-blown dementia, depression, or psychosis, secondary to progression of the underlying brain disease.

With respect to the locus of brain damage, Blumer and Benson (1975) have noted that damage to the prefrontal convexities is associated with apathetic withdrawal, psychomotor slowness, and social indifference. In contrast, damage to the orbital surface of the frontal lobe is more commonly associated with anger, poor impulse control, and socially inappropriate behavior (Spar and LaRue 1990). Lesions of the temporal lobes (e.g., gliomas) produce a high incidence of psychiatric symptoms; however, there is no particular personality disturbance specific for temporal lobe tumors (Lishman 1987). Psychopathic,

Table 3–11.   Medical causes of personality disturbance

Trauma to frontal lobes	Neurotoxin exposure (e.g., mercury)
Demyelinating disease (e.g., multiple sclerosis)	HIV infection (AIDS)
Ruptured cerebral aneurysm	Endocrine disorders
Parkinson's disease	Lupus cerebritis
Normal-pressure hydrocephalus	Brain tumor, abscess, granuloma
Temporal lobe epilepsy	Tertiary syphilis

Source. Extensively modified from Kaplan and Sadock 1988.

paranoid, hypochondriacal, and irritable features have all been reported. Temporal lobe epilepsy has been associated with interictal traits ranging from aggression and anger to "hyperreligiosity" and hyposexuality (McNeil and Soreff 1987).

Consider the following vignette, adapted from Welch and Bear (1990).

Vignette

A 38-year-old engineer was known as "Mr. Compulsive" by his subordinates because of his perfectionism, preoccupation with detail, strict punctuality, and anger with those who did not meet his "standards." The patient had had a strict "Protestant ethic upbringing" (as he himself put it), and he attributed his habits and behavior to this. However, a careful neurological and psychological history revealed that his obsessive-compulsive personality traits developed in midlife, associated with his documented temporal lobe epilepsy. In his early 20s, he had been, as his brother noted, "pretty laid back." A diagnosis of "interictal personality syndrome" was eventually established.

The moral here: Do not accept so-called Axis II pathology at face value. A diagnosis of, for example, "borderline personality traits" may tell you more about the diagnostician than the patient. As we will see in Chapter 9, the diagnosis of borderline personality disorder—and other "primitive character disorders"—is fraught with the perils of countertransference. Moreover, such personality disorders may represent the final common pathway for a number of etiologies, including brain trauma and attention-deficit disorder (with and without hyperactivity).

Management of Organic Personality Disorders

The management and treatment of organic personality disorders must be tailored to the specific disorder (e.g., the use of anticonvulsants for patients with epilepsy-related personality changes) (Welch and Bear 1990). But can we formulate some general guidelines applicable to most or all of the organic personality disorders? First, behavioral modification programs may be helpful, regardless of the specific syndrome. Second, working with the patient's family may be essential in the long-term care of the patient; averting anger and "burnout" in caregivers may spell the difference between home care and nursing home placement. Third, the judicious use of psychotropic medication can play an important role in reducing the disinhibited behaviors associated with many organic personality disorders. Anticonvulsants, trazodone, beta-blockers, and antipsychotics have been of use in the behavioral dyscontrol syndromes associated with organic personality disorders; benzodiazepines, though sometimes helpful, may lead to further disinhibition in many patients with brain damage.

Conclusion

The essence of this chapter is simply the following: Remember that hallucinations, delusions, anxiety, and depression are symptoms, not diagnoses. Remember also that at least 1 in 20 patients who receive an initial "psychiatric" diagnosis will be shown to have an underlying medical illness accounting for their symptoms (La Bruzza 1981). Finally, avoid the temptation of "premature closure" when confronting psychiatric symptoms; patients have an uncanny knack for refuting simplistic formulations, whether biological or psychosocial in nature.

References

American Psychiatric Association: Diagnostic and Statistical Manual of Mental Disorders, 3rd Edition, Revised. Washington, DC, American Psychiatric Association, 1987

American Psychiatric Association: Diagnostic and Statistical Manual of Mental Disorders, 4th Edition. Washington, DC, American Psychiatric Association, 1994

Anderson WH, Tesar G: The emergency room, in Massachusetts General Hospital Handbook of General Hospital Psychiatry, 3rd Edition. Edited by Cassem NH. St Louis, MO, Mosby Year Book, 1991, pp 445–464

Binder RL: Organic mental disorders, in Review of General Psychiatry, 2nd

Edition. Edited by Goldman HH. Norwalk, CT, Appleton & Lange, 1988, pp 252–265

Blumer D, Benson DF: Personality changes with frontal and temporal lobe lesions, in Psychiatric Aspects of Neurologic Disease, Vol 1. Edited by Benson DF, Blumer D. Orlando, FL, Grune & Stratton, 1975, pp 151–170

Cassem NH: Depression, in The Massachusetts General Hospital Handbook of General Hospital Psychiatry. Edited by Cassem NH. St Louis, MO, Mosby Year Book, 1991, pp 237–268

Chaisson RE, Griffin DE: Progressive multifocal leukoencephalopathy in AIDS. JAMA 264:79–82, 1992

Consensus Conference: Differential diagnosis of dementing diseases. JAMA 258:3411–3415, 1987

Cummings JL: Clinical Neuropsychiatry. New York, Grune & Stratton, 1985

Cummings JL: Depression and Parkinson's disease: a review. Am J Psychiatry 149:443–454, 1992

Drooker MA, Byck R: Physical disorders presenting as psychiatric illness: a new view. Psychiatric Times, July 1992, pp 19–24

Fornazzari L, Farcnik K, Smith I, et al: Violent visual hallucinations and aggression in frontal lobe dysfunction: clinical manifestations of deep orbitofrontal foci. J Neuropsychiatry Clin Neurosci 4:42–44, 1992

Greenblatt DJ, Harmatz JS, Shapiro L: Sensitivity to triazolam in the elderly. N Engl J Med 324:1691–1698, 1991

Harnett DS: Psychopharmacologic treatment of depression in the medically ill, in Recent Advances in Psychiatric Medicine. Edited by Hall RCW. Ryandic, 1989, pp 91–105

Jenike M: Handbook of Geriatric Psychopharmacology. Littleton, MA, PSG Publishing, 1985

Kaplan HI, Sadock BJ: Synopsis of Psychiatry, 5th Edition. Baltimore, MD, Williams & Wilkins, 1988

Koran LM, Sox HC Jr, Marton KI, et al: Medical evaluation of psychiatric patients, I: results in a state mental health system. Arch Gen Psychiatry 46:733–740, 1989

La Bruzza AL: Physical illness presenting as psychiatric disorder: guidelines for differential diagnosis. Journal of Operational Psychiatry 12:24–31, 1981

Lipowski ZJ: A new look at organic brain syndromes. Am J Psychiatry 137:674–678, 1980

Lishman WA: Organic Psychiatry, 2nd Edition. Boston, MA, Blackwell Scientific, 1987

McAllister TW: Neuopsychiatric aspects of delusions. Psychiatric Annals 22:269–277, 1992

McNeil GN: Depression, in Handbook of Psychiatric Differential Diagnosis. Littleton, MA, PSG Publishing, 1987, pp 57–126

McNeil GN, Soreff SM: Violence, in Handbook of Psychiatric Differential Diagnosis. Littleton, MA, PSG Publishing, 1987, pp 404–417

Moldofsky H: Sleep and musculoskeletal pain. Am J Med 81 (suppl 3a):85–89, 1986

Murray GB: Confusion, delirium, and dementia, in Massachusetts General Hospital Handbook of General Hospital Psychiatry, 3rd Edition. Edited by Cassem NH. St Louis, MO, Mosby Year Book, 1991, pp 89–120

Pies RW: The organic disorders (letter). Hosp Community Psychiatry 42:199, 1991

Pies RW: Geriatric psychopharmacology: an overview. Res Staff Physician 38(January):59–66, 1992

Pies RW, Weinberg AD: Quick Reference Guide to Geriatric Psychopharmacology. Branford, American Medical Publishing, 1990

Pies R[W], Adler DA, Ehrenberg BL: Sleep disorders and depression with atypical features: response to valproate. J Clin Psychopharmacol 9:352–357, 1989

Rundell JR, Wise MG: Causes of organic mood disorder. J Neuropsychiatry Clin Neurosci 1:398–400, 1989

Soreff SM: Hallucinations, in Handbook of Psychiatric Differential Diagnosis. Littleton, MA, PSG Publishing, 1987, pp 164–194

Spar JE, LaRue A: Concise Guide to Geriatric Psychiatry. Washington, DC, American Psychiatric Press, 1990

Tucker G, Popkin M, Caine E, et al: Reorganizing the "organic" disorders. Hosp Community Psychiatry 41:722–724, 1990

Weissberg MP: Emergency room medical clearance: an educational problem. Am J Psychiatry 136:787–790, 1979

Welch LW, Bear D: Organic disorders of personality, in Treating Personality Disorders (New Dir Ment Health Serv 47). Edited by Adler D. San Francisco, CA, Jossey-Bass, 1990, pp 87–101

Westreich L: AIDS dementia complex for the primary care physician. Res Staff Physician 36(June):47–53, 1990

4

Mood Disorders

> There's a certain Slant of light
> Winter Afternoons—
> That oppresses, like the Heft
> Of Cathedral Tunes—
> Emily Dickinson

Emily Dickinson was certainly on to something. Although DSM-III-R—with its "mood disorders, seasonal pattern"—didn't quite match the poet's language, it at least took her point. Indeed, DSM-III-R was the first major diagnostic system to recognize seasonal affective disorder, albeit only as a subtype.

"Mood," DSM-III-R told us, "refers to a prolonged emotion that colors the whole psychic life; it generally involves either depression or elation" (American Psychiatric Association 1987, p. 213). (In the "ancient" tome known as DSM-III [American Psychiatric Association 1980], you may recall, this diagnostic category was called affective disorders.) The principal division in DSM-IV (American Psychiatric Association 1994), the current classification, is again between bipolar and unipolar mood disorders. To oversimplify, within each of these categories, we can pick out a "major league" and a "minor league" disorder. Thus, cyclothymic disorder is a sort of low-grade bipolar disorder, and dysthymic disorder is typically viewed as a milder form of major depression. I'm speaking, of course, from a descriptive standpoint—we don't know the precise genetic or biochemical relationships between the full-blown mood disorders and their milder alter-egos. Even descriptively, there may be very little clinical difference between a "mild" major depressive episode and a dysthymic disorder that fulfills all of the nine symptomatic criteria listed in DSM-IV; both conditions can result in significant disability.

In DSM-III-R, so-called bipolar II disorder was relegated to the NOS (not otherwise specified) category; now, in DSM-IV, it has achieved the status of full-fledged disorder (i.e., recurrent major depressive episodes with hypomania). In DSM-IV, three "course specifiers" may be applied to bipolar I and II disorders: "with rapid cycling," "with seasonal pattern," and "with postpartum onset." The last two course specifiers may also be applied to major depressive disorder.

In DSM-IV, in accordance with its general philosophy, "medically based" mood disorders are now classified within the mood disorders category (i.e., mood disorder due to a general medical condition). Similarly, substance-induced mood disorder is now included among the mood disorders, rather than under the rubric of organic mental disorder. Both types of mood disorder—those due to a general medical condition (such as hyperthyroidism) or those due to substance intoxication/withdrawal—may present with manic, depressed, or mixed features. We will discuss these disorders in the sections below on pitfalls in differential diagnosis.

Of great interest to both nosologists and clinicians are those forms of mood disorders that, in much of the literature, have been termed "atypical." These conditions were placed in the NOS category in DSM-III-R. In DSM-IV, "atypical features" are now one of three sets of "cross-sectional symptom features" that may be applied to major depressive episodes occurring in major depressive disorder, bipolar I disorder, and bipolar II disorder. Other cross-sectional symptom features include melancholic and catatonic features—the latter having found their way into the mood disorders category after recognition that "catatonia" is actually more common in mood disorders than in schizophrenia.

Bipolar Disorder

DSM-IV recognizes three major types of bipolar disorder: bipolar I disorder, bipolar II disorder, and cyclothymic disorder. Bipolar I disorder has five major subdivisions: 1) single manic episode, 2) most recent episode hypomanic, 3) most recent episode manic, 4) most recent episode mixed, and 5) most recent episode depressed. Bipolar II disorder may present either as "hypomanic" or "depressed." There is also a bipolar NOS category to encompass difficult-to-classify conditions, such as recurrent hypomanic episodes without intercurrent depressive symptoms.

Bipolar I Disorder

The Central Concept

Patients with true bipolar I disorder give a history of one or more episodes of mania and usually one or more bouts of major depression. Let's consider the following vignette.

Vignette

G.F.H., a 46-year-old male, gave a history of "mood swings" going back to age 24. He described his "high" periods as "times when I feel like a cross between King Kong and Einstein." During these "high" periods—which typically lasted 3 or 4 weeks—G.F.H. reported "a tremendous surge of energy . . . I feel like I could make love five times a day and write two or three symphonies at night. I don't need more than two or three hours of sleep, and I run around the house like I'm on speed." In fact, the patient was a talented composer who got most of his creative work done during the early, "mellower" phase of his "highs." During this phase, G.F.H. typically became more talkative, experienced "racing thoughts," and took on an excessive number of tasks at once. Over a period of 2 or 3 days, the "mellower" phase of his illness gave way to a period of "being totally off the wall," in which the patient developed "crazy ideas . . . like that I was the Messiah of the musical world." During this second phase, G.F.H. would often "wind up in trouble with the cops . . . [with the patient] running around outside yelling and laughing, and ending up in the emergency room." In marked contrast to these bouts of elevated mood, G.F.H. also experienced longer periods of severely depressed mood. "It's like I shrivel up and die inside . . . I don't want to talk, or compose, or even eat. I wind up sleeping 15 hours a day and feeling lousy about myself—like I'm totally worthless. I get to the point of feeling like jumping out of a window." Sometimes, during these depressed phases, G.F.H. would develop the idea that his body was "rotting away . . . like God was causing some kind of worm to just eat away at my insides."

There was no history of any serious medical disorder, and the patient denied any alcohol or other substance abuse. Laboratory testing and the physical examination were completely within normal limits.

The case of G.F.H. is fairly typical of bipolar I patients. The early phase of our patient's illness—when delusional beliefs and severe social impairment were absent—is referred to as *hypomania*. As we will see, hypomania may exist "on its own" in other bipolar disorders, without progression into frank mania. G.F.H.'s depressed phase is representative of what DSM-IV calls, generically, a *major depressive episode*. Although in DSM-IV, the depressed phase of bipolar I disorder is indistinguishable from major depression of the unipolar type (discussed later in this chapter), some clinicians believe that the two conditions differ. The depressed phases of bipolar illness, for example, may involve hypersomnia and psychomotor retardation more frequently than do unipolar major depressive episodes, in which insomnia and agitation predominate (Akiskal 1983; Akiskal et al. 1983).

In recent years, the importance of "mixed" bipolar states and "dysphoric mania" has been clearly recognized—more than 70 years after Kraepelin tipped us off (Calabrese et al. 1993). A mixed state may occur as a transitional phase in classic bipolar I disorder or as a syndrome in its own right. Mixed states are more likely to become chronic, recurrent, lithium nonresponsive, and associated with substance abuse than are their "classical" cousins (Calabrese et al. 1993). As we will see, mixed states have important implications for somatic therapy.

By the way, another G.F.H., also a composer, may well have suffered from bipolar illness: George Frideric Handel (1685–1759). Yet nearly a century passed between Handel's death and Falret's description of "circular insanity"—the first clearly articulated account of bipolar illness.

Historical Development of the Disorder

The notion that extreme excitement and severe depression might be two sides of the same coin dates from antiquity. The physician Aretaeus (A.D. 50–130) described patients who would laugh, play, and dance night and day, only later to appear "torpid, dull, and sorrowful" (Sedler 1983, p. 1127). Aretaeus also noted that lucid intervals occur between these manic and depressive extremes—a critical observation utilized to this day (Alexander and Selesnick 1966). It took a leap of some 17 centuries before Falret provided us with the first clearly detailed description of bipolar affective illness (Sedler 1983). Falret described patients who live out their lives in a never-ending circle of depression and elation, interrupted by variable periods of lucidity. Falret even recognized the features of hypomania, which may begin with nothing more ominous than feelings of happiness or well-being (Sedler 1983).

By about 1896, Emil Kraepelin had legitimized the concept of manic-depressive illness as a distinct diagnostic entity. He also made the critical distinction between "dementia praecox" (schizophrenia) and manic-depressive psychosis on the basis of prognosis—the former having a far more morbid outcome. Although today we are less pessimistic about schizophrenia, Kraepelin's basic dichotomy has held up. Moreover, Kraepelin's observation that "slight colorings of mood" often overlap with "personal predisposition" anticipated our modern notion of the "bipolar spectrum" (Goodwin and Jamison 1987), which we will discuss later in this section. Sigmund Freud and Karl Abraham made important contributions to our understanding of bipolar illness, and we shall discuss these in the next subsection.

The Biopsychosocial Perspective

Biological factors. The "bio-" part of our model is a rapidly expanding area of research. Six classes of biological findings have been scrutinized in an attempt to distinguish "normal" subjects from depressive subjects, and unipolar from bipolar depressive subjects (Potter et al. 1987). This classification entails differences in electrolytes, membrane transport, neuropeptides, neuroendocrine factors, neurotransmitter receptors, and neurotransmitters per se. The bottom line, unfortunately, consists mostly of question marks. Nevertheless, there are some intriguing leads pointing to biological factors in bipolar disorder.

The three electrolytes reported to be abnormal in bipolar illness are sodium, magnesium, and calcium (Potter et al. 1987). Despite the methodological problems in interpreting the studies in this area, it is intriguing to speculate on these electrolytes, because lithium salts may operate through such endogenous ions (Baldessarini 1985). Taken as a whole, the studies to date suggest that some bipolar patients have an abnormality in the cell membrane processes that move sodium into, and lithium out of, the cell. A major cell membrane enzyme—Na-K ATPase—may be relatively less active in depression than in euthymia or mania, at least within a given patient (Nurnberger et al. 1982). Perhaps this seems a little removed from what even biologically oriented psychiatrists usually deal with. But consider that the neurotransmitter serotonin (5-hydroxytryptamine) is coupled to Na-K ATPase. Could a sluggish enzyme lead to reduced amounts of serotonin in the brains of bipolar patients? This is still a speculation, but there is some evidence behind it (Meltzer et al. 1981). Still other studies point to elevated plasma magnesium levels in both depressed and manic patients (Frazer et al. 1983), and elevated cerebrospinal fluid (CSF) calcium levels in bipolar depressed patients. The latter finding is especially interesting, because calcium channel blockers are now finding a role in the treatment of bipolar disorders (see discussion of treatment later in this section).

Perhaps you remember from basic physiology a gut peptide called somatostatin. This peptide has long been known to inhibit certain functions of the hypothalamic-pituitary-adrenal (HPA) axis. Now it turns out that somatostatin is present in neurons containing norepinephrine and may regulate noradrenergic function in depression and mania (Potter et al. 1987). In particular, some evidence suggests decreased somatostatin in the depressed phase of bipolar illness, as compared with euthymia or hypomania. Research is continuing on the role of other neuropeptides, including vasopressin, oxytocin, and thyrotropin-releasing hormone (TRH), in the genesis of mood disorders.

Neuroendocrine factors have been suspected in mood disorders at least since Hippocratic physicians ascribed "melancholia" to the accumulation of "black bile" (Alexander and Selesnick 1966). More recently, evidence has accumulated that most depressed patients have one or more abnormalities in the HPA axis. These abnormalities appear to be state dependent, often reverting to normal during periods of euthymia. We will discuss some of these when we take up the topic of unipolar depression. With respect to bipolar disorder, surprisingly few neuroendocrine factors seem to be specific. Some very preliminary evidence points to abnormalities in the release of growth hormone and thyroid-stimulating hormone (TSH) in bipolar patients, and there is a very high incidence of hypothyroidism in rapid-cycling bipolar patients (Potter et al. 1987).

Perhaps the "hottest" area of biological psychiatry research involves the study of neurotransmitters and neurotransmitter receptors. But again, the relationship between these factors and the unipolar-versus-bipolar dichotomy is far from clear. Perhaps the outstanding finding so far is that in bipolar depression, when compared with unipolar depression, one or more indices of norepinephrine output are reduced (Potter et al. 1987). For example, CSF and/or urinary MHPG (a metabolite of central norepinephrine) tend to be reduced in bipolar depression.

Research into the biology of bipolar disorder is also occurring on a more macroscopic level. The pioneering work of Flor-Henry (1983) has uncovered a number of neuropsychiatric variables that may characterize bipolar disorder. A variety of electroencephalographic and BEAM (brain electrical activity mapping) studies, for example, suggest that mania is associated with abnormal left hemisphere activation, possibly due to loss of inhibition originating in the right hemisphere (Flor-Henry 1983). Abnormalities on the sleep electroencephalogram (EEG) may also be found in bipolar patients, though these abnormalities may overlap with those seen in unipolar depressive patients (Wehr et al. 1987). Most intriguing are the data showing that in rapid-cycling bipolar patients, changes in REM sleep latency, sleep duration, first REM period duration, and slow-wave sleep actually parallel changes in clinical state. In some cases, sleep EEG changes appear to anticipate the switch from mania into depression (Post et al. 1977; Wehr 1977). There are also some positron-emission tomography (PET) scan data suggesting that unipolar and bipolar depressive patients utilize glucose differently (Schwartz et al. 1987). We will return to this point when we examine adjunctive testing in bipolar disorders.

Finally, Post (1993) and his colleagues have elaborated a "kindling" model of bipolar disorder that may help explain the accelerating course one often sees over the years in a bipolar patient. In effect, the "kindling" model holds that "with sufficient numbers of episodes the illness may . . . become progressively more 'well grooved' or autonomous" (Post 1993, p. 88). Presumably, changes in synaptic connections, receptor sensitivity, or secondary messengers such as cyclic AMP underlie this phenomenon. In any event, kindling may not only worsen the bipolar patient's course but also decrease responsiveness to somatic treatments (see discussion of treatment later in this section).

Psychological factors.   Do bipolar patients have specific psychodynamic characteristics? What about their premorbid personality and ego defenses? In the years before lithium treatment, a great deal was made of these questions. However, even in the lithium era, psychodynamic concerns are quite important in the understanding and treatment of bipolar disorder (Jamison 1987). As a point of departure, then, let's consider the following vignette.

Vignette

Craig was a 23-year-old single male who had begun to experience "amazing mood swings" at age 16. He described his childhood as one of "always being the star of the show . . . but if I messed up, someone would always smack me down." Craig was an extremely good student from elementary school until his junior year in high school, when his mood swings began to interfere with his performance. He described his parents as "Mr. and Mrs. Straightarrow," and added, "My father is so uptight he photocopies the Christmas cards he sends." Craig described himself as "very sociable, you know, the class clown," but at the same time "kinda guilty when I carry things too far . . . like with girls." Craig presented as a meticulously groomed, carefully controlled young man with many obsessional traits. He acknowledged, "Performance is everything with me," and added, "In my house, if you weren't the best, you weren't even there."

Craig epitomizes the classic dynamic description of the manic-depressive individual: a person with excessively high moral goals and an early childhood history of extreme discipline. Premorbid personality traits are said to include inordinate preoccupation with success, a high degree of extroversion, and a rigid superego (Akiskal et al. 1979). Manic-depressive individuals are also said to "externalize control"—to place responsibility for their well-being upon others, often resulting in intense anger when the individual's needs are not met (Waters and Calleia 1983). Another view of the manic-depressive person is that he or she has an underlying or premorbid "cyclothymic temperament"—a view we shall examine more closely in our discussion of cyclothymic disorder. At this juncture, let's reserve final judgment on these developmental and dynamic notions, except to say that they evolved more from theory and clinical extrapolation than from well-designed empirical studies. Moreover—as we will see over and over in this manual—it's often hard to know whether the supposed "psychodynamics" of a given disorder are truly causal, or merely the effects of having a biologically based disorder.

Karl Abraham (1877–1925), Sigmund Freud (1856–1939), and Franz Alexander (1891–1964) all made important contributions to our psychodynamic concept of manic-depressive illness. Abraham—comparing normal grief with "melancholia"—argued that in the latter, unconscious hostility toward a lost object becomes directed at the self. Expanding on this, Freud suggested that in melancholia the ambivalently regarded lost object is incorporated into the ego (introjection). The hostility once present in the actual relationship is then directed against the incorporated love object. This is experienced as self-hatred and the usual signs and symptoms of major depression. The superego, too, flails out at the psychic representation of the lost object—in effect, making war on the ego. Freud eventually explained mania as a fusion of the ego and superego, freeing up the energy previously used in the conflict between these two parts of the psyche (Arieti 1974). Alexander developed an interesting variant on the views of Abraham and Freud. He believed that in the depressed phase of manic-depressive illness the individual punishes himself or herself for supposed transgressions. When this self-punishment begins to feel excessive, the individual again feels free to behave uninhibitedly and becomes manic. Thus, "in the depressive phase he overpays his debts to his conscience, so that he has moral capital to spend" in the manic phase (Alexander and Selesnick 1966, p. 299).

Aside from these theoretical complexities, many psychiatrists would agree that mania is often an unconscious means of avoiding a "creeping" sense of depression. I recall a bipolar patient who would fly into a manic episode every time she ran into her "hated" ex-husband! On the whole, however, the view of manic-depressive illness as primarily "psychological" has given way to a more biologically based view.

Sociocultural factors. Although the incidence and prevalence of bipolar disorder do not seem related to marital status, religion, or race, some evidence exists for an increased rate of bipolar disorder in the upper socioeconomic classes. In the 1950s, Freida Fromm-Reichmann and her colleagues suggested that manic-depressive patients tend to come from upwardly mobile families in which discipline was strict but inconsistent—not unlike Craig's background in the vignette above (Cohen et al. 1954). Cancro (1985) hypothesizes that periods of hypomania may actually spur the bipolar individual "upward" socioeconomically, because such periods are often intensely productive. Ambelas (1987), working in England, found that two-thirds of patients hospitalized with their first manic episodes reported significant "life-events" within the 4 weeks preceding admission. Interestingly—and reminiscent of my divorced patient mentioned at the end of the preceding subsection—"pleasant" events rarely preceded manic episodes. Indeed, deaths accounted for the greatest percentage of presumed precipitating events.

In concluding our discussion of the biopsychosocial model and bipolar disorder, we should look with great interest at a more recent study by Thomas Wehr (see Wehr et al. 1987). Wehr describes four cases in which mania, indeed, seemed to be precipitated by life events: events that prevented sleep! In light of our earlier comments on the sleep-wake cycle, Wehr's findings suggest that "bio-" and "psychosocial" factors often interact in the onset of mania.

Pitfalls in the Differential Diagnosis

To put it succinctly, all that cycles is not DSM-IV 296.4. A great many medical ("organic") and nonmedical conditions can mimic bipolar disorder, especially its more moderate variants. Restricting our discussion now to the more classical type I bipolar disorder, let's consider a clinical vignette.

Vignette

> Emily was a 43-year-old married mother of two who presented in the ER with markedly pressured speech, flight of ideas, inappropriate sexualizing with staff, and the idea that "I'm the reincarnation of Emily Dickinson." According to her husband, Emily had no previous psychiatric history and no family history of mania or depression, and had been acting normally until 4 days prior to evaluation. At that time, the patient—an asthmatic—began to increase her dose of oral prednisone from 15 mg/day to 80 mg/day. She stated that she had experienced difficulty breathing prior to the increase and decided that she "had to do something to preserve the Belle of Amherst, whose spirit resides in my breast." Tapering the patient's prednisone back down to 15 mg/day, and her use of chlorpromazine 150 mg po qd and at hs, resulted in complete remission within 5 days.

Emily's case illustrates only one of the medical causes of manic and hypomanic symptoms—sometimes referred to as "secondary mania" (Krauthammer and Klerman 1978). Note, in Emily's case, the absence of past history of mood disorder, the absence of family history, and the relatively sudden onset of illness in a well-functioning individual—all clues to the "organic" origin of her mania. Other common medical causes of mania and hypomania are listed in Table 4–1.

What about other psychiatric disorders that can resemble bipolar disorder? In asking this question, we are focusing on conditions that may produce manic-like symptoms, since we will discuss the differential diagnosis of depression per se later in this chapter.

There are seven main conditions that can be confused with the manic phase of bipolar disorder:

- Schizophrenia (especially paranoid type)
- Schizoaffective disorder
- Borderline personality disorder
- Histrionic personality disorder
- Adolescent conduct disorder
- Attention-deficit/hyperactivity disorder
- Hypomania

Vignette

Howard was a 24-year-old male graduate student who presented with marked agitation, pacing, and loud, pressured speech. According to his roommate, Howard had begun "to lose it" approximately 2 weeks ago, when he became increasingly suspicious of one of his professors, accusing him in class of "threatening my territorial integrity by means of covert electronics." Howard had become increas-

Table 4–1.   Organic causes of mania and hypomania

Drug-related

Steroids, adrenocorticotropic hormone (ACTH)

L-Dopa

Antidepressants

Sympathomimetics (amphetamine, methylphenidate)

Anticholinergics (benztropine, trihexphenadyl)

Neurological conditions

Brain tumors

Epilepsy (especially temporal lobe)

Multiple sclerosis

Encephalitis

Metabolic conditions

Hyperthyroidism

Cushing's disease

Postdialysis state

Source.   Extensively modified from Keller 1987.

ingly hostile toward his roommate, insisting that he, Howard, deserved "the adulation befitting a minion of the archangel Irving." In the ER, Howard denied auditory hallucinations or the belief that others could control his thoughts, but added, "Not that they haven't tried." His thought processes were disorganized, with both tangential responses and periods of blocking. Howard's affect was generally constricted, despite his apparent irritability. The resident in the ER described his own response to Howard as one of "talking to someone from another planet . . . this guy was locked inside his own little world."

So what's with Howard? It's easy to see how he might be diagnosed as "manic"—he has the hyperactivity, pressured speech, and grandiosity of the manic patient. But other pieces of the puzzle don't fit with manic-depressive illness. Howard's affect is constricted, unlike the typical manic person, who is usually either euphoric or irritable. Furthermore, Howard's delusions include more bizarre and paranoid ideas than those of the typical manic (e.g., being influenced by "covert electronics"). Although he denies having his thoughts controlled, Howard acknowledges that people have "tried." This sort of passive idea of influence is not typical of mania, in which delusions tend to be more "active" (e.g., the manic person believes he or she has some special power or important position). The manic person "does unto others" rather than being "done unto." The resident's countertransference to Howard is also revealing: his lack of empathic "connectedness" to Howard and his feeling that Howard was from "another planet" are not a typical reaction to a manic patient. Generally, the manic individual is felt to be amusing, ingratiating, or at least "human." Finally, although "thought process disorder" is commonly seen in mania, the presence of "blocking" and tangentiality raises doubts about the diagnosis of mania.

By now, you've probably begun to decipher the clues. Most of the features just discussed are more consistent with paranoid schizophrenia than with mania. But the differential diagnosis of these two conditions is tricky, as Pope and Lipinski (1978), in their classic paper, make clear. Indeed, it is sometimes impossible to distinguish the hyperactive paranoid schizophrenic patient from the irritable, suspicious manic patient without a longitudinal history or observation—that is, without knowing the patient's clinical course over a period of years. The bipolar patient, of course, typically has relative or complete remissions between bouts of illness, whereas the schizophrenic patient usually shows significant "inter-morbid" dysfunction (Pope and Lipinski 1978).

What about the other six disorders that can mimic mania? As we will see in Chapter 5, the diagnosis of schizoaffective disorder is fraught with uncertainty. In particular, the "manic" subtype of this condition seems to share some genetic and clinical features with true bipolar disorder. In contrast, schizoaffective depressive patients probably constitute a mixed group of patients, including schizophrenic patients with depression, major depressive patients with psychotic features, and patients with other psychiatric disorders who have developed a psychotic depression (Clayton 1982; Keller 1987). As we will see, the distinction between "true" bipolar mania and schizoaffective mania becomes somewhat less important when the practicalities of treatment arise.

Borderline personality disorder can sometimes present with a manic-like picture. The patient may appear irritable, angry, and impulsive, sometimes giving a history of excessive spending or sexual activity. However, the borderline patient's mood is more labile than that of the manic patient. Grandiose delusions are less common in borderline personality disorder, in which psychotic symptoms (if present) tend to be more paranoid in nature. Furthermore, the borderline patient tends to show more intermorbid impairment than does the bipolar patient. Finally, one's countertransference toward the borderline patient is generally more negative than that toward the manic patient. On the other hand, manic patients sometimes play provocative and annoying "games" that feel much like those of the borderline patient, as Janowsky et al. (1970) have pointed out.

Histrionic personality disorder can occasionally present with manic-like features (see Chapter 9). The histrionic patient may be, for example, inappropriately sexual or seductive, or excessively emotional, self-centered, and demanding, thus mimicking some of the features of the manic patient. Differential diagnosis rests on obtaining a good recent history and observing the individual for a sufficient length of time. The histrionic patient does not typically give a history of acutely decreased need for sleep, racing thoughts, or self-defeating actions (such as wild spending sprees) that have compromised social or vocational function. Moreover, the histrionic patient will not demonstrate the persistently elevated energy level or rapid, pressured speech of the genuinely manic patient. Instead, he or she (more commonly she) will exhibit rapidly shifting and shallow expressions of emotion.

The adolescent with conduct disorder may sometimes present with a manic-like picture, and because bipolar disorder definitely does occur in this age group, the differential diagnosis is important. The essential feature of conduct disorder is "a repetitive and persistent pattern of behavior in which the basic rights of others or major age-appropriate societal norms or rules are violated" (American Psychiatric Association 1994, p. 85). (You can think of this disorder as the precursor, in some cases, of the adult's antisocial personality disorder [see Chapter 9], which can also at times be confused with mania.) The adolescent with conduct disorder may show irritability, temper outbursts, and reckless or aggressive behavior. Unlike the manic patient, however, the adolescent with conduct disorder has manifested these features over the course of many months or years, in the absence of typical manic neurovegetative signs and symptoms. Nevertheless, antisocial behaviors in an adolescent may herald the onset of a manic episode (Tyrer and Shopsin 1982), and bipolar disorder should always be considered in the assessment of "bad" or "wild" adolescents.

Attention-deficit/hyperactivity disorder (ADHD) may sometimes be confused with mania, particularly when it appears in an adult whose childhood ADHD has gone undiagnosed. (These same "grown-up ADHD" patients may be misdiagnosed as having borderline personality disorder.) In the hyperactive ADHD patient, as opposed to the manic patient, mood is not abnormally expansive or euphoric, and the disturbance lacks the relatively acute onset seen in mania. The ADHD patient is also less likely than the manic patient to exhibit thought process disorder such as flight of ideas. By the way, ADHD in adults—as in children—may respond well to stimulant medication (Wender and Klein 1981).

Finally, the differential diagnosis of mania forces us to confront the related condition of hypomania. As we will see, hypomania serves both as a clinical and as a conceptual bridge between the classical bipolar disorders on the one hand and the less dramatic cyclothymic disorder on the other. Taken together, these cyclical mood disorders constitute what Akiskal and others have termed "the bipolar spectrum" (Akiskal 1983). Hypomania is defined in DSM-IV as a distinct period of sustained elevated, expansive, or irritable mood lasting at least 4 days that, although sharing some features of mania, is not severe enough to cause marked impairment in social or occupational functioning or to require hospitalization (American Psychiatric Association 1994).

Hypomania is clearly different from the individual's usual non-depressed mood, and this change is observable by others. Unlike mania, hypomania is not associated with psychotic features. Hypomania may be a welcome relief to some patients, whose depressive bouts smother creativity and productivity. The hypomanic patient—unlike the manic patient—often accomplishes a tremendous amount of useful work during this "up" period and may strenuously resist medication that "takes away the highs." The hypomanic patient typically exhibits inflated self-esteem, decreased need for sleep, increased talkativeness, "racing" thoughts, distractibility, increased level of activity, and "excessive involvement in pleasurable activities that have a high potential for painful consequences" (American Psychiatric Association 1994, p. 338).

Adjunctive Testing

There is no single test—whether of the blood, the psyche, or the brain—that can "make" the diagnosis of bipolar disorder. Nevertheless, as our discussion of biological factors has suggested, one's clinical judgment may be supplemented by a number of adjunctive tests. In a tricky case, such tests may provide that final bit of evidence needed to "swing" toward or away from a diagnosis of bipolar disorder.

Neuroendocrine tests. As discussed earlier, there is accumulating evidence that, in comparison with unipolar depressive patients, bipolar depressive patients may show reduction in several indices of norepinephrine output. Therefore, it may be useful to obtain a urinary

MHPG (3-methoxy-4-hydroxyphenylglycol) and a supine plasma norepinephrine sample on a patient suspected to have bipolar disorder. If both are far below normal values, one's suspicion of bipolar disorder may be slightly increased (Potter et al. 1987).

Brain imaging techniques. Buchsbaum et al. (1986) and others have provided evidence that PET can help distinguish unipolar from bipolar depression. In these studies, the unipolar patients tended to show a higher frontal cortex metabolic rate than did the normal control subjects. In contrast, patients with bipolar affective illness had metabolic rates in their frontal cortex that were lower than those of normal control subjects. Metabolic rates in the basal ganglia were also higher in unipolar than in bipolar patients. Interesting as these results are, further research is required before one considers PET as critically important in diagnosing bipolar disorder.

Neuropsychological testing. Although the data are complex, Flor-Henry (1983) has presented evidence pointing to nondominant hemisphere dysfunction in bipolar patients, especially of the frontotemporal region. (In contrast, schizophrenic patients tend to show more impairment on neuropsychological variables that tap dominant hemisphere function, as we will note in Chapter 5.)

Psychological testing. The depressed bipolar patient shows patterns similar to those of the unipolar depressive patient, whom we will discuss in the section on depressive disorders. Although psychological testing is rarely necessary to diagnose the truly manic patient, it is worth mentioning some of the classical findings in mania. On the Minnesota Multiphasic Personality Inventory (MMPI), the 46 items on scale 9 are a direct measure of energy level, varying quantitatively from depression through hypomania to mania (Newmark 1985). The majority of medicated manic patients obtain scores of 75 to 90 on scale 9. Elevated scores on scales 4, 6, and 8 may also be seen in mania, and there is some evidence that the 9-6 code type discriminates manic from schizophrenic patients (Meyer 1983; Winters et al. 1981). However, an elevated scale 9 is not pathognomonic for mania, with the former being present in other conditions manifesting high energy levels.

On the Wechsler Adult Intelligence Scale (WAIS), the manic patient's inability to check and modify performance results in lower scores on block design, picture arrangement, and object assembly. On the Rorschach, the manic patient shows numerous poor quality W (i.e., whole blot) responses, with attention to details that normal subjects usually ignore. A high number of confabulation responses and/or shading responses, in combination with a high percentage of W, C, CF, S, and Dd responses, is indicative of mania (Meyer 1983; Wagner and Heise 1981).

Treatment Directions and Goals

Somatic approaches. By now, even the general public is aware of the use of lithium in manic-depressive illness. Indeed, lithium is the cornerstone of treatment for bipolar patients and has utility in both the acute and chronic, manic and depressed phases of the illness. (We shall use the designation "lithium," because the carbonate and citrate salts are both effective.) A few basic principles regarding the use of lithium should be kept in mind (Goodwin and Roy-Byrne 1987). The gap between therapeutic and toxic levels is narrow and is influenced by sex, age, weight, salt intake, sweating, renal function, and other medications. Moreover, more lithium is needed to achieve a given blood level during mania than during euthymia or depression; conversely, downward adjustment in dose may be necessary as a manic patient begins to "come down" toward normal mood. Generally speaking, blood levels above 1.5 mEq/L are not recommended, and considerable care is required when levels are in the 1.2 to 1.5 mEq/L range. Stable, euthymic bipolar patients can often be maintained on levels in the range of 0.6 to 0.7 mEq/L. Some data suggest that giving lithium as a single nighttime dose decreases renal and other side effects in stable patients on "lithium maintenance" (Goodwin and Roy-Byrne 1987). Periodic monitoring of renal and thyroid function is important.

In recent years a variety of new pharmacological treatments have arisen for the lithium-intolerant or -resistant bipolar patient (Post et al. 1987). Carbamazepine (Tegretol) and valproate (Depakote)—both anticonvulsants—have proved particularly useful in rapid-cycling and "mixed" bipolar patients. While there is no well-established "therapeutic" plasma level for either of these agents, most clinicians aim for carbamazepine levels of around 4 to 12 μg/ml, and valproate levels of roughly 50 to 125 μg/ml (Shader 1994). Either of these agents can be used adjunctively with lithium, or with each other, but such combinations can produce complex interactions that must be monitored closely. Electroconvulsive therapy (ECT) may be quite effective for both the acute manic and depressive phases of bipolar disorder, but the beneficial effect is usually transient. The use of antidepressants in the depressed bipolar patient is both tricky and somewhat controversial (Post 1993). Virtually all the currently available antidepressants are capable of inducing mania in such patients and perhaps of "accelerating" their intrinsic cycling frequency—and the latter effect can create a very refractory, "lithium-resistant" patient. Some evidence suggests that the MAOIs, bupropion (Wellbutrin), and the SSRIs may be less likely than tricyclics to induce mania (Simpson and DePaulo 1991; Wright et al. 1985), but this observation rests on rather modest data. My own practive is to make minimal use of antidepressants in bipolar patients, except during the worst part of the depressed phase of illness; after the patient begins to emerge from this phase, I attempt to taper and discontinue the antidepressant. Good recent reviews of somatic treatments of bipolar disorder are provided by Post (1993) and Shader (1994).

Psychosocial approaches. Despite the "biological" substratum in bipolar illness, a psychological approach to the patient is essential and may critically affect compliance with lithium treatment (Jamison 1987). In the first place, there are some general psychotherapeutic issues that practically all bipolar patients must confront: fears of recurrent mood swings, denial of serious illness, difficulty in discriminating normal from pathological mood swings, problems arising in interpersonal relationships as a consequence of illness, disruption of normal developmental stages by the illness, and concerns about transmission of bipolar illness to offspring (Jamison 1987).

The key elements of psychotherapy with bipolar patients may be summarized as follows: 1) education as to the nature of bipolar illness, 2) realistic reassurance and reality testing, 3) assessment and management of suicidality, and 4) management of countertransference. To understand how these elements coalesce in the clinical situation, let's consider the following vignette.

Vignette

Janet was a 34-year-old single female with a long history of bipolar I illness. Her therapist, a young male resident whom the patient described as a "dreamboat," had worked with Janet for a period of 3 months, during which time she had remained euthymic. During her last appointment, Janet began addressing the therapist by his first name; previously she had always addressed him as "Doctor." The resident found this a bit odd but assumed it was part of the "growing therapeutic alliance" between the patient and himself. In supervision, he also acknowledged feeling "somehow a little flattered" at the new form of address. During the session, Janet asked the therapist whether her recent difficulty sleeping could be treated with a "sleeping pill." The resident replied that insomnia "happens to everyone now and then" and that no specific treatment was necessary. Janet replied, "I appreciate your leveling with me, Jim," and seemed satisfied. She added, "You're one of the reasons I go on with life, even with this damn illness." The session ended routinely. Two days later, the resident received a call from the ER, reporting that Janet was being admitted for a florid manic episode along with some suicidal ideation.

As you can see, Murphy's Law sometimes exerts its influence on psychotherapy—in this case, everything that could have gone wrong did so. First, the resident failed to recognize that the sudden change in form of address signified a subtle but important mood swing—and probably symbolized the erotized component of Janet's hypomania. (The author himself has fallen into this tender trap.) Second, the resident missed the additional clue of Janet's insomnia and failed to educate her about the premonitory significance of this symptom. Instead, he gave Janet some false reassurance about the insomnia, possibly as a result of his own erotized countertransference. (The forest, in this case, was obscured by some rather seductive trees.) Finally, Janet's seemingly innocent remark about "going on with life" should have alerted the therapist to some covert suicidal ideation—ideation that may coexist with hypomania or mania in so-called mixed bipolar states.

The issue of "explorative" or "uncovering" psychotherapy in the treatment of bipolar illness is complicated and beyond the scope of our discussion. However, most clinicians agree that such an approach is not useful for the average bipolar patient without concomitant character pathology—especially during the depressed phase of illness (Jamison 1987). Manic patients, of course, are hardly in a position to process dynamically oriented interpretations. Instead, therapy with the bipolar patient tends to be more "supportive" and directive than might be the case with many unipolar depressive patients. This is not to say that the therapist can ignore dynamic issues in understating the patient; but understanding and intervention are two different things.

Cyclothymic Disorder

The Central Concept

We discussed earlier the notion of a "bipolar spectrum" and suggested that cyclothymic disorder may represent the "lower end" of this spectrum—that is, it produces mood swings of a lesser magnitude than those seen in either classical (type I) bipolar disorder or in type II bipolar illness. In DSM-III-R, cyclothymia (as it was termed then) was described as a "chronic mood disturbance, of at least 2 years' duration . . . involving numerous hypomanic episodes and numerous periods of depressed mood . . . of insufficient severity or duration to meet the criteria for a major depressive or a manic episode" (American Psychiatric Association 1987, p. 226). The concept required that during a 2-year period of the disturbance (1 year in children and adolescents), the patient was never without hypomanic or depressive symptoms for more than 2 months at a time. DSM-III-R also gave its usual exclusionary criteria, such as no evidence of a chronic psychotic disorder or organic factors.

DSM-IV has "tightened up" the earlier criteria in one respect. DSM-III-R stipulated that in cyclothymia there was no evidence of a major depressive episode or manic episode during the first 2 years of the disturbance (or 1 year in children and adolescents). DSM-IV stipulates that the patient "has never met criteria for a major depressive episode" (American Psychiatric Association 1994); this modification helps avoid confusion with type II bipolar disorder. DSM-IV, like its predecessor, requires that in cyclothymic disorder there is no clear evidence of a manic episode during the first 2 years of the disturbance. After this initial 2-year period (1 year in children or adolescents), there may be superimposed manic episodes, in which case both bipolar I disorder and cyclothymic disorder may be diagnosed. While the diagnosis of cyclothymia excludes known organic factors, many cyclothymic patients may abuse sedatives or stimulants to mitigate their mood swings.

Historical Development of the Disorder

The term "cyclothymia" was coined by Kahlbaum in the mid-19th century. However, it was Kraepelin who first recognized cyclothymia as a forme fruste of manic-depressive illness, contending that certain temperaments are "rudiments" of manic-depressive insanity (Kraepelin 1921). Kraepelin's notion of "temperament" colored our thinking about cyclothymia for many years—indeed, most classifications viewed cyclothymia as a personality disorder. To this day, as we will see below, it is often difficult to distinguish the cyclothymic patient from, for example, the labile borderline patient. As Akiskal and his colleagues have argued, the patient's "tempestuous" lifestyle, the repeated pattern of failed relationships, the unstable employment record, and the frequent abuse of drugs may all camouflage the affective basis of the patient's disorder (Akiskal et al. 1979). Unfortunately, unless this basic affective "drive" is recognized, treatment may be only partially successful.

Although DSM-III-R stipulated the occurrence of hypomanic episodes in the cyclothymic individual, most workers in the area of the "bipolar spectrum" disorders have evolved a somewhat broader notion of cyclothymic disorder. Indeed, DSM-IV requires only "numerous periods with hypomanic symptoms," rather than clear-cut hypomanic episodes, in cyclothymic disorder. Akiskal and colleagues

(1979) apply the term cyclothymia to persons with lifelong traits of emotional instability and abrupt mood shifts that lack the duration and severity of full-blown bipolar mood swings.

The Biopsychosocial Perspective

Biological factors. The biology of cyclothymic disorder is—guess what—largely unknown. However, it is noteworthy that the condition appears to occur more often in women than men, in contrast to full-blown bipolar disorder, which affects both sexes equally (Keller 1987). Perhaps this indicates a slightly less "biologically driven" condition, in which sociocultural factors account for the higher incidence in women. Alternatively, hormonal factors specific to women may account for the difference. In any event, cyclothymic disorder is more common in families of patients who have a major mood disorder, and, conversely, cyclothymic patients show a greater-than-expected family history of bipolar illness (Akiskal 1983; Akiskal et al. 1979). These data suggest, but do not prove, that cyclothymic disorder is a biological variant of bipolar illness. If so, we would expect that similar neurochemical mechanisms underlie cyclothymic and classical bipolar disorder. However, research in this area is scant. Perhaps the most persuasive—albeit indirect—evidence is the relatively good response to lithium shown by cyclothymic patients (Akiskal 1983). Interestingly, Akiskal and colleagues (1979) observed one drug-free cyclothymic patient shift overnight from hypomania to depression, with an accompanying change in REM latency from 170 minutes to 35 minutes. This, too, suggests a biological affinity with classical bipolar disorder.

Psychosocial factors. Cyclothymia has been explained psychodynamically in terms of trauma and fixation during the early oral stages of development (Cohen et al. 1954; Jacobson 1971). However, the evidence for these claims rests mainly on observation of patients in long-term psychotherapy and does not really distinguish cyclothymic from other bipolar states. Akiskal and his colleagues (1979) have argued persuasively that cyclothymia is best understood as a subsyndromal form of manic-depressive illness, manifested as a secondary disturbance in "personality." On this view, the cyclothymic individual's irritability, marital failures, uneven work record, and alcohol or drug abuse are manifestations not of a developmental problem but of an often unrecognized affective disorder. Akiskal and his colleagues have argued that dynamically oriented psychotherapy does not seem to affect the cyclothymic individual. Moreover, such patients can seldom relate their mood fluctuations to concomitant stressors (Akiskal et al. 1979). Indeed, some cyclothymic patients report going to bed in a cheerful mood and waking up "down in the dumps." It is also of note that cyclothymic patients experience their irritable, angry episodes as ego-dystonic—something one would not expect in, say, a sociopathic personality (Akiskal et al. 1979). Although all of these findings strongly suggest that cyclothymic persons are "born, not made," we cannot rule out the role of early developmental influences in this disorder. And as we shall see below, cyclothymic persons are often difficult to distinguish from individuals in whom developmental factors undoubtably are important.

Pitfalls in the Differential Diagnosis

Many of the diagnostic problems we discussed in relation to classical bipolar I disorder arise again when considering cyclothymic disorder. Cyclothymic disorder is rarely confused with schizophrenia or schizoaffective disorder, as was the case with the manic phase of bipolar I disorder. However, cyclothymic disorder may be hard to distinguish from borderline or histrionic personality disorder, adolescent conduct disorder, and ADHD. Drugs such as steroids, amphetamines, and alcohol can also produce "secondary cyclothymia," just as we saw in our discussion of secondary mania. Let's consider the following vignette.

Vignette

Vinny was a 22-year-old single male who was employed as a grocery-store clerk. He gave a 3-year history of "real bad mood swings," characterized by occasional wrist cutting or violence directed at others. As Vinny put it, "When I feel down, I cut. When I feel high, I punch." He did not seem to feel much remorse over his violence toward others, stating, "People have to learn they can't push me around or I'm gonna push back." On the other hand, Vinnie often spoke of himself in very derogatory terms, once stating, "Sometimes I think I'm just a walking piece of crap . . . like, why do I even bother trying? I don't even know who I am sometimes." Although Vinny dates his problems to the preceding 3 years, interviews with family members revealed a much longer history. His mother reported that Vinny's father had abused him as a child, sometimes "beating him up real bad." When Vinnie was 10 years old, his father left the family and had not been heard of since. Vinny's mother described his childhood as "a real roller coaster," characterized by Vinny's frequent angry outbursts and fits of crying. A school psychologist had wondered if Vinny was "a little hyperactive," but this was never pursued. In junior high school, Vinny began to use "speed, pot, whatever he could get his hands on." However, Vinny repeatedly denied current drug abuse. Recently, Vinny had gotten into trouble for "messing around" with a 13-year-old boy, about whom Vinny commented, "You gotta understand, this kid is really queer."

Vinny's psychiatrist made a diagnosis of "cyclothymic disorder" and recommended to the patient a trial on lithium carbonate. Vinny had an almost immediate response, stating, "Two days after I started it, I felt great." However, Vinny's serum lithium level after 5 days was only 0.1 mEq/L. On close questioning, he admitted he had tried only "a few tablets" because "I'm not the one who needs a shrink—its the jerks that keep hassling me."

At first blush, we can understand why Vinny's psychiatrist diagnosed cyclothymic disorder—and perhaps the diagnosis was correct. But Vinny's history and presentation revealed significant borderline and sociopathic personality traits (e.g., externalization of blame, projection, poor self-concept, self-damaging acts, drug abuse, and perhaps some sexual identity confusion). Even if—following Akiskal's thesis—these traits are "secondary" to Vinny's underlying cyclothymia, the issue is rendered moot by the patient's poor medication compliance. Nevertheless, as we will see in the treatment subsection below, a trial on medication is often warranted in patients like Vinny.

Adjunctive Testing

Neuroendocrine and brain imaging. Neuroendocrine and brain imaging data are lacking in strictly defined cyclothymic disorder, though we might expect results to parallel those seen in bipolar disorder. Although we usually do not think of pharmacologically induced hypomania as an ethically permissible "test," it is nevertheless true that some cyclothymic patients may be "unmasked" by this phenomenon (Akiskal et al. 1979).

Psychological testing. In our discussion of mania, we mentioned scale 9 of the MMPI as a direct measure of "energy level" (Newmark 1985). T (i.e., true) scores greater than 90 usually indicate mania. Scores between 75 and 90 often pick up patients described as restless, enthusiastic, impatient, energetic, gregarious, and having an exaggerated sense of self-worth who are, however, not delusional—in short, patients who may be hypomanic (Newmark 1985). Unfortunately, the MMPI is probably not sensitive enough to distinguish the various gradations between "high energy" and frank mania.

In our discussion of mania, we alluded to the psychodynamic hypothesis that mania is a "reaction formation" to an underlying depression. Hypomanic individuals may show an interesting 2-point code type on the MMPI that suggests such a mechanism. The 2-9/9-2 code type often reflects an agitated depression in which tension is discharged through heightened motor activity. These patients "are denying underlying feelings of inadequacy and worthlessness and may be attempting to use a variety of manic mechanisms, such as hyperactivity, denial of poor morale, and over-involvement with others to avoid focusing on their depression" (Newmark 1985, p. 43). However, this code type may be seen in other conditions, such as the "identity crisis" of adolescence.

Treatment Directions and Goals

In many instances, the elevated mood swings of cyclothymic disorder do not require psychiatric intervention; indeed, because the patient often experiences these "up" periods as a relief, engagement in psychotherapy may be minimal (Meyer 1983). When the upward shift in mood approximates the manic state, the principles discussed earlier (in relation to mania) apply. The depressed phases of cyclothymic disorder may benefit from supportive or cognitive-behavior therapy (Meyer 1983), but systematic research is lacking in this area. However, if Akiskal et al. (1979) are correct regarding the "affective core" of cyclothymia, psychotherapy in general and "depth interpretations" in particular may not be especially useful in treating the cyclothymic individual.

In contrast, there is growing evidence that lithium may be useful in the treatment of cyclothymia and other hypomanic states (Akiskal et al. 1979; Gershon and Shopsin 1973). Generally, however, lithium should be reserved for those cyclothymic patients whose mood swings cause significant incapacity or disruption in their lives. Blood levels should probably be kept lower (0.6–0.9 mEq/L) than those sought in the treatment of frank mania (Akiskal et al. 1979). Indeed, it seems as if a sort of "lithium space" exists in the cyclothymic or bipolar individual, such that the higher the mood, the bigger the "space" for lithium. A bipolar patient in the manic phase may tolerate a lithium level of 1.2 mEq/L but may be uncomfortable with this level when euthymic.

It remains to be seen whether other mood-stabilizing agents, such as carbamazepine, clonidine, or calcium channel blockers, will find a role in treating cyclothymic disorder.

Bipolar Disorder Not Otherwise Specified

In DSM-IV, the residual category of bipolar disorder NOS contains three main syndromes: recurrent hypomanic episodes without intercurrent depressive symptoms; a manic episode superimposed on delusional disorder or residual schizophrenia; and situations in which the clinician cannot decide whether the bipolar disorder is primary, due to a general medical condition, or substance induced. Some workers (Akiskal 1983) have described a disorder labeled either bipolar III or unipolar II. It is similar to bipolar II disorder, except that the hypomania occurs only upon "pharmacologic challenge" (e.g., after the use of a tricyclic or stimulant). There is some evidence that patients with such a pattern are biologically related to the other bipolar types we've discussed and that they may benefit from lithium.

Depressive Disorder (Unipolar)

In a sense, we've already covered some of this ground—at least, it would seem so. After all, DSM-IV uses the umbrella concept of "major depressive episode" to cover the depressive phase of both unipolar and bipolar I mood disorders. You may recall our manic-depressive composer, G.F.H., and the symptoms of his depressed phase. They are quite similar to those we shall describe in a unipolar patient. Nevertheless, genetic, biochemical, and even clinical differences between unipolar and bipolar depressive individuals warrant our discussing these conditions separately.

Major Depression

The Central Concept

In major depression there is a loss of interest or pleasure in all, or nearly all, activities for a period of at least 2 weeks. In addition, a set of rather stereotyped symptoms are present and represent a change from previous functioning. These symptoms occur for most of the day, nearly every day, and include appetite disturbance, change in weight, sleep disturbance, psychomotor agitation or retardation, decreased energy, feelings of worthlessness, excessive guilt, difficulty concentrating, and recurrent thoughts of death or suicide. Psychotic features—either mood congruent or mood incongruent—may be present. A particularly severe form of major depression is the melancholic type, in which neurovegetative features (such as early morning awakening and significant weight loss) are especially prominent.

In our discussion of the differential diagnosis, we shall outline some differences between these unipolar depressive bouts and those of bipolar illness.

Historical Development of the Disorder

Severe depression has been known and described at least since the eighth century B.C. King Saul was apparently subject to such severe bouts of (possibly psychotic) depression that he attempted to kill both his son Jonathan and his servant David, of David and Goliath fame (Andreasen 1982).

"Melancholia" as a distinct disease is noted in Hippocratic writings at least as early as the fifth century B.C. It was associated with "aversion to food, despondency, sleeplessness, irritability, [and] restlessness" (qtd. in Jackson 1986, p. 30). Interestingly, the Hippocratic writers seemed to distinguish "melancholia" from depression per se in a manner akin to our own, stating that "fear or depression that is prolonged means melancholia" (qtd. in Jackson 1986, p. 30). Even more intriguing was the humoral theory put forward by Hippocratic writers. Disease was attributed to a disturbance in the equilibrium of four bodily humors: blood, yellow bile, black bile, and phlegm. Each humor was thought to be dominant in one of the four seasons: spring, summer, autumn, and winter, respectively. Furthermore, each humor was paired with "qualities" such as warmth or moisture. Melancholia was associated with cold, dry, black bile, and autumn was the season of particular risk (Jackson 1986). Without too much of a stretch, it may be seen that the Hippocratics anticipated not only the catecholamine theory of depression but the existence of seasonal affective disorder!

A complete historical discussion of melancholia would take us far afield; the interested reader should consult Stanley W. Jackson's masterful work, *Melancholia and Depression* (1986). However, no survey should omit mention of Robert Burton's classic work, *The Anatomy of Melancholy*, first published in 1621. In Burton's description of melancholia as occurring "without any apparent occasion," we see the attempt to distinguish between severe depression and "ordinary passions" of fear or sorrow (Jackson 1986). The latter conditions are the ancestors of our modern-day "adjustment disorders."

Perhaps the most radical conceptualization of depression is that which distinguishes unipolar from bipolar types. Kraepelin, you may recall, distinguished manic-depressive illness from dementia praecox. However, he did not distinguish unipolar and bipolar depression. Instead, he grouped all depressive syndromes together under the rubric of manic-depressive psychosis (Andreasen 1982). It fell to Leonhard, Angst, and others to propound the unipolar-bipolar distinction. Subsequently, a number of genetic and biochemical variables were identified as distinguishing these two types of depression (see next subsection). Despite some opinion to the contrary, the unipolar-bipolar dichotomy persists as one of the strongest distinctions in psychiatry.

Of course, other ways of understanding depression have been put forth (Andreasen 1982). The most prominent dichotomies are summarized in Table 4–2. Although DSM-IV does not make direct use of these concepts, it does incorporate elements of each. For example, the notion of "secondary" affective illness finds its way into the DSM-IV category of "Mood Disorder Due to a General Medical Condition." And although the words "endogenous" and "reactive" have disappeared as etiologic terms—suggesting, respectively, depression arising "from within" or "from without"—they have strongly influenced the DSM-IV concept of "melancholia" and the diagnosis of "adjustment disorder with depressed mood." Nevertheless, the three classifications presented below are of largely historical interest, because each has serious conceptual and empirical flaws (Andreasen 1982).

Table 4–2.   Depression: alternate classifications

Primary vs. secondary

Primary: Not associated with antecedent medical or psychiatric illness.

Secondary: Occurs in patient with antecedent medical/psychiatric illness.

Endogenous vs. reactive

Endogenous: No recent history of severe stress or loss; prominent neurovegetative features.

Reactive: Occurs in response to recent loss, disappointment; neurovegetative features are less prominent.

Psychotic vs. neurotic

Psychotic: Hallucinations, delusions, and confusion are present; there is severe impairment of psychosocial functioning.

Neurotic: No hallucinations or delusions are present; there is long-standing characterological problems and modest impairment of functioning.

Source.   Extensively modified from Andreasen 1982.

The Biopsychosocial Perspective

Biological factors. In our discussion of bipolar depression, we listed six areas of biological research: electrolytes, membrane transport, neuropeptides, neuroendocrine factors, neurotransmitter receptors, and neurotransmitters per se. Research into the causes of unipolar major depressive episodes has focused on similar areas and has yielded some interesting results. But before discussing these, let's ask a more basic question: Why suppose that unipolar major depression has a biological basis at all? First, both unipolar and bipolar affective illness show a pattern suggesting familial and genetic influences (Nurnberger and Gershon 1982). Studies looking at monozygotic and dizygotic twins—in order to separate genetic from familial influences—have shown significantly greater risk of concordance for depression in monozygotic twins. Generally speaking, unipolar illness and bipolar illness "breed true"—that is, if one monozygotic twin has unipolar illness, the other twin, if affected, is also likely to have unipolar illness (Nurnberger and Gershon 1982). However, some twin pairs show a unipolar-bipolar pattern, suggesting that unipolar and bipolar illnesses are sometimes associated with the same genetic makeup. Winokur and his colleagues (Van Valkenburg and Winokur 1979) have presented evidence suggesting that unipolar depressive patients may be divided according to family history. Those with alcoholic or sociopathic first-degree relatives form a group having "depression spectrum disease." Those unipolar depressive patients with depressed first-degree relatives (lacking alcoholism or sociopathy) form a group characterized by "familial pure depressive disease." A number of genetic markers (such as alpha-haptoglobin) appear to distinguish these two groups (Tanna et al. 1976). Furthermore, over 80% of the "pure depression" group failed to suppress dexamethasone in the dexamethasone suppression test (DST), versus only 4% in the "depressive spectrum" group (Schlesser et al. 1979). We will look more closely at neuroendocrine function a little later.

There is another a priori reason for suspecting biological factors in unipolar depression—namely, the surprisingly stereotyped clinical presentation of this illness. This is not to suggest that one depressed patient is "the same" as another—far from it. But the symptomatic picture is strikingly similar from patient to patient. Whatever the psychosocial components of the major depressive episode, the patient is very likely to show a disturbance in appetite, sleep, and psychomotor function. The classic pattern in the most severe cases—those of DSM-IV melancholia—usually involves loss of appetite, significant weight loss (more than 5% body weight in a month), early morning awakening, and psychomotor agitation. The "cognitions" of these patients are also quite stereotyped and differ little from those noted by Robert Burton more than three centuries ago. The patient almost always exhibits ideas of self-worthlessness, guilt, sinfulness, or bodily decay (sometimes reaching delusional proportions). None of these stereotyped features "proves" that major depression has a biological basis, but they surely lead one to suspect such a basis. What, then, do we know about the biochemistry and neurophysiology of unipolar major depression?

Most of the research in this area has focused on neurotransmitters and neurotransmitter receptors. It seems clear that the catecholamine theory of depression as initially formulated just doesn't explain the data; that is, major depression isn't due simply to "not enough" norepinephrine or serotonin. Rather, depression seems to result when the overall balance of neurotransmitter quantity and function is disturbed. It's not necessarily that the neurochemical "orchestra" is missing musicians, but rather that the musicians are playing out of tune.

True, there are some data suggesting deficient norepinephrine or serotonin in the blood, urine, or CSF of depressed patients (Zis and Goodwin 1982). But other data suggest that overactivity of the cholinergic system may also predispose to depression; indeed, McCarley (1982) has proposed a unitary hypothesis taking into account adrenergic function, cholinergic function, and their relationship to REM sleep. In essence, McCarley hypothesizes that depression may result from adrenergic underactivity, cholinergic overactivity, or a relative imbalance of both systems.

Neurotransmitter receptors may also be deficient, in excess, or "out of tune" in some depressed patients. For example, the alpha$_2$-adrenergic receptor is a presynaptic inhibitory receptor that normally mediates inhibition of norepinephrine release. Too many of these receptors might result in deficient release of norepinephrine. In one study of radioligand binding of an alpha2 agonist to the platelets of depressed patients and control subjects, the depressed patients showed 21% more alpha2 binding sites than did the control subjects (García-Sevilla et al. 1981). However, other studies have not confirmed the importance of alpha2 mechanisms in depression. Much of the recent work in depression has focused on the role of the postsynaptic beta receptors. It has long been known that centrally active beta-blockers (such as propranolol) can cause or exacerbate depression in susceptible individuals (Petrie et al. 1982). It is tempting to infer that a deficiency of beta receptors—or beta-receptor hypofunction—leads to depression. Although this may be so, curiously, almost all known antidepressants seem to down-regulate beta receptors. Whether this is a primary effect or merely the compensatory effect of increased norepinephrine release is not precisely known. Moreover, the serotonergic system appears necessary for the down-regulation of beta receptors in response to antidepressants (Sulser 1991). If you are a little confused by now, you are resonating with the existing literature.

Neuroendocrine factors also seem important in the etiology, or at least the phenomenology, of severe depression. For example, roughly 50% of patients with severe depression (most studies utilized pre-DSM-III criteria) have elevated baseline cortisol secretion (Sachar 1982). Roughly the same percentage—though not necessarily the same individuals—show early escape of cortisol secretion from suppression by dexamethasone (B. G. Carroll et al. 1976). These abnormalities may indicate a release of HPA function from normal corticolimbic inhibition. This, in turn, may be due to underlying abnormalities in neurotransmitter function. Some recent data suggest that high circulating levels of corticosteroids may exacerbate or perpetuate behavioral symptoms of depression (Wolkowitz et al. 1993)—a claim that has clear therapeutic implications, as we will see below.

A good deal of research has focused on thyroid abnormalities in patients with major depression—for example, blunted TSH response to TRH, or elevated levels of antithyroid antibodies (Gold et al. 1988; Nemeroff et al. 1985). In a recent study of eight inpatients with refractory major depression, Hatterer et al. (1993) found low levels of the protein that transports thyroid hormone from the blood to the brain (transthyrenin). If this finding is borne out in larger studies, this may mean that some patients with major depression do not have enough thyroid hormone "on the brain," despite apparently adequate plasma hormone levels. Finally, some research suggests a blunted growth hormone response to hypoglycemia in patients with major depression (Sachar 1982).

Sleep disturbance is common in depression, and this may not be simply the effect of the depression itself. The principal EEG abnormalities noted in major depression include shortened REM latency (i.e., time between sleep onset and first REM period), reduced delta sleep, and increased total REM and percentage of REM sleep during the early REM periods of the night (Gillin et al. 1979). A "phase advance" of REM sleep could explain the decreased REM latency; in effect, depressed patients are getting their first REM period too soon. Such phase changes and desynchronization of other important biorhythms (such as temperature and cortisol secretion) may actually be causal in depression and mania (Wehr et al. 1987). Interestingly, the decreased REM latency and higher REM density found in depressed patients are often reversed by tricyclic antidepressants.

Finally, we should mention some recent studies (using PET) of cerebral glucose metabolism in depressed patients. Most studies have shown relative hypometabolism in the frontal regions, and in some cases the alterations are more severe in the left hemisphere (Buchsbaum et al. 1984; Phelps et al. 1984). This distribution of metabolic change correlates well with the production of depression by focal left anterior lesions resulting from cerebrovascular disease (Cummings 1985; Robinson et al. 1984).

Psychological factors.   We have already discussed a number of psychodynamic theories of manic-depressive illness. The psychodynamics of depression per se have been reviewed at length (Mendelson 1982), and we shall not attempt to cover the entire literature. However, we can summarize the principal psychodynamic theories (including object-relations views) as follows.

Psychoanalytic theories.   Freud and Abraham emphasized, respectively, the depressive person's loss of an ambivalently regarded object and his or her regression to "oral phase" gratification. Freud believed that in "melancholia" (as opposed to ordinary "mourning"), hostile feelings that were once directed against the lost object become directed at the self, which—through introjection—has subsumed the lost object. Abraham believed that early and repeated disappointments in childhood—such as the discovery that one is not mother's favorite—predispose one to later depression in the face of similar disappointment, with the ego then retreating from its mature functioning state to the oral phase of development. (One wonders if the hyperphagia seen in some depressed patients is a manifestation of this.)

Object-relations theories. Melanie Klein (1934) was probably the earliest analyst to focus on object relations in the etiology of depression (Mendelson 1982). Klein posited that the child normally goes through phases comparable to those of mourning in the adult, and that this early mourning is revived whenever grief is experienced in later life (Jackson 1986). Normally the infant learns that the mother he sometimes hated (the frustrating, or "bad," object) and the mother he loved (the rewarding, or "good," object) are one and the same person (the "whole" object). This normal child thus develops a "good internal object" that becomes the basis for a stable sense of self. Such a child is less likely to suffer severe depressions as an adult. But if the child fails to integrate these two (good and bad) "part objects," the stage is set for depression later in life; the individual has never really worked through what Klein called the "infantile depressive position." Klein's thinking strongly influenced the theories of Kernberg and other object-relations theorists, especially in their understanding of narcissism.

In concluding the psychological portion of our discussion, we should mention the work of Aaron Beck, Albert Ellis, and other "cognitive-behavioral" theorists (Beck 1967; Ellis 1962). These workers hold that depression is essentially the result of irrational and self-defeating cognitions that lead to decreased self-esteem. The depressed individual "indoctrinates" himself or herself with "all-or-none" statements such as "I must succeed at everything or I am worthless," "I must be loved by everyone or I can't go on," and so forth. Natually, neither this view nor the psychoanalytic ones rule out the influence of biological factors in the etiology of depression.

Sociocultural factors.   It is difficult to separate the earliest "social" factors impinging on the individual from that person's "psychology." Thus, the finding that early loss of a parent predisposes to later depression (Bowlby 1980) can easily be linked with object-relations theories. Nevertheless, it is convenient to speak of such losses under the rubric of "psychosocial" factors. Many such factors have been invoked to explain the onset of depression, although it is always difficult to prove causal relationships. Let's look at a clinical vignette that draws together some of the main psychosocial factors in depression.

Vignette

Karen was a 38-year-old married mother who presented with symptoms of major depression. Her four children were aged 2, 4, 7, and 9. Karen had been working as a computer programmer until 2 years prior to her current psychiatric evaluation. After the birth of her youngest child, Karen left her job to "do the whole motherhood trip again." In the month prior to evaluation, Karen had been arguing more frequently with her husband, who had diabetes and had "not been taking real good care of himself." Her husband had "run out" on Karen several times in the past year, and the family finances were under considerable strain. At the time of presentation, Karen was preoccupied with thoughts of her deceased mother, who had died at the same time of year when Karen was 10. "I got to feeling like there was no one to take care of me anymore," Karen stated, adding, "All I do is have to take care of other people."

Karen's situation embodies the chief psychosocial factors associated with serious depression (Brown and Harris 1978; Paykel 1974). The word "associated" is really as strong a term as we may use, because depression may actually precede so-called psychosocial precipitants. In any case, the factors correlated with the onset of depression (particularly in women) are summarized in Table 4–3. This brief list does not do justice to the many complex psychosocial variables implicated in depression. For example, what other factors might lead to the higher prevalence of depression among women? Gove (1972) concludes that being married has a protective effect for men but a detrimental effect for women. If this is true, is it due to marriage per se or to the lack of stimulation and support for women within the marriage?

The role of social class and race in depression is also a bit unclear and may depend, in part, on how "depression" is defined. The New Haven epidemiologic survey suggested that major depression is highest in whites and upper-class individuals (Weissman and Myers 1978). Other investigators have not confirmed this relationship between depression and class, and Zung et al. (1988) found no significant difference between blacks and whites in prevalence or severity of depressive symptoms.

Finally, ethnic factors may shape the specific presentation of depression. Thus, blacks with affective disorders may be more likely than whites to have hallucinations or delusions, even when economic status has been taken into account (Welner et al. 1973). Hispanic patients with bipolar disorder may also show more hallucinations than non-Hispanic patients, possibly leading to the misdiagnosis of schizophrenia (Lawson 1986).

Pitfalls in the Differential Diagnosis

Organic factors. Major depression may be mimicked by a multitude of organic factors and physical disorders (Table 4–4). The most important organic causes include antihypertensive agents (notably alpha-methyldopa and propranolol), steroids, cimetidine, various hypnotics and tranquilizers, hyper- or hypoadrenalism, hypercalcemia, perni-

Table 4–3. Factors correlated with onset of depression

Absence of close social ties

Marital discord and separation

Absence of employment outside home

Loss of mother prior to age 11

Presence of more than three children under age 14 living at home

Death or illness in family

Source. Extensively modified from Brown and Harris 1978; Paykel 1974.

cious anemia, pancreatic carcinoma, viral infections, systemic lupus erythematosus, hypothyroidism, stroke, and the subcortical dementias (Cassem 1988; Dubovsky 1988). Let's consider the following vignette.

Vignette

Jim was a 45-year-old married male who presented to his family physician with a complaint of "feeling down." He described a 6-month history of general weakness, loss of appetite, a 10-pound loss in weight, and an inability to maintain erections. He also described "fainting spells" and wondered if he had "hypoglycemia." The physical examination was notable for subnormal temperature of 96.5° and significant hypotension. Exposed skin surfaces showed abnormal pigmentation. Plasma cortisol measurements at 9 A.M. and 11 P.M. strongly suggested Addison's disease.

Functional disorders.   Major depressive episode in "pure culture" is rather tough to miss. However, there are muted, atypical, or "masked" forms of this disorder that sometimes stymie the clinician.

Table 4–4.   Medical conditions associated with depression

Drugs and toxins: reserpine, alpha-methyldopa, propranolol, cimetidine

Infectious disease: mononucleosis, influenza, viral pneumonia

Neoplasm: pancreatic, bronchogenic carcinoma, brain tumor, lymphoma

Cardiovascular: hypoxia, mitral valve prolapse

Endocrine: hyper-/hypothyroidism, hyper-/hypoparathyroidism, hyper/hypo adrenal function

Metabolic: uremia, hyponatremia, hypokalemia

Nutritional: pellagra, thiamine deficiency, B_{12}/folate deficiency

Collagen-vascular: systemic lupus erythematosus, rheumatoid arthritis, giant cell arteritis

CNS disease: Parkinson's disease, Huntington's disease, chronic subdural hematoma, temporal lobe epilepsy, stroke

Miscellaneous: Wilson's disease, psoriasis, amyloidosis

But before discussing psychiatric disorders that may be confused with major depression, let's return to a loose thread we tugged on earlier: namely, the distinction between unipolar and bipolar depressive episodes. To repeat, the "orthodox" view of DSM-IV does not distinguish between these two conditions. Nevertheless, clinicians over the years have amassed data that may help differentiate them. The major differential features are summarized in Table 4–5.

Recently, some studies have cast doubt on the last two differential features listed in Table 4–5, suggesting that suicide attempts are no more common in bipolar patients than in unipolar patients (Black et al. 1988) and that tricyclic-induced hypomania may not distinguish bipolar (at least type II) from unipolar depression (Kupfer et al. 1988).

A number of other psychiatric disorders may be confused with a major depressive episode (McNeil 1987). Among the most important

Table 4–5.   Differences between unipolar and bipolar depression

Unipolar depression	Bipolar depression
Psychomotor agitation	Psychomotor retardation
Initial/middle insomnia	Hypersomnia
Decreased appetite	Hyperphagia
Weight loss	Weight gain
Onset often after age 35	Onset often before age 35
Untreated episodes lasting 3 to 6 months	Untreated episodes lasting 6 to 9 months
Psychosis less likely	Psychosis more likely
+/- Postpartum association	Commonly postpartum
+/- Seasonal association	Bipolar II often seasonal
+/- Family history of bipolarity	Family history of bipolarity common
Less education	Higher degree common
Premorbid "introversion"	Premorbid "extroversion"
? Fewer suicide attempts	? Suicide attempts common
? Pharmacological hypomania rare	? Pharmacological hypomania common

Note.   +/− = may or may not be associated; ? = conflicting data.
Source.   Extensively modified from Maxmen 1986.

are dysthymic disorder, various personality disorders, normal bereavement, adjustment disorder with depressed mood, schizoaffective disorder, and depression secondary to schizophrenia, anxiety disorders, or somatoform disorders. Keep in mind, of course, that many patients in a major depressive episode will also have an Axis II personality disorder diagnosis.

We will examine dysthymic disorder in detail later in this chapter. With respect to distinguishing dysthymic disorder from major depression, the chief issues are severity and chronicity. The dysthymic patient generally does not have the profound neurovegetative changes seen in major depression. For example, he or she lacks significant weight loss, autonomy of mood, early morning awakening, and psychomotor retardation/agitation. Moreover, the dysthymic individual has had symptoms for at least 2 years, and often for a lifetime. McNeil (1987) gave us a good tip when he suggested that the depressed patient be asked, "When was the last time you did not feel depressed?" Unlike the patient with "simple" major depression, the dysthymic patient often cannot remember when he or she was not depressed. Remember, however, that the "rules" of DSM-IV permit both a major depressive episode and dysthymic disorder to coexist—so-called double depression. If, on the other hand, the initial onset of dysthymic disorder directly follows a major depressive episode, the correct diagnosis may be "major depression, in partial remission."

Among the personality disorders that may be confused with a major depressive episode are borderline, narcissistic, avoidant, dependent, and obsessive-compulsive personality disorders. We will examine these conditions in detail in Chapter 9. For our present purposes, keep in mind that personality disorders are diagnosed "only when the characteristic features are typical of the person's long-term functioning and are not limited to discrete episodes of illness" (American Psychiatric Association 1987, p. 335). Severely depressed patients sometimes develop secondary adaptations or apparent personality traits that annoy or distress others; such patients often end up being described by staff as "definitely Axis II." You may translate this into the staff member's (unconscious) countertransference statement, "I really don't like this patient. He drives me nuts!" The following vignette is based on a patient I have treated.

Vignette

A 70-year-old married female complained of persistent tingling of her extremities, depressed mood, initial and middle insomnia, poor appetite, and moderate weight loss, all having occurred over the past 2 years. Prior to that, the patient described herself as "a happy person . . . I never needed a psychiatrist." Her husband essentially confirmed this. A thorough organic workup revealed a mild peripheral neuropathy, attributed to slight vitamin B_{12} deficiency. Vitamin supplementation mitigated the patient's "tingling" but did not affect her overall mood. Successive trials on a variety of tricyclic and monoamine oxidase inhibitor antidepressants, with adequate blood levels and durations of treatment, produced very little improvement. Staff members on the inpatient unit often spoke disparagingly of the patient's "passive-dependent, passive-aggressive" style and wondered, "What's the point of treating someone with that much character pathology?" The unit director decided to begin the patient on a course of ECT. After six treatments, the patient's subjective feeling of depression and her vegetative features were essentially gone. More striking was the change in her "personality." The "passive-dependent, passive-aggressive" woman was now an active, cooperative, and autonomous individual.

Normal bereavement is sometimes confused with a major depressive episode, and sometimes with good reason: the line between normal grief in bereavement and the pathological mourning characteristic of major depression is not so clear as psychoanalytic theory might suggest. Nevertheless, some differences are summarized in Table 4–6.

These differential features, of course, aim at the general case. There are many exceptions among individuals and cultures (Clayton 1982). Thus, some "normal" mourners may have a variety of depressive symptoms for a year following the loved one's death—including hallucinations of the deceased. (In the Jewish tradition, mirrors are covered during the immediate postdeath period, ostensibly to guard against vanity, but probably to protect the bereaved from just such hallucinations, as well.) Most of the differential features we have discussed also apply to the distinction between a major depressive episode and adjustment disorder with depressed mood. Further, in the latter, the symptoms remit after resolution of the stressful precipitant.

To distinguish schizoaffective disorder (see Chapter 5) from a major depressive episode (with psychotic features), the central question is whether there have been delusions or hallucinations in the absence of prominent mood disturbance for a period of at least 2 weeks. If so, the diagnosis would be schizoaffective disorder. Of course, schizoaffective disorder probably is quite heterogeneous (Levitt and Tsuang 1988). The "depressive type" may embrace patients whose condition is biologically similar to that in a major depressive episode and who respond to treatments (such as ECT) for psychotic depression (Maj 1987).

A major depressive episode may sometimes be confused with depression secondary to schizophrenia, anxiety disorders, or somatoform disorders. Correct diagnosis clearly depends on teasing out the "core" features of the particular underlying condition. (In the case of the anxiety disorders, this can be quite difficult; anxiety and depression may be interwoven in so-called atypical depression. We will discuss this condition under the rubric of depressive disorder NOS.) An important diagnostic issue is the longitudinal course of the illness; for

Table 4–6.   Differences between normal grief in bereavement and a major depressive episode

Normal grief	Major depressive episode
Follows recent major loss	Loss not always evident
Self-esteem preserved	Feeling "worthless" common
Functioning moderately impaired	Functioning markedly impaired
Realistic sense of lost person	Faults of lost person idealized or denied
Neurovegetative signs may or may not be present	Neurovegetative signs present to a marked degree
Subsides after 3 to 4 months	Unchanged or worse after 3 to 4 months
Suicide intent rare	Suicide intent common

Source. Extensively modified from Clayton 1982.

example, did the patient's problem begin as panic attacks, which—left untreated—led to demoralization and hopelessness? If so, one would not diagnose major depressive episode. If, on the other hand, the patient met the criteria for major depression, this diagnosis would be given on Axis I along with panic disorder. Some research has shown that major depression plus panic disorder is associated with increased psychiatric morbidity in first-degree relatives, when compared with major depression alone (Leckman et al. 1983).

Adjunctive Testing

Neuroendocrine tests.   Despite the volumes of data amassed in this area over the past 10 years, there is still no "blood test" for major depression. Nevertheless, when diagnosis is uncertain, the summation of certain neuroendocrine tests may be helpful. The best known, of course, is the DST. Although the sensitivity and specificity of this test have been eroded over the years, it still retains some utility (Allen et al. 1987). An abnormal DST may occur in several psychiatric disorders besides major depression and may result from several medical conditions as well (Table 4–7).

Although it appears quite unlikely that DST can serve as a validating criterion for major depressive episode, it may be predictive of clinical course and outcome. An abnormal DST often precedes the onset of depressive episodes, and normalization heralds clinical recovery. A persistently positive DST despite clinical improvement is predictive of rapid relapse (Allen et al. 1987).

Table 4–7.   Medical and psychiatric conditions yielding false positive results in the dexamethasone suppression test

Cushing's syndrome	Bulimia without depression
Pregnancy	Primary degenerative dementia
Estrogen use	Schizophrenia
Anticonvulsant use	Alcoholism (abstinent period)
Cardiac, renal disease	"Neurotic depression"

Source. Extensively modified from Allen et al. 1987.

Another important neuroendocrine test is the thyrotropin-releasing hormone test. Essentially, the maximum TSH response to administered TRH is diminished (i.e., blunted) in patients with unipolar or bipolar depression, mania, or mixed manic-depressive illness. In contrast, normal responses are obtained in patients with so-called reactive, or neurotic, depression, or reactive paranoid schizophrenia (Allen et al. 1987). Clearly, this test cannot help one distinguish unipolar from bipolar depression, but it might help one distinguish dysthymic disorder from major depression. Keep in mind, however, that responsiveness to TRH declines in elderly men and may also be affected by a variety of drugs and hormones.

A less commonly used neuroendocrine test is the growth hormone response to a variety of stimuli. Thus, a normal response of growth hormone to insulin is a rise of at least 5 mg/ml. However, growth hormone response to insulin-induced hypoglycemia may be diminished in major depression (B. J. Carroll 1978). This test has been used primarily in research settings thus far.

Sleep studies.   We have alluded to some of the sleep EEG findings in bipolar illness. So far, we don't have a very clear idea of the differences between sleep abnormalities in unipolar and bipolar illness. But if, for a moment, we consider "major depression" without regard to polarity, we can summarize the main sleep abnormalities as follows: 1) short REM sleep latency (i.e., time from sleep onset to REM sleep onset), 2) reduced slow-wave sleep, 3) increased frequency of rapid eye movements during REM sleep (i.e., REM density), and 4) decreased sleep efficiency (e.g., more awakenings and early awakening) (Ballenger 1988). With respect to polarity, some evidence suggests that in unipolar depression, REM sleep is less fragmented than in bipolar depression (Duncan et al. 1979). We have already noted that insomnia (as opposed to hypersomnia) is more characteristic of unipolar depression.

Brain imaging techniques.   The rapidly expanding field of brain imaging is producing new studies almost every day, but the data are still inconclusive. In one intriguing study by Baxter et al. (1989), PET scans of unipolar and bipolar depressive patients revealed significant differences in glucose metabolism. The bipolar patients showed greater whole-brain reduction of glucose metabolism compared with the unipolar patients and normal control subjects. The unipolar patients showed a decreased ratio of caudate-to-hemisphere metabolism compared with the bipolar patients and normal control subjects. The suggestion, in effect, of hypometabolism in the caudate of unipolar depressive patients is intriguing because the caudate is part of the basal ganglia and rich in dopaminergic pathways. Could the dopaminergic system be specifically involved in some types of depression and not others?

Another burgeoning area is the application of magnetic resonance imaging (MRI) to affective disorders. Krishnan et al. (1992) have summarized the evidence implicating basal ganglia abnormalities in depressive illness and have added an important finding: subjects with major depression show smaller right and left caudate nucleus volumes on MRI, when compared with normal control subjects. This study complements the PET studies cited above and again focuses our attention on the increasingly interesting basal ganglia. Krishnan et al. point out that "the caudate is interconnected with several cortical and limbic areas implicated in the regulation of mood" (p. 557). Another recent MRI study by Rabins et al. (1991) examined elderly patients with major depression. Greater cortical and subcortical atrophy, as well as more basal ganglia pathology, was seen in the depressed patients compared with age-matched control subjects. The meaning of these findings is not yet clear, but the study raises important questions about the relationship of major depression to the traditional category of "dementia."

Psychological testing. On the MMPI, scale 2 is consistently elevated in chronic depressive disorders (Meyer 1983). There is some evidence suggesting that elevation on scale 2 correlates with increased risk of suicide, and the 2-7/7-2 code seems especially correlated with suicidal ideation (Meyer 1983). An elevated scale 8 may also be correlated with increased suicide risk as well as with schizoaffective illness (Meyer 1983).

On the revised WAIS (WAIS-R), the classic sign of depression is an overall performance scale score significantly lower than the verbal scale score. (This situation, however, may be seen in various "organic" conditions and in certain learning disabilities.) Depressed patients typically give up on WAIS-R items or answer "I don't know" (Meyer 1983). On the Rorschach, long reaction times to the cards and rejection of several cards are typical. The patient—not surprisingly—is self-critical while responding to the cards, and there is a high F or FY% (Newmark 1985). (Remember, F relates to form and Y relates to variations in shading, and that Y responses often correlate with a sense of helplessness in the face of stress.) Because depression is often described in terms of "darkness," it is intuitively gratifying that chromatic color (C) responses are rare in major depression (Meyer 1983). Finally, on the Thematic Apperception Test (TAT), the depressed patient usually shows short, stereotyped responses that amount to mere descriptions of the cards.

Treatment Directions and Goals

The treatment of major depression usually involves an integration of psychological and somatic approaches; indeed, there is evidence that an integration of these approaches works better than either one alone (Conte et al. 1986). Psychotherapy may have its effects primarily on depressed mood, suicidal ideation, guilt, and social engagement; medication primarily affects sleep difficulty, poor appetite, and somatic complaints (DiMascio et al. 1979). There is very little evidence to suggest that medication interferes with the effects of psychotherapy in treating depression (Klerman and Schechter 1982).

Somatic approaches. The mainstay of somatic treatment is still the use of tricyclic antidepressants, despite the plethora of "new, improved" agents now available (see Pies and Shader 1994 for review). On the whole, the second- and third-generation agents have not quite lived up to the initial "hot" reviews. In particular, amoxapine, maprotiline, and trazodone have all proved to have their Achilles' heels. Amoxapine may cause extrapyramidal effects and even tardive dyskinesia; maprotiline is associated with a higher-than-expected incidence of seizures; and trazodone, aside from its occasional association with priapism, may produce dizziness, orthostatic hypotension, and ventricular dysrhythmias (Bernstein 1991). For the average patient with major depressive episodes, the newer agents probably offer few advantages over desipramine and nortriptyline, both of which have reasonably good side-effect profiles. Nortriptyline may be especially useful in the elderly patient, because it is associated with a low incidence of cardiovascular and hypotensive side effects. Nortriptyline also has a well-defined therapeutic range (50–150 ng/ml), which aids in dosing strategy. Of course, the tricyclics are extremely toxic in "overdose" situations, and in this respect they are at a real disadvantage compared with newer agents.

One addition to the field does deserve special mention: the selective serotonin reuptake inhibitor (SSRI) fluoxetine. This agent, so far, seems to have a more benign toxicity/side-effect profile than do the tricyclics and may prove to be useful in psychomotorically retarded hypersomnic patients. However, fluoxetine is commonly associated with insomnia, nausea, anxiety, and headache, at least in the early phase of treatment, and may produce sexual dysfunction in more than 5% of cases (Bernstein 1991). Because of its long half-life (3–5 days), fluoxetine may prove feasible on a twice- or thrice-weekly basis (DeVane 1992). On the other hand, this long half-life forces one into a 5-week "wash out" period when changing from fluoxetine to a monoamine oxidase inhibitor (MAOI), because of the risk of a "hyperserotonergic" syndrome (i.e., hyperthermia, confusion, myoclonus) when these agents are used in close temporal proximity.

There has been concern in recent years—mainly in the lay press—about fluoxetine's potential for "inducing" suicidal or homicidal ideas or behavior. Despite some alarming anecdotal reports of such reactions, the overwhelming epidemiological data do not support this claim (Fava and Rosenbaum 1991). In a recent unpublished study by my own group, we found no difference in suicidal ideation between fluoxetine-treated depressed outpatients ($n = 17$) and control subjects treated with other antidepressants ($n = 11$). However, if patients develop severe motor restlessness or akathisia on fluoxetine, they may become extremely distressed and perhaps suicidal; this problem may be avoided by dosage reduction or by adjunctive use of a beta-blocker (Rothschild and Locke 1991). Contrary to early opinion, fluoxetine may be effective in doses of as low as 5 mg/day; such low doses may be appropriate in elderly depressed patients and in depressed patients with panic attacks. The latter group often shows a heightened sensitivity to fluoxetine's excitatory effects. A number of other SSRIs are now available, including sertraline (Zoloft) and paroxetine (Paxil). These agents have a shorter half-life than fluoxetine, and they may also be associated with somewhat less psychomotor agitation.

Although the SSRIs avoid most of the "old tricyclic" side effects (e.g., postural hypotension, blurry vision, constipation, significant sedation), they have their own side-effect profile: principally, gastrointestinal distress, loose stools, tremor, increased sweating, and a rather high incidence of sexual dysfunction. The SSRIs do appear to be much safer than the tricyclics in overdose and have a more benign cardiovascular profile. They may yet prove to be the antidepressants of choice in elderly patients, medically ill patients, and cardiac-impaired patients, but—in my experience—nortriptyline yields good results in all these populations, with few serious side effects. (All tricyclics, however, may aggravate cardiac conduction abnormalities and should generally be avoided in patients with preexisting degrees of heart block.)

Bupropion (Wellbutrin) is a new, nonsedating dopaminergic antidepressant that bears some structural and functional similarities to amphetamine. Like fluoxetine, bupropion has very little anticholinergic activity, little tendency to promote weight gain or sexual dysfunction, and very few cardiovascular effects. A recent report suggests that optimal response to bupropion occurs at plasma levels between 10 and 29 ng/ml (Goodnick 1992). Side effects with bupropion include mild agitation, headache, and insomnia. Although the overall incidence of seizures is probably similar in patients on bupropion versus tricyclics, doses of bupropion exceeding 450 mg/day may be associated with increased seizure risk. There have also been reports of bupropion-induced psychosis, but it is not clear that this occurs more frequently than with standard antidepressants (Ames et al. 1992). Finally, there is modest evidence suggesting that bupropion may be useful in stabilizing bipolar patients, as discussed earlier in this chapter, but this claim has been challenged recently.

The MAOIs are said to be the drugs of choice for "atypical depression," but this diagnostic term is used in so many ways that the claim becomes a bit confusing (Pies 1988). There are reasonably good data showing that patients with panic attacks and the pattern termed "hysteroid dysphoria" may do better on MAOIs than on standard antidepressants (Liebowitz et al. 1985). Patients with the "atypical" features of hypersomnia and hyperphagia may do well on an MAOI, or possibly fluoxetine. Remember, however, that such patients may turn out to have bipolar disorder.

For depressed patients with clear-cut melancholia and psychotic features, ECT is probably the treatment of choice—especially if the patient is noncompliant with medication or is extremely suicidal (Welch 1987). Some patients with recurrent major depression may require "maintenance" ECT, perhaps on a once-monthly basis.

A variety of "potentiation" strategies for so-called treatment-resistant major depression have been summarized in recent reviews (American Psychiatric Association 1993; Osser 1993; Pies and Shader 1994). Potentiation strategies include the addition of lithium or thyroid hormone to a tricyclic or other antidepressant; the use of psychostimulants (usually in combination with a standard antidepressant); and the combination of a tricyclic with an SSRI (e.g., imipramine plus fluoxetine). Naturally, the risks of polypharmacy must be weighed carefully when such combination strategies are employed; for example, fluoxetine can elevate plasma levels of tricyclics substantially.

We noted earlier that hypercortisolemia is common in major depression, and suggested that this has therapeutic implications. Recently, Wolkowitz et al. (1993) described the use of the anti-glucocorticoid agent ketoconazole in depressed patients with hypercortisolemia. Although their results were encouraging, the authors caution against use of this agent at the present time, given its potential for hepatotoxicity.

We can look forward to the introduction of several new agents in the near future. For example, venlafaxine (Effexor), a phenethylamine agent that strongly inhibits reuptake of both norepinephrine and serotonin, may be the harbinger of a whole new class of agents, the "SNRIs" (serotonin/norepinephrine reuptake inhibitors). Nefazodone (Serzone) is structurally similar to trazodone (Desyrel), but appears less likely to induce hypotension or priapism (Pies and Shader 1994).

Psychosocial approaches.   There may be as many psychotherapies for depression as there are psychotherapists. Nevertheless, these therapies can be boiled down to three main approaches: psychodynamic, experiential-expressive, and cognitive-behavioral. None of these has proved consistently more effective than the others (Smith et al. 1980), and the approaches are not mutually exclusive. Moreover, to repeat an important point, psychotherapy does not preclude the use of antidepressants, nor is there reason to fear that one will interfere with the other.

Bellak (1981) has nicely summarized the principles of brief psychoanalytic psychotherapy of nonpsychotic depression; however, the principles he elucidates apply quite well to longer-term psychodynamic approaches. Based on general psychoanalytic theory, Bellak lists 10 main problem areas and accompanying therapeutic approaches to the depressed patient, as summarized in Table 4–8.

By the way, Arieti (1982) has stated that orthodox psychoanalytic therapy—with the use of "the couch" and free association—is not indicated in the treatment of severe depression. Rather, by becoming a significant, new and reliable object for the patient, the therapist must actively help the depressed individual live more autonomously (Arieti 1982). Lesse (1975) has gone so far as to contend that "*one cannot deal with the psychodynamics of depression until the actual depression has been greatly ameliorated.* The patient's ego capacities in this particular phase are too fragile to accept discussion of any unconscious mechanisms . . ." (p. 320). Lesse advocates a sort of "ego transfusion" during the initial treatment of severe depression, with the therapist providing active reassurance and support.

Experiential-expressive approaches to severe depression have their roots in the work of Carl Rogers, Abraham Maslow, and Fritz Perls. These clinicians emphasized the importance of releasing pent-up emotions, dealing with the here and now, and minimizing the role of the "unconscious" (Frances et al. 1984). In his "client-centered" therapy, for example, Carl Rogers emphasized the critical role of the therapist's attitudes: those of empathic understanding, unconditional positive regard for the patient, and genuineness. If this sounds a little vague, keep in mind that the experiential-expressive philosophy deliberately avoids sharp definitions of "techniques," feeling that "a description might be regarded as a rigid rule that would limit the necessary flexibility required to be as open and receptive . . . as possible when interacting with a client" (Frances et al. 1984, p. 134). Nonetheless, the following therapeutic dialogue may help elucidate this approach. Let's set up the case example as follows:

Jonathan is a 40-year-old business executive who has just begun client-centered therapy for treatment of a major depressive episode. The relevant history is that Jonathan was fired from his most recent job and subsequently "broke up" with his fiancée. For the 2 months prior to treatment, Jonathan had experienced early morning awakening, a loss of appetite, weight loss (i.e., 10 pounds), and suicidal ideation. He was begun on nortriptyline 50 mg at hs by his internist,

Table 4–8. Brief psychotherapy of nonpsychotic depression

Problem area	Approach
Low self-esteem	Explore recent insults to self-esteem; relate recent precipitants to past traumata.
Punitive superego	Explore superego formation and relation to current problems; facilitate catharsis.
Aggression against self	Make patient aware of aggression by one part of self on another part.
Feeling of loss	Examine early losses in relation to present; examine passive-dependent demands.
Feeling of disappointment	Deal with anger toward disappointing love object; relate this to transference, if appropriate.
Feeling of being deceived	Examine past "broken promises"; work through paranoid feelings.
Oral demands	Examine history of depression secondary to unmet demands; relate to transference.
Narcissism	Explore excessive need to be loved.
Denial of pain	Facilitate catharsis of covert rage.
Object relations	Explore overly critical parenting and excessive need to please others; relate to transference.

Source. Extensively modified from Bellak 1981.

who subsequently referred him for psychotherapy. Jonathan began to sleep and eat better after 10 days of treatment with nortriptyline, but still felt "like a total washout." Here is an "excerpt" from the second session between Jonathan and his psychiatrist:

Jonathan: I don't know . . . it's like there's nothing left to me . . . the job, I mean . . . that's what defined me, you know? That and Karen [his ex-fiancée).

Psychiatrist: It's as if all of your value as a human being came from those two things.

J.: Yeah. Intellectually, I know that's dumb, but I just feel that way. And like, if I hadn't screwed up the job in the first place, I never would have lost Karen. And yet I feel pissed off at everyone around me . . . looking for someone to kick."

P.: So on the one hand, you blame yourself for all the losses, and yet you keep searching for someone, anyone, to pin the blame.

J.: That's it. So how do I get myself out of this?

P.: It would be great, wouldn't it, if I could just tell you how to do that?

J.: Well, maybe you can. Maybe you just don't want to.

P.: It feels as if I'm holding out on you, punishing you, in a way.

J.: Yeah, maybe.

P.: No, I don't have any miracles up my sleeve, Jonathan. But it's O.K. to be a little angry at me for not having them.

J. (*beginning to cry*): I guess I just want to depend on you to rescue me like I wanted to with my job and Karen.

P. (*moving his chair closer to Jonathan*): This is really painful to talk about.

J.: Yeah . . . to need so much from people.

P.: It's O.K., right now, to need me.

In this highly condensed dialogue I have tried to demonstrate the Rogerian use of accurate empathic understanding, unconditional positive regard, and therapeutic "genuineness" (Rogers 1980). These elements of therapy, however, are not the exclusive property of any one therapeutic approach and are important, to some degree, in the success of any psychotherapy. Nonetheless, the "surface features" of other types of therapy look quite different from what we have just seen. The cognitive-behavioral approach to depression, for example, sounds a bit harsh after hearing the Rogerian method. But in fact, the cognitive-behavioral approach has a good deal of empirical support (Rush et al. 1977; Smith et al. 1980) and certainly can be done empathically. It emphasizes the irrational and self-defeating cognitions that often underlie severe depression. The cognitive-behavioral therapist, for example, might focus on Jonathan's deeply held belief that his self-worth depends on external trappings such as a job or a fiancée. Instead of simply empathizing with Jonathan's inordinate need for love or approval, the cognitive-behavioral therapist would "attack" these ideas actively. The patient might also be given "homework assignments" such as seeking out negative criticism from his boss—the idea being that the patient can be "desensitized" to such previously threatening stimuli. The depressed patient eventually learns to substitute more rational beliefs for the "depressogenic" irrational ones; for example, Jonathan might learn to internalize the statement, "Just because I lost my job, doesn't make me a bad person." One note of caution with the cognitive-behavioral approach: In the early stages of treating depression, an "attack" on the patient's irrational beliefs may be perceived as an attack on the patient. Careful and empathic preparation is needed before the depressed patient can make use of such a direct approach. In my experience, the cognitive-behavioral approach is extremely useful when used with care.

A form of "interpersonal psychotherapy," based in part on the theories of Harry Stack Sullivan, has been systematized by Klerman et al. (1984) and has proved effective in several controlled studies of major depression. Full discussion of this and other psychotherapeutic approaches to depression may be found in the review by Shea et al. (1988).

Although we have emphasized the "individual" format in discussing psychotherapy, the depressed patient may benefit from other formats (e.g., group, family, or marital counseling), depending on the circumstances of the depression (Frances et al. 1984). Finally, the integration of psychotherapy and pharmacotherapy is an increasingly important area of research and practice; some helpful guidelines are provided by a recent APA work group (American Psychiatric Association 1993). Such a combined approach can be seen in the following integrated case history.

Integrated Case History

Mr. Alghieri, a 28-year-old graduate student in literature, presented to a psychiatrist with the chief complaint that "it feels like everything is over for me . . . like I'm in a dark woods with no way out." The patient gave a history, over the past 3 months, of decreased appetite, weight loss of more than 10 pounds, early morning awakening, loss of pleasure in his usual activities, inability to concentrate, and suicidal ideation. There was no clear precipitant that the patient could point to at first, but further exploration revealed the breakup of a long relationship with a female colleague, some 5 months prior to evaluation. The patient gave this assessment of the breakup: "I was an idiot . . . Beatrice was such a jewel, and I couldn't appreciate her. If I hadn't been so arrogant and so stupid, she would have stayed." The patient had no history of episodes similar to the current one, no history of suicide attempts, and no history of sustained episodes of euphoria or irritability. Family history was positive for depression in the patient's maternal grandmother and in a first cousin, who had attempted suicide.

The patient was admitted to the inpatient psychiatric unit. On mental status examination, the patient appeared malnourished and in considerable distress. He continually ran his hands through his hair and tugged at his beard. He was oriented to day and date but had trouble with short-term memory, usually responding, "I'm sorry . . . I don't know." There was no evidence of frank delusions, but the patient's thinking revealed a punitive, all-or-none quality (e.g., "Anybody who did what I did to screw up his life deserves what he gets"). He acknowledged feeling that he "might be better off dead" but denied any suicidal plans.

Physical examination was within normal limits, except for recent weight loss. Laboratory studies were unremarkable, except for nonsuppression on the DST. A subsequent TRH stimulation test showed blunted TSH response. A polysomnogram showed markedly decreased REM latency (16 minutes). Because of the patient's memory problems, a computed tomography scan of the brain (with contrast) was obtained and was interpreted as "normal."

Psychological testing yielded the following: on the WAIS-R, the patient's verbal score exceeded his performance score (115 vs. 86); on many of the WAIS items, the patient had "given up." On the Rorschach, the patient demonstrated a long reaction time, with rare C (chromatic color) responses. He tended to be highly self-critical in response to the cards ("I should be able to tell what that is, but I'm so damn out of it").

Neuropsychiataric testing (including the Bender-Gestalt) showed no evidence of organicity, but rather, "a pattern of inconsistent responses suggesting diminished effort or concentration."

The admitting diagnosis was "major depressive episode, unipolar, nonpsychotic." The patient was begun on nortriptyline 25 mg at hs, which was rapidly increased to 75 mg. After 1 week, a plasma level came back as 78 ng/ml. The patient was seen by the resident in twice-weekly sessions aimed at 1) establishing a "safe," supportive therapeutic alliance; 2) gradually and gently examining cognitive distortions; 3) dealing with covert anger toward the patient's former lover; and 4) relating the present episode to earlier losses, including, the resident soon learned, an unresolved grief reaction related to the death of the patient's mother, some 10 years earlier.

Over the ensuing month, the patient showed significant improvement. However, he remained moderately depressed at therapeutic levels of nortriptyline. (The Beck Depression Inventory [short-form] showed a score of +12.) Tri-iodothyronine (Cytomel) 15 μg/day was added to the tricyclic. The patient improved further over the next 2 weeks, with the Beck score dropping to +6 (mild depression).

A repeat DST showed normal suppression. The patient was discharged with outpatient follow-up arranged in 1 week.

Dysthymic Disorder (Dysthymia)

Dysthymic disorder is to major depression as cyclothymia is to bipolar disorder—it is, in effect, an attenuated form of major depression. The "old" term for dysthymic disorder—safely surrounded by parentheses in DSM-III-R—was "depressive neurosis." We will say more about this in our historical perspective, below. In moving from DSM-III-R to DSM-IV, an attempt was made to "sharpen up" the criteria for dysthymic disorder in order to reduce overlap with major depression; hence, some of the "vegetative" symptom criteria (poor appetite, insomnia) in DSM-III-R dysthymia have been replaced with more "intrapsychic" symptoms in DSM-IV dysthymic disorder.

We will use the more general term "dysthymia" interchangeably with the official term dysthymic disorder.

The Central Concept

Vignette

Mr. Cansado, a married 27-year-old, had moved to the United States from Peru 12 years prior to evaluation. The patient's chief complaint was that "I just don't enjoy life . . . I don't have any interest in doing things, and I have no energy even if I wanted to do them." These symptoms had been present for at least the past 5 years, but the patient added, "I really can't remember the last time I felt happy."

There was no history of "mood swings," psychiatric hospitalization, or bouts of depression resulting in missed work, suicide attempt, or severe weight loss.

Although he was functioning as a salesperson in an electronics store, Mr. Cansado felt like he had to "drag myself through the day." He had few friends at work and remained socially isolated even from his wife and two children. At times, he would "snap" at them for "absolutely nothing." He had difficulty making decisions at work and had lost the chance of a promotion recently. This prompted feelings of intense guilt on the patient's part and the belief that "I've never amounted to anything and I never will." However, the patient denied suicidal ideation or intent. His appetite was "fair," and there was no history of significant weight loss or gain. His sleep was "usually O.K.," with no pattern of early morning awakening.

On mental status examination, the patient appeared "sad looking," but was well groomed and "pleasant." There was no significant psychomotor retardation or agitation, although the patient showed some inattentiveness to questions. A full physical and laboratory examination revealed no significant abnormality.

Historical Development of the Disorder

Yerevanian and Akiskal (1979) found six overlapping meanings to the term "neurotic depression": mild depression, nonpsychotic depression, nonendogenous depression, depression coexisting with neurotic symptoms, reactive or psychogenic depression, and characterological depression. These workers pointed out that none of the operational features of neurotic depression defined above was useful in assuring a homogeneous outcome. Put a bit more bluntly, the diagnosis of "neurotic depression" doesn't tell you beans about what will happen to your patient. For example, some will go on to develop psychotic or manic symptoms (Yerevanian and Akiskal 1979). Nevertheless, our present notion of dysthymia has its roots in this rather boggy historical soil. Yerevanian and Akiskal noted that the characterological dimension of the old term "neurotic depression" may, indeed, be worth preserving: patients who truly have lifelong histories of depression with few if any remissions may constitute a distinct population.

Yerevanian and Akiskal went on to make an important discovery: that characterological depression could be subdivided into two clinically relevant groups—subaffective dysthymia and character spectrum disorder. Some of the differences between these subgroups are summarized in Table 4–9. Note that some subaffective dysthymic patients may be "fair" responders to antidepressants. The "take home" message: Don't abandon the idea of treating so-called chronic depressives or assume that such patients will "never" get better.

The Biopsychosocial Perspective

Biological factors. If dysthymia is an attenuated form of major depression, we might expect to find similar biochemical factors in the etiology and expression of these two disorders. Although the biology of dysthymia is largely unknown, there are some data to support our expectation. We have already mentioned Yerevanian and Akiskal's finding that some of their characterologically depressed patients had unusually short REM latencies—a finding also seen in many patients with major depression. Roy et al. (1985), however, in studying a group of early-onset dysthymic patients and nondepressed control subjects, found no differences between groups on either the DST or the TRH stimulation test—impugning but not refuting the hypothesis that dysthymic disorder is biologically related to major depression. Of course, an entirely different pathophysiology may underlie dysthymic disorder. Finally, Klerman (1980) pointed out that some chronic depression may represent the residual effects of chronic substance abuse, or the complications of long-standing medical illness such as arthritis or the more recently described "fibrositis syndrome" (Gupta and Moldofsky 1986).

Psychological factors.   We noted earlier that dysthymic disorder has its roots in the old notion of "depressive neurosis." In their review of dysthymic disorder, Kocsis and Frances (1987) note that chronically depressed individuals, in the traditional psychoanalytic view, have been characterized by "oral dependency," "object hunger," "super-ego pathology," and "pathological narcissism." These traits, presumably, leave such individuals vulnerable to intermittent or chronic bouts of depressed mood. Clearly, such lifelong impairment has much in

Table 4–9.   Characterological depression: subaffective dysthymia and character spectrum subgroups

	Subaffective dysthymia	Character spectrum
Family history	Affective disorder	Alcoholism
Personality	Stable	Unstable
Response to tricyclics	Fair	Poor
Prognosis	Fair	Poor
REM latency	Short	Normal
Pharmacological hypomania	Common	No

Source.   Extensively modified from Yerevanian and Akiskal 1979.

common with so-called personality disorder—and, indeed, some in-vestigators have asked whether dysthymic disorder properly belongs on Axis II. Unfortunately, depressed mood may itself confound eval-uation of personality disorder, as we saw earlier in our "passive-dependent" depressed woman who responded dramatically to ECT. The issue of nosology aside, let's try to get the psychological "flavor" of dysthymic disorder by considering the following vignette.

Vignette

Herb was a 37-year-old single male who presented to the outpatient clinic with the complaint of "feeling like ending it all." He described his mood as "bleak," stating that he had felt this way most of his life. He held a middle-level job with an engineering firm and found only "a scintilla of satisfaction" in the work he did. However, he was regarded as something of a "wimp" by his co-workers, and stated, "Of course, they're undoubtedly right." Herb went on to describe himself as a "loser's loser," adding, "I'm the kind of guy who would have been a lookout at Pearl Harbor." Despite his gloom, Herb maintained his sense of humor throughout much of the interview, although at times he seemed on the verge of tears. He had never been able to form satisfactory relationships with women, although he very much wanted to. He described some difficulty falling asleep for many years and occasional midcycle awakening. His appetite had "never been robust," but there was no recent history of weight loss. Herb had a number of chronic physical complaints, such as head-aches, muscular cramps, and nausea, that had never been explained on an organic basis. "They think I'm a crock," Herb noted, "and they're probably right." Herb then presented the interviewer with a detailed list of all the "physical and emotional perturbations" he had undergone on a daily basis over the preceding month. Herb gave a family history that appeared to be positive for major depressive illness.

Herb fits into the general category of subaffective dysthy-mia, described by Yerevanian and Akiskal (1979). He shows the "obsessoid-introverted" personality style typical of this group, as well as the somatic features sometimes associated with hypochondriasis and "atypical" depression. Also striking are Herb's low self-esteem and his "negative filter," which seems to transform all of life's colors into shades of gray.

Sociocultural factors.   We have already discussed the role of parental deprivation and life stress in the etiology of major depressive illness. What role these factors play in dysthymic disorder is not clearly known. DSM-III-R maintained that in children and adolescents, predisposing factors for dysthymia include an "inadequate, disorganized, rejecting, and chaotic environment" (American Psychiatric Association 1987, p. 231). Yerevanian and Akiskal (1979) note that unstable parenting is a reasonable hypothesis for the entire character spectrum subgroup of characterological depressions. Klerman (1980) has noted that "divorce, unemployment, and business or professional failure may often be the consequence of dysthymic disorder" (p. 1334); but clearly, these same occurrences can worsen or precipitate depressive downswings in dysthymic individuals. On the other hand, in their community survey of depression, Hornstra and Klassen (1977) found no relationship between life stress and chronic depressive symptoms.

Pitfalls in the Differential Diagnosis

Dysthymia presents the clinician with a difficult and often frustrating differential diagnosis because "mild depression" is so ubiquitous. We have already reviewed the medical and organic factors that may cause or exacerbate major depression; the same list applies now to dysthymia. Therefore, let's focus on the various functional psychiatric diagnoses that may be confused with dysthymia.

We have already alluded to the difficulty in distinguishing major depression from dysthymic disorder. Indeed, in an important paper, Osser (1993) notes the "syndromal fogginess" of this dichotomy and offers a nosologic alternative: he divides depression into mood-nonreactive (autonomous) and mood-reactive types (Osser 1993). Osser points out that loss of mood-reactivity—that is, the patient feels depressed even when distracted, socially stimulated, and so forth—is highly correlated with "endogenous" or "melancholic" depression across many diagnostic approaches.

Such "autonomous" depression is also correlated with psycho-motor agitation or retardation, which in DSM-IV is a common feature in major depression but not in dysthymic disorder.

To mention another very rough guideline, most patients with dysthymia or its variants—as opposed to major depression—do not experience strong suicidal ideation on a frequent basis and do not lose the ability to function socially or vocationally. Rather, like our Mr. Cansado, dysthymic patients present as the "walking wounded"—that is, significantly impaired but generally not incapacitated. Of course, as DSM-IV notes, the diagnosis of dysthymic disorder should not be used if the patient's symptoms are better explained as "major depressive disorder in partial remission"—a very tough call in some cases.

Next in line are the personality disorders, with histrionic, narcissistic, borderline, avoidant, dependent, and obsessive-compulsive personality disorders leading the way (Klerman 1980). If you're thinking that these just about cover the whole spectrum of personality disorders, you'd be very nearly right. But note that these personality disorders fall into DSM-IV Clusters B and C, entailing, respectively, individuals who are "dramatic, emotional, or erratic" and those who are "anxious or fearful." Note that the Cluster A personality disorders are missing from the differential diagnosis: the paranoid, schizoid, or schizotypal disorders, which are associated with "odd or eccentric" behavior.

It may seem surprising that chronically depressed individuals could also appear, at times, "dramatic" or histrionic, but they often do (Plutchik and Platman 1977). Indeed, we will see that so-called hysteroid dysphoria serves as a "bridge" between dysthymic disorder and histrionic personality disorder. The principal clues in distinguishing dysthymia from the Cluster B personality disorders—including histrionic, narcissistic, and borderline personality disorders—have to do with the onset, pervasiveness, and intermorbid dysfunction of the condition. But having said that, remember that dysthymic disorder may coexist with any of the Axis II personality disorders. (The empirical evidence is sparse, but Kocsis and Frances [1987] conclude that dependent and mixed personality disorders may be the most commonly diagnosed personality disorders in states of chronic depression.)

But back to the issues of onset, pervasiveness, and intermorbid functioning. How might these factors permit the differential diagnosis of dysthymia from the aforementioned personality disorders? First, recall that personality disorders, by definition, are often recognizable by adolescence or earlier and continue throughout most of adult life. In contrast, dysthymic disorder may or may not begin prior to age 21. DSM-III-R distinguished early-onset (i.e., age at onset before age 21 years) from late-onset dysthymia. The former, it is true, has its onset in the same years as the personality disorders; the latter, however, may begin at age 25 or later—quite unlike the personality disorders. Second, personality disorders are grounded in maladaptive, inflexible personality traits that are exhibited in a wide range of social and personal contexts and that result in significant functional impairment (DSM-III-R). Dysthymia, in partial contrast, may result in only "mild or moderate" impairment in social or occupational function. Finally, some (though not all) individuals with dysthymia may experience at least partial spontaneous remission—though not for more than 2 months at a time within a 2-year period of the disorder. Individuals with personality disorder would not be expected to show such fluctuation in impairment. We shall also see, in our discussion of treatment, that some dysthymic patients respond well to antidepressants; this has yet to be demonstrated for most of the aforementioned personality disorders.

What about the specific features of the Cluster B personality disorders, as compared with dysthymia? Broadly speaking, individuals with histrionic, narcissistic, or borderline personality disorder, though often presenting with depressive symptoms, have a much more "unstable" history. Individuals with borderline personality disorder, especially, differ from dysthymic individuals in their greater frequency of self-damaging acts, impulsivity, and often primitive negative rage. Narcissistic individuals, though often concealing a profoundly negative self-image, frequently present with extravagant claims of self-importance and self-entitlement. This is less likely in the dysthymic individual. Similarly, the individual with histrionic personality disorder is likely to be more flamboyant and seductive than the typical dysthymic individual, who is more likely to show obsessional traits. Finally, remember that the dysthymic individual is more likely than the individual with personality disorder (Cluster B) to show a persistent disturbance in appetite, energy, sleep, and concentration.

The "anxious and fearful" individuals with Cluster C personality disorders (i.e., avoidant, dependent, obsessive-compulsive) may pose a greater diagnostic challenge. After all, it stands to reason that a chronically timid, easily embarrassed individual will often become depressed over his or her plight; thus, avoidant personalities often present with symptoms of dysthymia. However, the avoidant individual is more likely than the "pure" dysthymic individual to experience marked anxiety in front of other people; indeed, the avoidant patient often goes on to develop a full-fledged social phobia (on Axis I). The dependent personality tends to feel uncomfortable or helpless when alone and, as DSM-III-R phrased it, "will go to great lengths to avoid being alone" (American Psychiatric Association 1987, p. 353). In contrast, the dysthymic individual, though often dependent on others for self-esteem, usually becomes socially withdrawn. The individual with an obsessive-compulsive personality is commonly depressed but, unlike the typical dysthymic individual, shows a "pervasive pattern of perfectionism and inflexibility" and a preoccupation with rules, efficiency, and trivial details. (Of course, as Yerevanian and Akiskal [1979] have shown, the "subaffective dysthymic" individual often shows obsessional traits.) Finally, like individuals with Cluster B personality disorders, Cluster C individuals will usually lack the disturbance in sleep, appetite, energy, and concentration commonly seen in dysthymic individuals.

The differential diagnosis of dysthymia, unfortunately, includes other psychiatric illnesses beside the personality disorders. Let's consider the following vignette.

Vignette

Ms. Schmertz was a 35-year-old divorced female with a 3-year history of severe neck pain. Extensive orthopedic and neurological evaluation had turned up no evidence of organic pathology. The patient also gave a history of decreased pleasure in most activities, poor appetite, and initial insomnia over the same time period. There was, however, no significant weight loss, midcycle insomnia, or psychomotor abnormality. The patient's family history was positive for depression, alcohol dependence, and "lots of low back pain."

The diagnosis in this case is technically "somatoform pain disorder." But as you can see, the patient might very well merit a concomitant diagnosis of dysthymia. Indeed, the relationship between chronic depression and chronic pain is still unclear. Blumer and Heilbronn (1982) have described what they call "pain-prone disorder" and note that complaints of somatic pain are very common in depressed patients. Furthermore, chronic pain may mask clinical depression and may represent an unconscious defense against depression.

Finally, we should take note of the important finding of Sanderson et al. (1990) that 65% of patients with dysthymia receive at least one additional Axis I diagnosis—usually social phobia or generalized anxiety disorder. Furthermore, just over 10% of patients with dysthymia receive additional diagnoses of alcohol abuse or dependence. This study points out the vexing problem of comorbidity in the depressive disorders, as well as the interaction between depression and substance abuse.

Adjunctive Testing

Neuroendocrine.   As yet, there are no reliable neuroendocrine correlates of dysthymia. We have already mentioned Roy et al.'s (1985) finding that early-onset dysthymic patients did not differ from nondepressed control subjects on either the DST or the TRH stimulation test.

Psychological testing.   On the MMPI, dysthymia shows a lower overall profile than does major depression, because the dysthymic patient's' anxiety, agitation, and psychoticism scores are lower. The overall pattern is one of introversion, dependency, and obsessional traits (Yerevanian and Akiskal 1979). Scale 2 is elevated but is not as high as in major depression. A 2-0 profile, indicating chronic depression, may be seen (Meyer 1983). If scale 4 (psychopathic deviance) is elevated, a passive-aggressive use of the depression may be present. If somatization is a major factor, scale 1 (hypochondriasis) should be high. Performance on other tests is similar to that described for major depression, although the findings are less pronounced.

Treatment Directions and Goals

Somatic approaches.   As we have noted, some dysthymic patients—particularly those with a family history of affective illness, short REM latency, and relatively "stable" personality—will respond fairly well to tricyclic antidepressants (Yerevanian and Akiskal 1979). Those chronically depressed patients with a family history of alcoholism, normal REM latency, and "unstable" personality—Yerevanian and Akiskal's "character spectrum" group—tend to have a poor response to tricyclics. Preliminary results of a double-blind, placebo-controlled study by Kocsis et al. (1985) suggest that imipramine is significantly more effective than placebo in relieving dysthymia. However, this study used subjects who met DSM-III criteria for both dysthymia and major depression; we know little about the response to medication among patients with "pure" dysthymia.

Kocsis and Frances (1987), having reviewed the rather scant literature on this topic, concluded that "chronically depressed patients" of various types ("characterological," "neurotic dysphoria," etc.) may be helped by antidepressant medications. Osser (1993, p. 136) believes that "there is no basis to favor" one antidepressant over another for the treatment of mood-reactive depression, which overlaps significantly with dysthymic disorder. However, Osser suggests, based on "clinical experience," that SSRIs work at least as well in this population as do tricyclics and MAOIs. I would agree with this, based on my own clinical experience, though I have found many so-called dysthymic patients to be quite refractory to somatic treatment—perhaps raising the issue of "chronic characterological depression."

We will consider dysthymic patients with histrionic features in our discussion of hysteroid dysphoria in the section "Depressive Disorder Not Otherwise Specified."

Psychotherapeutic approaches.   Many of the therapeutic approaches we discussed in relation to major depression are applicable to the treatment of dysthymia. However, the "chronic characterological" quality of dysthymia may present some complications. After all, to the extent that patterns of feeling, thinking, and behaving have become "ingrained" over the years, the dysthymic patient may be relatively more resistant to change than is the patient with major depression alone. Thus, Bonime (1976) calls attention to the "manipulative" quality in the chronically depressed individual's manner of relating to others. By manipulating others to meet his or her needs, the dysthymic individual may build up a wall of protection against self-change. Attempts to promote change may be met with increased symptoms and veiled threats of suicide (Klerman 1980), reminding us that borderline personality disorder is in the differential diagnosis of dysthymia.

There is no single "proven" approach to treatment of the dysthymic patient. Among the shorter-term approaches, cognitive-behavioral techniques may be useful (Beck 1976), as may assertiveness training and "re-education" techniques aimed at improving stress tolerance and interpersonal relationships (Kiev 1975). As Kiev notes, "Treatment moves most rapidly when patients can focus on concrete problems in work, at home, or in interpersonal relationships, for these areas offer the greatest opportunity for trying out new ways of dealing with others" (p. 347).

Longer-term psychoanalytically oriented approaches emphasize the analysis of character structure—or what Wilhelm Reich called "character armor"—in addition to the analysis of depressive symptoms.

Depressive Disorder Not Otherwise Specified

In DSM-III, the category depressive disorder NOS was called "atypical depression." This was probably an unfortunate term, as it defined something quite unlike the "atypical depression" described in the British literature of the late 1950s and early 1960s (Sargant 1961; West and Daly 1959). In DSM-III, atypical depression was simply a residual category; any illness that could not be placed into the other specific categories of depression was placed in the "atypical" category. In DSM-IV, we can specify "with atypical features" if a patient with a depressive disorder shows mood reactivity, weight gain, hypersomnia, and so forth.

In effect, the conditions in the DSM-IV category "depressive disorder NOS" are defined with respect to other DSM-IV categories into which they do not fit! But we have already alluded to conditions that appear to exist in the "real world" and that have been independently defined by certain investigators. It is appropriate to consider them under the rubric of depressive disorder NOS. Examples cited in DSM-IV include "premenstrual dysphoric disorder," "minor depressive disorder," "recurrent brief depressive disorder," and "postpsychotic depression of schizophrenia," among others. No doubt the most controversial of these is premenstrual dysphoric disorder—popularly referred to as PMS (or premenstrual syndrome). Valuable reviews of this complex condition and its possible treatment are provided by Rubinow and Roy-Byrne (1984) and by Stone et al. (1991).

Seasonal Affective Disorder

In DSM-IV, the specifier "with seasonal pattern" may be appended to either unipolar or bipolar mood disorders, as a "course specifier." But there is modest evidence that seasonal affective disorder (SAD) may be a syndrome in its own right—albeit related, in a large number of cases, to bipolar disorder (Rosenthal et al. 1985). The original defining criteria for SAD were as follows (Rosenthal et al. 1984): 1) a history of at least one episode of major depression by Research Diagnostic Criteria; 2) recurrent fall-winter depressions, at least two of which occurred during successive years, separated by nondepressed periods in spring and summer; 3) no other DSM-III Axis I psychopathology; and 4) the absence of regularly occurring psychosocial variables that might account for the regular seasonal depression. The symptomatology of SAD, which should remind you of a syndrome we looked at earlier, is delineated in the following vignette.

Vignette

Marjorie was a 35-year-old married female who gave a 4-year history of "bad depression every time it starts getting cold out." Marjorie, who lived in New England, began to experience her depression in mid-November. During one winter when she and her husband had spent 2 weeks in Florida, the depression had temporarily lifted. Each depressive bout was characterized by excessive eating (especially "cake and cookies"), excessive sleeping, and what Marjorie called "a bad habit of biting people's heads off when they cross me." Marjorie noted that many of these symptoms also occurred during the 4 or 5 days prior to her menstrual flow, although less consistently.

Seasonal affective disorder appears to resemble the depressed phase of bipolar illness to the extent that hyperphagia, carbohydrate craving, and hypersomnia are often present in both. Interestingly, around 80% of SAD patients are bipolar II patients—that is, they have periods of hypomania (usually in the summer months) alternating with their winter depressions. And as suggested in the vignette, many persons with SAD have PMS, alluded to earlier. Biologist Judith Wurtman (1988) has suggested that the "sweets craving" seen in SAD and PMS may be related to altered serotonin metabolism, and in one study (O'Rourke et al. 1989), the serotonin agonist D-fenfluramine improved the mood of SAD patients.

Hysteroid Dysphoria

We have alluded several times to the syndrome of hysteroid dysphoria and have stated that it serves as a "bridge" between dysthymic disorder and histrionic personality disorder. We shall see now that it also overlaps with SAD and the "British" notion of "atypical depression" mentioned earlier. But first, what is hysteroid dysphoria? Donald Klein and colleagues (Liebowitz and Klein 1979) have defined hysteroid dsyphoria as

> chronic nonpsychotic disturbance involving repeated episodes of abruptly depressed mood in response to feeling rejected. Individuals with this disorder, who are usually but not exclusively women, characteristically spend much of their time seeking approval, applause, attention, and praise, especially of a romantic nature, to which they respond with elevation of mood and energy. (p. 555)

Hysteroid dsyphoria patients, like SAD patients, tend to overeat and oversleep when depressed, experiencing a kind of "leaden paralysis." Typically, these patients abuse various substances (both sedatives and stimulants) to mitigate their depressive bouts, and diet chronically to maintain normal weight. When euthymic, hysteroid dsyphoria patients tend to be histrionic, flamboyant, intrusive, seductive, self-centered, or demanding in their interpersonal style—hence, their "overlap" with histrionic personality disorder. Liebowitz and Klein speculate that hysteroid dsyphoria patients suffer from a deficiency of a neuromodulator called phenylethylamine (PEA), a substance found plentifully in chocolate!

Individuals with hysteroid dysphoria share a number of features with the "British" atypical depressive individuals we mentioned earlier. The latter were characterized by prominent anxiety, emotional overreactivity, lethargy, reversed diurnal variation in mood, and numerous somatic complaints. Indeed, Liebowitz and Klein (1979) consider hysteroid dsyphoria a subtype of atypical depression in this "British" sense. Both hysteroid dsyphoria patients and those with the "British" atypical features respond quite well to MAOIs. The presence of panic attacks in atypically depressed patients may also predict preferential response to MAOIs as opposed to tricyclics (Liebowitz et al. 1984).

We should note that the very diagnosis of hysteroid dysphoria is controversial (Spitzer and Williams 1982). My colleagues and I (Beeber et al. 1984) found considerable overlap between hysteroid dysphoria and borderline personality disorder. We were also unable to detect differences in severity, premorbid adjustment, number of "atypical" features, or presence of melancholia between hysteroid dysphoria patients and other inpatients with major depression. However, in my clinical experience, hysteroid dysphoria patients do exist, and relatively recent pharmacological studies seem to support the validity of the diagnosis (Liebowitz et al. 1984, 1988). I have found MAOIs quite useful in depressed patients with prominent hypersomnia, weight gain, worsening in winter, and "hysteroid dysphoric" features; however, these may be the very patients who "test out" the MAOI diet, make dosage changes on their own, and so forth.

Conclusion

We have now been through the marketplace of mood disorders and found it to be a crowded and often confusing place. Where are we headed in our diagnosis and treatment of these disorders? As we gain genetic, biochemical, and epidemiological data, we shall probably move toward increasing subcategorization of the mood disorders. At the same time, we may come to recognize the "phenotypic" or phenomenological overlap among seemingly diverse groups of de-pressed patients (e.g., among SAD, hysteroid dysphoria, "atypically" depressed, and bipolar patients). Whether genotypic similarities will be found in these disorders remains to be seen. I believe we will also come to discover that many "depressed" patients are suffering from more specific neurophysiological disorders, such as specific sleep dis-orders (Pies et al. 1989). As we refine our understanding, more specific psychological and biological treatments will become possible. The SSRIs and "polyblockers" such as venlafaxine promise improved treatment of some refractory mood disorders. Finally, we need to learn more about the successful integration of somatic and psychotherapeu-tic treatments.

References

Akiskal HS: The bipolar spectrum: new concepts in classification and diagno-sis, in Psychiatry Update: American Psychiatric Association Annual Re-view, Vol 2. Edited by Grinspoon L. Washington, DC, American Psychiatric Association, 1983, pp 271–292

Akiskal HS, Khani MK, Scott-Strauss A: Cyclothymic temperamental dis-orders. Psychiatr Clin North Am 2:527–554, 1979

Akiskal HS, Walker P, Puzantian VR, et al: Bipolar outcome in the course of depressive illness: phenomenologic, familial, and pharmacologic predic-tors. J Affect Disord 5:115–128, 1983

Alexander FG, Selesnick ST: The History of Psychiatry: An Evaluation of Psychiatric Thought and Practice From Prehistoric Times to the Present. New York, Harper & Row, 1966

Allen CB, Davis BM, Davis KL: Psychoendocrinology in clinical psychiatry, in American Psychiatric Association Annual Review, Vol 6. Edited by Hales RE, Frances AJ. Washington, DC, American Psychiatric Press, 1987, pp 188–209

Ambelas A: Life events and mania: a special relationship? Br J Psychiatry 150:235–240, 1987

American Psychiatric Association: Diagnostic and Statistical Manual of Mental Disorders, 3rd Edition. Washington, DC, American Psychiatric Association, 1980

American Psychiatric Association: Diagnostic and Statistical Manual of Mental Disorders, 3rd Edition, Revised. Washington, DC, American Psychiatric Association, 1987

American Psychiatric Association: Practice guideline for major depressive disorder in adults. Am J Psychiatry 150(No 4, Suppl):1–26, 1993

American Psychiatric Association: Diagnostic and Statistical Manual of Mental Disorders, 4th Edition, Revised. Washington, DC, American Psychiatric Association, 1994

Ames D, Wirshing WC, Szuba MP: Organic mental disorders associated with bupropion in three patients. J Clin Psychiatry 53:53–55, 1992

Andreasen NC: Concepts, diagnosis and classification, in Handbook of Affective Disorders. Edited by Paykel ES. New York, Guilford, 1982, pp 24–44

Arieti S: Affective disorders: manic-depressive psychosis and psychotic depression, in American Handbook of Psychiatry, 2nd Edition, Vol 3. Edited by Arieti S. New York, Basic Books, 1974, pp 449–490

Arieti S: Individual psychotherapy, in Handbook of Affective Disorders. Edited by Paykel ES. New York, Guilford, 1982, pp 297–306

Baldessarini RJ: Chemotherapy in Psychiatry: Principles and Practice. Cambridge, MA, Harvard University Press, 1985

Ballenger JC: Biological aspects of depression: implications for clinical practice, in American Psychiatric Press Review of Psychiatry, Vol 7. Edited by Frances AJ, Hales RE. Washington, DC, American Psychiatric Press, 1988, pp 169–187

Baxter LR Jr, Schwartz JM, Phelps ME, et al: Reduction of prefrontal cortex glucose metabolism common to three types of depression. Arch Gen Psychiatry 46:243–250, 1989

Beck AT: Depression. New York, Harper & Row, 1967

Beck AT: Cognitive Therapy and the Emotional Disorders. New York, New American Library, 1976

Beeber AR, Kline MD, Pies RW, et al: Hysteroid dysphoria in depressed inpatients. J Clin Psychiatry 45:164–166, 1984

Bellak L: Brief psychoanalytic psychotherapy of nonpsychotic depression. Am J Psychother 35:160–172, 1981

Bernstein JG: Psychotropic drug prescribing, in Massachusetts General Handbook of General Hospital Psychiatry, 3rd Edition. Edited by Cassem NH. St Louis, MO, Mosby Year Book, 1991, pp 527–569

Black DW, Winokur G, Nasrallah A: Effect of psychosis on suicide risk in 1,593 patients with unipolar and bipolar affective disorders. Am J Psychiatry 145:849–852, 1988

Blumer D, Heilbronn M: Chronic pain as a variant of depressive disease: the pain-prone disorder. J Nerv Ment Dis 170:381–406, 1982

Bonime W: The psychodynamics of neurotic depression. J Am Acad Psychoanal 4:301–326, 1976

Bowlby J: Attachment and Loss, Vol 3: Loss: Sadness and Depression. New York, Basic Books, 1980

Brown GW, Harris T: Social Origins of Depression: A Study of Psychiatric Disorder in Women. London, Tavistock, 1978

Buchsbaum MS, DeLisi LE, Holcomb HH, et al: Anteroposterior gradients in cerebral glucose use in schizophrenia and affective disorders. Arch Gen Psychiatry 41:1159–1166, 1984

Buchsbaum MS, Wu J, DeLisi LE, et al: Frontal cortex and basal ganglia metabolic rates assessed by positron emission tomography with [^{18}F]2-deoxyglucose in affective illness. J Affect Disord 10:137–152, 1986

Calabrese JR, Woyshville MJ, Kimmel SE, et al: Mixed states and bipolar rapid cycling and their treatment with divalproex sodium. Psychiatric Annals 23:70–78, 1993

Cancro R: Overview of affective disorders, in Comprehensive Textbook of Psychiatry/IV, 4th Edition, Vol 1. Edited by Kaplan HI, Sadock BJ. Baltimore, MD, Williams & Wilkins, 1985, pp 760–763

Carroll BJ: Neuroendocrine procedures for the diagnosis of depression, in Depressive Disorders (Symposia Medica Hoechst 13). Edited by Carattini S. New York, Schattauer Verlag, 1978, pp 231–236

Carroll BJ, Curtis GC, Mendels J: Neuroendocrine regulation in depression, I: limbic system–adrenocortical dysfunction. Arch Gen Psychiatry 33:1039–1044, 1976

Cassem EH: Depression secondary to medical illness, in American Psychiatric Press Review of Psychiatry, Vol 7. Edited by Frances AJ, Hales RE. Washington, DC, American Psychiatric Press, 1988, pp 256–273

Clayton PJ: Bereavement, in Handbook of Affective Disorders. Edited by Paykel ES. New York, Guilford, 1982, pp 403–415

Cohen MB, Baker G, Cohen RA, et al: An intensive study of twelve cases of manic-depressive psychosis. Psychiatry 17:103–137, 1954

Conte HR, Plutchik R, Wild KV, et al: Combined psychotherapy and pharmacotherapy for depression: a systematic analysis of the evidence. Arch Gen Psychiatry 43:471–479, 1986

Cummings JL: Clinical Neuropsychiatry. Orlando, FL, Grune & Stratton, 1985

DeVane CL: Pharmacokinetics of the selective serotonin reuptake inhibitors. J Clin Psychiatry 53 (No 2, Suppl):13–20, 1992

DiMascio A, Weissman MM, Prusoff BA, et al: Differential symptom reduction by drugs and psychotherapy in acute depression. Arch Gen Psychiatry 36:1450–1456, 1979

Dubovsky SL: Concise Guide to Clinical Psychiatry. Washington, DC, American Psychiatric Press, 1988

Duncan WC Jr, Pettigrew KD, Gillin JC: REM architecture changes in bipolar and unipolar depression. Am J Psychiatry 136:1424–1427, 1979

Ellis A: Reason and Emotion in Psychotherapy. Seacaucus, NJ, Citadel Press, 1962

Fava M, Rosenbaum JF: Suicidality and fluoxetine: is there a relationship? J Clin Psychiatry 52:108–111, 1991

Flor-Henry P: Cerebral Basis of Psychopathology. Boston, MA, John Wright/PSG Publishing, 1983

Frances A, Clarkin J, Perry S: Differential Therapeutics in Psychiatry: The Art and Science of Treatment Selection. New York, Brunner/Mazel, 1984

Frazer A, Ramsey TA, Swann A, et al: Plasma and erythrocyte electrolytes in affective disorders. J Affect Disord 5:103–113, 1983

García-Sevilla JA, Zis AP, Hollingsworth PJ, et al: Platelet α_2-adrenergic receptors in major depressive disorder: binding of tritiated clonidine before and after tricyclic antidepressant drug treatment. Arch Gen Psychiatry 38:1327–1333, 1981

Gershon S, Shopsin B (eds): Lithium: Its Role in Psychiatric Research and Treatment. New York, Plenum, 1973

Gillin JC, Duncan W, Pettigrew KD, et al: Successful separation of depressed, normal, and insomniac subjects by EEG sleep data. Arch Gen Psychiatry 36:85–90, 1979

Gold MS, Potash ALC, Extein IL: "Symptomless" autoimmune thyroiditis in depression. J Psychiatr Res 6:261–269, 1988

Goodnick PJ: Blood levels and acute response to bupropion Am J Psychiatry 149:399–400, 1992

Goodwin FK, Jamison KR: Foreword: bipolar disorders, in American Psychiatric Association Annual Review, Vol 6. Edited by Hales RE, Frances AJ. Washington, DC, American Psychiatric Press, 1987, pp 5–9

Goodwin FK, Roy-Byrne P: Treatment of bipolar disorders, in American Psychiatric Association Annual Review, Vol 6. Edited by Hales RE, Frances AJ. Washington, DC, American Psychiatric Press, 1987, pp 81–107

Gove WR: The relationsip between sex roles, marital status, and mental illness. Social Forces 51:34–44, 1972

Gupta MA, Moldofsky H: Dysthymic disorder and rheumatic pain modulation disorder (fibrositis syndrome): a comparison of symptoms and sleep physiology. Can J Psychiatry 31:608–616, 1986

Hatterer JA, Herbert J, Hidaka C, et al: CSF transthyretin in patients with depression. Am J Psychiatry 150:813–815, 1993

Hornstra RK, Klassen D: The course of depression. Compr Psychiatry 18:119–125, 1977

Jackson SW: Melancholia and Depression: From Hippocratic Times to Modern Times. New Haven, CT, Yale University Press, 1986

Jacobson E: Depression: Comparative Studies of Normal, Neurotic, and Psychotic Conditions. New York, International Universities Press, 1971

Jamison DR: Psychotherapeutic issues and suicide prevention in the treatment of bipolar disorders, in American Psychiatric Association Annual Review, Vol 6. Edited by Hales RE, Frances AJ. Washington, DC, American Psychiatric Press, 1987, pp 108–124

Janowsky DS, Leff M, Epstein RS: Playing the manic game. Arch Gen Psychiatry 22:252–261, 1970

Keller MB: Differential Diagnosis, natural course, and epidemiology of bipolar disorders, in American Psychiatric Association Annual Review, Vol 6. Edited by Hales RE, Frances AJ. Washington, DC, American Psychiatric Press, 1987, pp 10–31

Kiev A: Psychotherapeutic strategies in the management of depressed and suicidal patients. Am J Psychother 29:345–354, 1975

Klein M: A contribution to the psychogenesis of manic-depressive states. Int J Psychoanal 16: , 1934

Klerman GL: Other specific affective disorders, in Comprehensive Textbook of Psychiatry/III, 3rd Edition. Edited by Kaplan HI, Freedman AM, Sadock BJ. Baltimore, MD, Williams & Wilkins, 1980, pp 1332–1338

Klerman GL, Schechter G: Drugs and psychotherapy, in Handbook of Affective Disorders. Edited by Paykel ES. New York, Guilford, 1982, pp 329–337

Klerman GL, Weissman MM, Rounsaville BJ, et al: Interpersonal Psychotherapy of Depression. New York, Basic Books, 1984

Kocsis JH, Frances AJ: A critical discussion of DSM-III dysthymic disorder. Am J Psychiatry 144:1534–1542, 1987

Kocsis JH, Frances AJ, Mann JJ, et al: Imipramine for the treatment of chronic depression. Psychopharmacol Bull 21:698–700, 1985

Kraepelin E: Manic-Depressive Insanity and Paranoia. Edinburgh, E & S Livingtone, 1921

Krauthammer CD, Klerman GL: Secondary mania: manic syndromes associated with antecedent physical illness or drugs. Arch Gen Psychiatry 35:1333–1339, 1978

Krishnan KRR, McDonald WM, Escalona PR, et al: Magnetic resonance imaging of the caudate nuclei in depression: preliminary observations. Arch Gen Psychiatry 49:553–557, 1992

Kupfer DJ, Carpenter LL, Frank E: Possible role of antidepressants in precipitating mania and hypomania in recurrent depression. Am J Psychiatry 145:804–808, 1988

Lawson WB: Racial and ethnic factors in psychiatric research. Hosp Community Psychiatry 37:50–54, 1986

Leckman JF, Weissman MM, Merikangas KR, et al: Panic disorder and major depression. Arch Gen Psychiatry 40:1055–1060, 1983

Lesse S: The range of therapies in the treatment of severely depressed suicidal patients. Am J Psychotherapy 29:308–326, 1975

Levitt JJ, Tsuang MT: The heterogeneity of schizoaffective disorder: implications for treatment. Am J Psychiatry 145:926–936, 1988

Liebowitz MR, Klein DF: Hysteroid dysphoria. Psychiatr Clin North Am 2:555–575, 1979

Liebowitz MR, Quitkin FM, Stewart JW, et al: Psychopharmacologic validation of atypical depression. J Clin Psychiatry 45 (No 7, Sec 2):22–25, 1984

Liebowitz MR, Quitkin FM, Stewart JW, et al: Effect of panic attacks on the treatment of atypical depressives. Psychopharmacol Bull 21:558–561, 1985

Liebowitz MR, Quitkin FM; Stewart JW, et al: Antidepressant specificity in atypical depression. Arch Gen Psychiatry 45:129–137, 1988

Maj M: Schizoaffective disorder, depressed type: clinical, biological, and neuropsychological aspects, in Anxious Depression: Assessment and Treatment. Edited by Racagni G, Smeraldi E. New York, Raven, 1987, pp 57–62

Maxmen JS: Essential Psychopathology. New York, WW Norton, 1986

McCarley RW: REM sleep and depression: common neurobiological control mechanisms. Am J Psychiatry 139:565–570, 1982

McNeil GN: Depression, in Handbook of Psychiatric Differential Diagnosis. Edited by Soreff SM, McNeil GN. Littleton, MA, PSG Publishing, 1987, pp 57–126

Meltzer HY, Arora RC, Baber R, et al: Serotonin uptake in blood platelets of psychiatric patients. Arch Gen Psychiatry 38:1322–1326, 1981

Mendelson M: Psychodynamics of depression, in Handbook of Affective Disorders. Edited by Paykel ES. New York, Guilford, 1982, pp 162–174

Meyer RG: The Clinician's Handbook. Boston, MA, Allyn & Bacon, 1983

Nemeroff CB, Simon JS, Haggerty JJ Jr, et al: Antithyroid antibodies in depressed patients. Am J Psychiatry 142:840–843, 1985

Newmark CS: Major Psychological Assessment Instruments. Boston, MA, Allyn & Bacon, 1985

Nurnberger JI, Gershon ES: Genetics, in Handbook of Affective Disorders. Edited by Paykel ES. New York, Guilford, 1982, pp 126–145

Nurnberger J Jr, Jimerson DC, Allen JR, et al: Red-cell ouabain-sensitive Na$^+$-K$^+$-adenosine triphosphatase: a state marker in affective disorder inversely related to plasma cortisol. Biol Psychiatry 17:981–992, 1982

O'Rourke D, Wurtman JJ, Wurtman RJ, et al: Treatment of seasonal depression with d-fenfluramine. J Clin Psychiatry 50:343–347, 1989

Osser DN: A systematic approach to the classification and pharmacotherapy of nonpsychotic major depression and dysthymia. J Clin Psychopharmacol 13:133–144, 1993

Paykel ES: Recent life events and clinical depression, in Life Stress and Illness. Edited by Gunderson EK, Rahe RH. 1974, pp 134–163

Petrie WM, Maffucci RJ, Woosley RL: Propranolol and depression. Am J Psychiatry 139:92–94, 1982

Phelps ME, Mazziotta JC, Baxter L, et al: Positron emission tomographic study of affective disorders: problems and strategies. Ann Neurol 15(suppl):149–156, 1984

Pies RW: Atypical depression, in Handbook of Clinical Psychopharmacology. Edited by Tupin JP, Shader RI, Harnett DS. New York, Jason Aronson, 1988, pp 329–356

Pies RW, Shader RI: Approaches to the treatment of depression, in Manual of Psychiatric Therapeutics, 2nd Edition. Edited by Shader RI. Boston, MA, Little, Brown, 1994, pp 217–246

Pies R[W], Adler DA, Ehrenberg BL: Sleep disorders and depression with atypical features: response to valproate. J Clin Psychopharmacol 9:352–357, 1989

Plutchik R, Platman SR: Personality connotations of psychiatric diagnoses. J Nerv Ment Dis 165:418–422, 1977

Pope HG Jr, Lipinski JF Jr: Diagnosis in schizophrenia and manic-depressive illness: a reassessment of the specificity of 'schizophrenic' symptoms in the light of current research. Arch Gen Psychiatry 35:811–828, 1978

Post RM: Issues in the long-term management of bipolar affective illness. Psychiatric Annals 23:86–93, 1993

Post RM, Stoddard FJ, Gillin JC, et al: Alterations in motor activity, sleep, and biochemistry in a cycling manic-depressive patient. Arch Gen Psychiatry 34:470–477, 1977

Post RM, Uhde TW, Roy-Byrne PP, et al: Correlates of antimanic response to carbamazepine. Psychiatry Res 21:71–83, 1987

Potter WZ, Rudorfer MV, Goodwin FK: Biological findings in bipolar disorders, in American Psychiatric Association Annual Review, Vol 6. Edited by Hales RE, Frances AJ. Washington, DC, American Psychiatric Press, 1987, pp 32–60

Rabins PV, Pearlson GD, Aylward E, et al: Cortical magnetic resonance imaging changes in elderly inpatients with major depression. Am J Psychiatry 148:617–620, 1991

Robinson RG, Starr LB, Price TR: A two year longitudinal study of mood disorders following stroke: prevalence and duration at six months follow-up. Br J Psychiatry 144:256–262, 1984

Rogers CR: A Way of Being. Boston, MA, Houghton-Mifflin, 1980

Rosenthal NE, Sack DA, Gillin JC, et al: Seasonal affective disorder: a description of the syndrome and preliminary findings with light therapy. Arch Gen Psychiatry 41:72–80, 1984

Rosenthal NE, Sack DA, Carpenter CJ, et al: Antidepressant effects of light in seasonal affective disorder. Am J Psychiatry 142:163–170, 1985

Rothschild AJ, Locke CA: Reexposure to fluoxetine after serious suicide attempts by three patients: the role of akathisia. J Clin Psychiatry 52:491–493, 1991

Roy A, Sutton M, Pickar D: Neuroendocrine and personality variables in dysthymic disorder. Am J Psychiatry 142:94–97, 1985

Rubinow DR, Roy-Byrne P: Premenstrual syndromes: overview from a methodologic perspective. Am J Psychiatry 141:163–172, 1984

Rush AJ, Beck AT, Kovacs M, et al: Comparative efficacy of cognitive therapy and imipramine in the treatment of depressed outpatients. Cognitive Therapy and Research 1:17–37, 1977

Sachar EJ: Endocrine abnormalities in depression, in Handbook of Affective Disorders. Edited by Paykel ES. New York, Guilford, 1982, pp 191–201

Sanderson WC, Beck AT, Beck J: Syndrome comorbidity in patients with major depression or dysthymia: prevalence and temporal relationships. Am J Psychiatry 147:1025–1028, 1990

Sargant W: Drugs in the treatment of depression. BMJ 1:225–227, 1961

Schlesser MA, Winokur G, Sherman BM: Genetic subtypes of unipolar primary depressive illness distinguished by hypothalamic-pituitary-adrenal axis activity. Lancet 1:739–741, 1979

Schwartz JM, Baxter LR Jr, Massiotta JC, et al: The differential diagnosis of depression. JAMA 258:1368–1374, 1987

Sedler MJ: Falret's discovery: the origin of the concept of bipolar affective illness. Am J Psychiatry 140:1127–1133, 1983

Shader RI: Approaches to the treatment of manic-depressive states, in Manual of Psychiatric Therapeutics, 2nd Edition. Edited by Shader RI. Boston, MA, Little, Brown, 1994, pp 247–258

Shea MT, Elkin I, Hirschfeld RMA: Psychotherapeutic treatment of depression, in American Psychiatric Association Annual Review, Vol 7. Edited by Frances AJ, Hales RE. Washington, DC, American Psychiatric Press, 1988, pp 235–255

Simpson SG, DePaulo JR: Fluoxetine treatment of bipolar II depression. J Clin Psychopharmacol 11:52–54, 1991

Smith ML, Glass GV, Miller TI: The Benefits of Psychotherapy. Baltimore, MD, Johns Hopkins University Press, 1980

Spitzer RL, Williams JBW: Hysteroid dysphoria: an unsuccessful attempt to demonstrate its syndromal validity. Am J Psychiatry 139:1286–1291, 1982

Stone AB, Pearlstein TB, Brown WA: Fluoxetine in the treatment of late luteal phase dysphoric disorder. J Clin Psychiatry 52:290–293, 1991

Sulser F: The neurochemistry of refractory depression: a molecular view on therapy-resistant signal transfer, in Refractory Depression. Edited by Amsterdam JD. New York, Raven, 1991, pp 13–21

Tanna VL, Winokur G, Elston R, et al: A linkage study of depression spectrum disease. Neuropsychobiology 2:52–62, 1976

Tyrer S, Shopsin B: Symptoms and assessment of mania, in Handbook of Affective Disorders. Edited by Paykel ES. New York, Guilford, 1982, pp 12–23

Van Valkenburg C, Winokur G: Depressive spectrum disease. Psychiatr Clin North Am 2:469–482, 1979

Wagner EE, Heise MR: Rorschach and Hand Test data comparing bipolar patients in manic and depressive phases. J Pers Assess 45:240–249, 1981

Waters B, Calleia S: The effect of juvenile-onset manic-depressive disorder on the developmental tasks of adolescence. Am J Psychother 37:182–189, 1983

Wehr TA: Phase and biorhythm studies of affective illness in the switch process in manic-depressive psychosis. Ann Intern Med 87:321–324, 1977

Wehr TA, Sack DA, Rosenthal NE, et al: Sleep and biological rhythms in bipolar illness, in American Psychiatric Association Annual Review, Vol 6. Edited by Hales RE, Frances AJ. Washington, DC, American Psychiatric Press, 1987, pp 61–80

Weissman MM, Myers JK: Affective disorders in a US urban community. Arch Gen Psychiatry 35:1304–1311, 1978

Welch CA: Electroconvulsive therapy in the general hospital, in Massachusetts General Hospital Handbook of General Hospital Psychiatry, 2nd Edition. Edited by Hackett TP, Cassem NH. Littleton, MA, PSG Publishing, 1987, pp 261–267

Welner A, Liss JL, Robins E: Psychiatric symptoms in white and black inpatients, II: follow-up study. Compr Psychiatry 14:483–488, 1973

Wender PH, Klein DF: Mind, Mood, and Medicine. New York, Farrar, Straus & Giroux, 1981

West ED, Daly PJ: Effects of iproniazid in depressive syndromes. BMJ 1:1491–1493, 1959

Winters KC, Weintraub S, Neale JM: Validity of MMPI codetypes in identifying DSM-III schizophrenics, unipolars, and bipolars. J Consult Clin Psychol 49:486–487, 1981

Wolkowitz OM, Reus VI, Manfredi F, et al: Ketoconazole administration in hypercortisolemic depression. Am J Psychiatry 150:810–812, 1993

Wright G, Galloway L, Kim J, et al: Bupropion in the long-term treatment of cyclic mood disorders: mood stabilizing effects. J Clin Psychiatry 46:22–25, 1985

Wurtman JJ: Carbohydrate craving, mood changes, and obesity. J Clin Psychiatry 49 (No 8, Suppl):37–39, 1988

Yerevanian BI, Akiskal HS: "Neurotic," characterological, and dysthymic depressions. Psychiatr Clin North Am 2:595–617, 1979

Zis AP, Goodwin FK: The amine hypothesis, in Handbook of Affective Disorders. Edited by Paykel ES. New York, Guilford, 1982, pp 175–190

Zung WWK, MacDonald J, Zung EM: Prevalence of clinically significant depressive symptoms in black and white patients in family practice settings. Am J Psychiatry 145:882–883, 1988

5

Schizophrenia and Related Disorders

That's my pudding, doctor. All God give forgiveness. Oh, mamma, why did they make expensive weddings? Why don't they stay home, mamma?

> A schizophrenic patient's interpretation of the proverb "The proof of the pudding is in the eating" (Benjamin 1964, p. 75)

Schizophrenia is among the most crippling of all mental illnesses, though recent evidence suggests that more optimism is warranted than heretofore believed. Studies in a variety of cultures have yielded a lifetime prevalence of between 0.2% to nearly 1%—perhaps higher in some urban populations. The nature of schizophrenia—if we may speak at all of a single diagnostic entity—remains obscure. Equally disappointing has been the absence—until quite recently—of any "revolutionary" breakthroughs in treatment. We had little more to offer schizophrenic patients in 1988 than we had in 1954—the year chlorpromazine was introduced in the United States. But in the period between 1988 and 1992, there was cause for renewed optimism. This was the period, in many American centers, during which the new antipsychotic clozapine (Clozaril) was introduced. As we will see in our treatment section, this medication is truly a "breakthrough" for many thousands of patients. In the past 10 years or so, there have been other important refinements in pharmacological treatment and real advances in our psychosocial approach to the families of schizophrenic individuals. Moreover, neurophysiological studies are beginning to reveal at least some of the underpinnings of this illness.

Schizophrenia

The Central Concept

Let's begin our examination of schizophrenia with the following vignette.

Vignette

Jim was a 19-year-old college student majoring in computer science. Although he and his family agreed that Jim had always been "a shy boy," he had had no significant psychiatric problems until 1 year prior to evaluation. At that time—during his freshman term—Jim began to withdraw from his friends and classmates. His roommate found him "real hard to live with," as Jim had begun to "let the room go to hell . . . like never cleaning up, leaving old food lying around, and not showering." He began to get involved in what he called "Tai Chi," but what his roommate described as "doing these weird postures . . . like posing in one position for 3 or 4 hours." Jim began to skip his classes and failed three of his five courses that semester. He grew increasingly suspicious of his roommate, accusing him of "spying on him in bed," and eventually moved into his own apartment off campus. On a trip home, Jim's parents found him extremely withdrawn, "paranoid," and ill-kempt. His thinking "didn't make sense . . . he'd skip from one thought to another, or else he'd stop in the middle and laugh." He spoke of the "Ganja gangsters" who were "trying to dope me up on bad reefer," but denied any actual use of marijuana or other drugs of abuse. His parents confirmed this, adding, "Basically, he stayed in his room night and day." His parents brought Jim to their family doctor, who diagnosed a "psychotic reaction" and hospitalized Jim the same day.

As our vignette shows, schizophrenia is an insidious and pervasive disturbance of thought content and process, affect, social function, and overall behavior. The "active" phase of the illness is usually preceded by a "prodromal phase," in which there is increasing social withdrawal, impairment in role functioning, peculiar behavior, poor hygiene, blunted or inappropriate affect, bizarre ideation (not yet reaching delusional proportions), and disturbed communication. During the active phase—which may follow a major stressor—psychotic symptoms such as frank delusions, hallucinations, and grossly incoherent thinking are prominent. DSM-IV (American Psychiatric Association 1994) requires continuous signs of the illness for at least 6 months, including at least 1 month of "active phase symptoms"—so-called criterion A. In order to meet criterion A, the patient should show at least two of the following features for most of a 1-month period: delusions, hallucinations, disorganized speech, grossly disorganized or catatonic behavior, or "negative symptoms" such as affective flattening. DSM-IV has given increased "weight" to Schneiderian features such as a voice keeping up a running commentary on the patient or two voices conversing with each other. Like DSM-III-R (American Psychiatric Association 1987), DSM-IV requires evidence of impaired social and occupational functioning for a significant period of time since the illness began.

A "residual phase" usually follows the active phase of schizophrenia and resembles the prodrome in its predominantly "negative" symptoms (i.e., social isolation, blunted affect, and marked lack of energy and initiative). The course of the illness is variable, with acute exacerbations and intermorbid residual impairment being most typical. Some patients with schizophrenia will completely recover, but these patients seem to be quite rare; perhaps some are actually patients with schizophreniform disorder, which we will discuss later in this chapter.

The delusions in schizophrenia are often of a bizarre or persecutory nature—for example, the belief that one is being poisoned by the KGB or that a "computer" has been implanted into one's brain. The hallucinations may occur in any modality but are most commonly auditory. They often entail the perception of two voices commenting on the sufferer in a threatening or derogatory way. One hallmark of schizophrenia is the relative preservation of purely "cognitive" abilities; for example, memory and calculation are often normal in the early stages of the illness. However, thought processes may show marked loosening of associations, "blocking" (i.e., intrusion of unconscious material into the stream of conscious thought), or "word salad."

DSM-III-R described five subtypes of schizophrenia, based on the cross-sectional clinical presentation; however, the genetic, prognostic, and treatment implications of these types are not clear. In *catatonic* schizophrenia, the patient shows some abnormality in psychomotor function such as extreme excitement, rigidity, "waxy flexibility," or mutism. A patient with the *disorganized* subtype of schizophrenia shows predominantly incoherence or grossly disorganized behavior. In *paranoid* schizophrenia, the patient presents with the familiar delusions of persecution or external control, and lacks the marked incoherence or gross disorganization of the aforementioned category. A patient with *undifferentiated* schizophrenia shows symptoms of criterion A but does not meet criteria for the paranoid, catatonic, or disorganized subtypes. Finally, in *residual* schizophrenia, the patient lacks prominent delusions, hallucinations, incoherence, or grossly disorganized behavior but shows such "negative" symptoms as emotional blunting and social withdrawal. DSM-IV has retained this basic schema of subtypes, despite questions as to their prognostic and therapeutic significance.

Let's consider the following vignette.

Vignette

Harry was a 53-year-old male with a long history of psychiatric hospitalizations. He presented in the emergency room mute and unresponsive to staff. He held his arms in a "praying" position, but when his arms were repositioned by the psychiatric resident, he assumed the new posture. He also raised and lowered his eyebrows in a coordinated, stereotyped manner. The physical examination was grossly normal. Harry was given lorazepam, 2 mg im, and became responsive and communicative for approximately 30 minutes. He revealed that he had recently been evicted from a "shelter" and had not been taking his medications.

Harry's presentation is typical of catatonic schizophrenia, a syndrome far less common these days than the paranoid or undifferentiated forms. The use of benzodiazepines (such as lorazepam) is discussed later in this chapter.

Historical Development of the Disorder

In his landmark work on schizophrenia, Silvano Arieti (1974) named Kraepelin, Bleuler, Meyer, Freud, Jung, and Sullivan as the workers most fundamentally responsible for developing our modern concept of schizophrenia. We shall say more about these individuals, but should first note that the clinical description of schizophrenia-like symptoms long antedates any of these 19th-century figures. In the 16th century, Felix Platter's (1536–1614) detailed descriptions of "melancholia" often sound more like our modern ones of schizophrenia (Jackson 1986). For example, Platter described a man who thought he had become an earthenware vessel. Other "melancholics" believed that they had devoured serpents or frogs and were bearing them alive in their bodies (Diethelm and Heffernan 1965). Of course, we can't rule out from afar such diagnoses as neurosyphilitis in Platter's patients—but it is hard to imagine that schizophrenia had its origins only in the minds of 19th-century psychiatrists.

Still, the concept of schizophrenia as we now know it arose in the 1890s, crystallizing with the appearance of Kraepelin's *Dementia Praecox and Paraphrenia* (ca. 1896). Kraepelin brought together the previously described phenomena of catatonia, hebephrenia, and paranoia under the rubric *dementia praecox*. Unlike the other main group in Kraepelin's scheme—the manic-depressive patients—schizophrenic patients had a relatively poor, "downhill" course. Kraepelin accurately described the syndrome as consisting typically of hallucinations, delusions, incongruous affect, impairment of attention, negativism, stereotyped behavior, and progressive deterioration in the presence of a relatively intact sensorium. Interestingly, Kraepelin hypothesized an organic etiology, perhaps of a metabolic nature (Arieti 1974).

In 1911, Eugen Bleuler (1857–1930) renamed dementia praecox "schizophrenia," emphasizing the "splitting" of various psychic functions rather than the progression toward a demented state. Bleuler classified the symptoms of schizophrenia into fundamental and accessory types. The former have become the famous "four A's": autism, (inappropriate) affect, ambivalence, and (loose) associations, in simplified terms. The accessory symptoms, in Bleuler's view, consisted of what we now refer to as the "active" or "positive" symptoms of schizophrenia—delusions and hallucinations—as well as catatonic postures. For Bleuler, schizophrenia was fundamentally a disorder of thought process (Arieti 1974).

Adolf Meyer (1866–1950) was skeptical of Kraepelin's "disease model" of schizophrenia and emphasized instead the adaptive use of fantasy—as opposed to action—in the illness. Meyer stressed the longitudinal, psychodynamic development of schizophrenia, arguing that the preschizophrenic individual begins with "trivial and harmless subterfuges," such as daydreaming or rumination, which eventually progress to frank delusions, hallucinations, thought blocking, and so forth. Thus, as Arieti (1974) puts it, "Meyer seems to believe that there is only a gradual or quantitative difference between faulty habits and clear-cut schizophrenic symptoms" (p. 17)—a view few psychiatrists today would support. Nevertheless, Meyer's focus on pre-psychotic habits of mind may have helped point the way to our current concept of schizophreniform disorder, discussed later in this chapter.

Although Sigmund Freud (1856–1939) is best known for his work on the "neuroses," he contributed some fundamental ideas in the area of paranoid psychoses and schizophrenia (see Arieti 1974 for a complete discussion). Essentially, Freud regarded schizophrenia as a regression to a primitive narcissistic state—one in which libido is "withdrawn" from objects (i.e., other people) and directed into the self. Clinically, Freud's hypothesis seems to fit the very regressed, uncommunicative schizophrenic patient, who spends all day rocking, muttering, and "responding to internal stimuli." Freud also delineated the role of projection in the development of paranoid states, although his focus on homosexual urges has not been borne out in all cases.

While we often associate Carl Jung (1875–1961) with "archetypal psychology," Arieti (1974) points out that Jung was the first author to suggest a "psychosomatic" mechanism in schizophrenia. Specifically, Jung hypothesized that a primary emotional disturbance in dementia praecox engendered some form of abnormal brain metabolism. This is consistent with more recent theories, in which "stress" is thought to induce changes in dopamine metabolism, perhaps precipitating a psychotic relapse in the chronic schizophrenic patient. (Jung, according to Arieti, also never ruled out a primary metabolic derangement in schizophrenia.)

Harry Stack Sullivan (1892–1949), according to Arieti (1974), contributed significantly to our understanding of schizophrenia as an *interpersonal* phenomenon. Indeed, Sullivan, Arieti notes, "demonstrated that schizophrenia . . . is engendered by poor interpersonal relations, especially parent-child relations" (Arieti 1974, p. 29). This claim may have had some inadvertent "negative" consequences; for example, encouraging Fromm-Reichmann's unfortunate notion of the "schizophrenogenic" mother (see Arieti 1974, pp. 81–82). However, Sullivan's thinking contributed positively to our current concept of the "high EE" (expressed emotion) family, discussed later in this chapter, and its role in precipitating relapse in schizophrenic patients.

Not mentioned in Arieti's pantheon is Kurt Schneider, who has contributed a good deal to our current DSM-III-R (American Psychiatric Association 1987) and DSM-IV (American Psychiatric Association 1994) concepts of schizophrenia (Lehmann 1980). Schneider developed a set of pragmatic criteria called "first-rank symptoms," which, when other pathology can be excluded, suggest a diagnosis of schizophrenia. These include the hearing of one's thoughts spoken aloud; auditory hallucinations that comment on one's behavior; the experience of having one's thoughts controlled; the spreading of one's thoughts to others; and the experience of having one's actions controlled or influenced from the outside. Schneider also believed that schizophrenia could be diagnosed exclusively on the basis of "second-rank" symptoms, along with an otherwise typical clinical picture (Lehmann 1980). These symptoms, which are reminiscent of Bleuler's "fundamental" ones, include perplexity and euphoric or blunted affect.

In recent years the concept of schizophrenia as a biological disorder has gained primacy (as discussed later in this chapter). Not unexpectedly, this view has influenced recent typologies of schizophrenia, most notable of which is that of Crow (1982). Crow has proposed that schizophrenia be divided into two distinct subtypes, as summarized in Table 5–1. We shall say much more about the role of dopamine in our discussion of the biopsychosocial perspective.

The Biopsychosocial Perspective

Biological Factors

No survey of this topic can do justice to the burgeoning literature of the past 10 years—at best, we can point out some of the most compelling recent findings. But first, let's drop back to the older literature on the genetics of schizophrenia. Kendler (1986), in reviewing this field, concluded that, indeed, "genetic factors play a major role in the familial transmission of schizophrenia" (p. 38). Perhaps the most comprehensive data come from adoption studies in which the separated (adopted-away) offspring of schizophrenic parents (usually mothers) are assessed for the development of schizophrenia. In one strategy, the rate of psychosis in these children is compared to the rate in adopted-away offspring of "normal" control parents. Most such studies (e.g., Heston 1966) showed a higher rate of psychosis in the offspring of schizophrenic mothers. Even more convincing are the twin studies, in which monozygotic (identical) twins not only show a higher concordance rate for schizophrenia than do dizygotic twins, but do so even when reared in separate homes (Gottesman and Shields 1982). Despite many methodological problems with such studies, the

Table 5–1.   Schizophrenia subtypes

Type 1 (positive schizophrenia)	Type 2 (negative schizophrenia)
Delusions, hallucinations, and thought process disorder prominent	Less prominent
Relatively acute onset	Insidious onset
Good premorbid functioning	Poor premorbid functioning
Exacerbations/remissions	Deteriorating course
Normal CT scan	Ventricular enlargement common
Good response to antipsychotics	More refractory to medication
Normal cognitive function	Cognitive impairment

Source. Extensively modified from Crow 1982.

preponderance of data supports the view that the concordance rate of schizophrenia is three to five times higher in monozygotic twins than in dizygotic twins (Kendler 1986).

Many studies of schizophrenia have focused on structural brain abnormalities, as we saw in Crow's (1982) scheme. Cortical atrophy and ventricular enlargement have been noted in chronic schizophrenia, and Golden et al. (1980) have correlated such changes with measurable disturbances in expression, reading, and arithmetic. However, not all studies have confirmed these findings. Recently, Shenton and colleagues (1992) found abnormalities of the left temporal lobe in schizophrenic patients and related these to the degree of thought disorder present. They have assimilated these findings into a larger hypothesis in which damage to interconnected structures such as the amygdal-hippocampal complex, parahippocampal gyrus, and superior temporal gyrus accounts for the impaired associational linkages ("loose associations") seen in schizophrenia. Shenton et al. also speculate on the role of NMDA (N-methyl-D-aspartic acid) receptors in schizophrenia (discussed later in this chapter). In a recent study of five schizophrenic patients, Akbarian et al. (1993a, 1993b) found some intriguing "immunocytochemical" abnormalities. They examined cortical neurons containing the enzyme NADPH-d, which appears to be a kind of "protective" enzyme that may, for example, help prevent certain types of cellular necrosis. Akbarian et al. detected a significant decline in NADPH-d neurons in the cortical gray matter of the schizophrenic subjects compared with matched control subjects. More important, these investigators went on to show that there is abnormal distribution of NADPH-d neurons in the brains of schizophrenic subjects, strongly suggesting impaired migration of neurons during early brain development.

Taken together with the work of Shenton et al., these data suggest that schizophrenia is, indeed, a neurodevelopmental disorder. This hypothesis has been thoroughly reviewed by Bloom (1993). We will defer further discussion of structural brain imaging until our discussion of adjunctive testing.

Of course, the leading biochemical hypothesis holds that schizophrenia involves a disorder of dopamine function. In the "old days"— about 15 years ago—schizophrenia was attributed, in part, to excessive dopamine in the limbic system. Since then, more subtle variations have been advanced, one of which dovetails with Crow's scheme. First of all, subpopulations of dopamine receptors have been identified, called D_1 and D_2; other subtypes (D_3, D_4, etc.) have also been identified, but we will focus on the first two for now. D_2 receptors seem to be responsible for mediating the therapeutic effect of most classic antipsychotic drugs, such as haloperidol. Crow et al. (1978) presented some postmortem evidence showing D_2 receptor up-regulation in schizophrenic patients—even in those not exposed to antipsychotic medication. On the other hand, MacKay et al. (1980) could not confirm this finding. To reconcile such conflicting data, Crow (1982) proposed that his type 1 schizophrenia is characterized by an increase in D_2 receptors, as contrasted with his type 2 ("negative") schizophrenia, which shows no such increase in D_2 receptors. When we discuss the new "atypical" antipsychotic clozapine, we will see that occupancy of D_1 receptors (or low D_2 receptor occupancy) may play an important role in the clinical and side-effect profiles of antipsychotic drugs (Farde et al. 1992).

As suggested above, dopamine is not the only neurotransmitter implicated in schizophrenia. Shenton et al. (1992) hypothesize that NMDA receptors—which are activated by the excitatory neurotransmitters aspartate and glutamate—may play a critical role in schizophrenia. They speculate that "overactivation" of these receptors may underlie "positive" symptoms such as hallucinations and thought process disorder. Postmortem studies examining serotonin and gamma-aminobutyric acid (GABA) function in schizophrenia have been suggestive but inconclusive (Weinberger and Kleinman 1986).

In Chapter 2, we discussed in vivo techniques such as positron-emision tomography (PET) scanning and regional cerebral blood flow (rCBF) studies. These techniques have been applied recently to the study of schizophrenia, with some exciting, if preliminary, results (Weinberger and Kleinman 1986). Using PET scanning, Buchsbaum et al. (1982) found decreased frontal cortical activity and decreased activity in the left contralateral gray matter in eight drug-free schizophrenic patients. Others have confirmed this so-called hypofrontality in both treated and untreated schizophrenic individuals (Wolkin et al. 1985). However, at least one study (Widen et al. 1984) found no differences in frontal glucose metabolism (i.e., no hypofrontality), and many methodological problems complicate the PET literature (Weinberger and Kleinman 1986). This is also true of the rCBF study. Weinberger et al. (1986) examined schizophrenic patients performing various cognitive tests. Dramatic differences between patients and control subjects were seen in dorsolateral prefrontal cortex rCBF studies, the findings of which, on the whole, seem to support the claim of frontal lobe dysfunction in schizophrenia.

Many other biological hypotheses have been generated in recent years, including those that attribute schizophrenia to autoimmune disease (Pandey et al. 1981) and to excessive or deficient endorphin activity (Kline et al. 1977; Terenius et al. 1976). Of course, it is possible that more than one biological factor is at work and that different subgroups of schizophrenia have different biochemical etiologies.

Psychological Factors

Arieti (1974) has written extensively on the psychodynamics of schizophrenia, and we cannot do justice to the richness of his thinking in so brief a discussion. But perhaps Arieti himself is most helpful in summarizing the psychodynamics felt by some to predispose toward schizophrenia:

> We have seen how an extreme state of anxiety, originating in early childhood, produces a vulnerability that in many instances lasts for the whole life of the individual. We have seen how desperately . . . the patient attempts to maintain contact with reality, to survive, and to grow. However, in dealing with new threats in adolescence and adult life, his defenses become increasingly inadequate. Confronted with overpowering anxiety, the patient finally succumbs, and the break with reality occurs. In other words, when he cannot change the unbearable vision of himself any longer, not even in prepsychotic ways, he has to change reality. But reality cannot change, and he has to change himself again in order to see "reality" in a different way. (Arieti 1974, p. 215)

We can think of Arieti's view as a "stress-adaptational defense" model of schizophrenia, and we are reminded of Meyer's views in this

regard. However, Arieti is inclined to see schizophrenia as a qualita-
tively different state—a "break," in effect, from the kind of "habits of
mind" postulated by Adolf Meyer. McNeil and Soreff (1987) have
formulated a position similar to Arieti's, as follows:

> The infant who is the victim of chaotic parenting may never develop
> the basic trust upon which later psychological growth depends.
> Under stress in later life, the fragile ego defenses of such a person
> may tumble like a house of cards, exposing the infantile psychotic
> core of the individual. (p. 133)

Although it isn't easy to separate psychological from biological
mechanisms when discussing schizophrenic "cognition," we shall discuss this topic here. Gur (1986) has reviewed the cognitive deficits
often found in schizophrenia and separated them into four areas:
intellectual functioning, attention, memory, and language/abstract
reasoning. Although the notion of "intellectual decline" in schizophrenia goes back to Kraepelin, the evidence is a bit ambiguous: some
studies document deterioration on standard IQ tests, whereas others
do not. However, there does seem to be a correlation between high
IQ and favorable prognosis (Gur 1986). With respect to attention,
schizophrenic individuals appear impaired in two main areas: sustained
attention and selective attention. Thus, studies of so-called smooth
pursuit eye movements in schizophrenia have suggested deficits in the
nonvoluntary, oculomotor aspects of attention (Holzman and Levy
1977). (One wonders whether the schizophrenic patient's difficulty in
carrying on conversations stems from such attentional deficits rather
than from thought process disorder per se.) Memory function may
also be impaired in schizophrenia, at least in more severe cases; however, memory is a complex function, requiring intact intellectual and
attentional abilities. Finally, language and thought are clearly disordered in many schizophrenic individuals. The early literature focused
on poverty of expression, idiosyncratic word association, confab-
ulations, neologisms, impaired abstraction, echolalia, and clanging
(e.g., "She's a deer, beer, clear, person"). One cautionary note:
Andreasen (1979) and others have shown that thought process disorder may be seen in conditions besides schizophrenia (see discussion of

the differential diagnosis), including mania.

Perhaps you have noticed an apparent disjunction in our discussion of "psychological" factors. We began by briefly summarizing some psychodynamic issues in the development of schizophrenia. We then launched into a more descriptive discussion of cognitive and psychological deficits. Fortunately, Arieti (1974) has provided us with an intriguing hypothesis that links these two realms. We may approach this by asking the following: Are there any psychodynamic factors that actually "explain" the apparent thought process disorder in schizophrenia? Arieti's answer is clearly yes. He states that "if, in a situation of severe anxiety, function at a certain level of psychological integration . . . does not bring about the desired results, a strong tendency exists toward functioning at lower levels of integration in order to effect those results" (Arieti 1974, p. 221). Stated more baldly: The schizophrenic "talks funny" because that is the best available way to get by. The patient's "thought process disorder" is a coping strategy whose goal is not always achieved—or is achieved but at the expense of normal interpersonal functioning. Perhaps we can understand Arieti's principle—known as "progressive teleologic regression"—by examining the following "dialogue":

> **Therapist:** You look a little upset today. Is anything wrong?
> **Patient:** Oh, Doctor, which set is the up set and which is the down set? Why don't you set down and talk?
> **T.:** Yes, I'd like to sit down and talk. How are you?
> **P.:** Well, the ink's running dry, you know, Doctor, the ink well, I mean. Do a thing here and there, grin and bear, you know.
> **T.:** So you're trying to grin and bear things these days? That sounds tough.
> **P.:** Oh, it's not tough, Doctor, it's just a factor of divine intervention and prevention, like a cardinal sin or the Virgin's holy affinity. Do you believe in infinity, Doctor?

Now you see why I put the work "dialogue" in quotation marks: this is really more of a double monologue. Arieti has compared the schizophrenic individual to one who would solve mathematical problems using an idiosyncratic system and who would consequently reach peculiar solutions. In the conversation above, the patient appears to be using his own system of language, thought, and logic. We see the classical schizophrenic features of clang associations ("here and there, grin and bear"), tangential responses, and idiosyncratic word usage (note the word play surrounding "up set," etc.). But note also the emotional context of the patient's remarks—the therapist began by observing that the patient looked "upset." In Arieti's formulation, we might posit that the patient became anxious at this and underwent, as it were, a protective regression. His language became a kind of smoke screen. Although the therapist tried to pursue the underlying affect ("That sounds tough"), the patient apparently could not tolerate it. Later, we will explore the therapeutic implications of such regression.

Sociocultural Factors

McGlashan (1986) has reviewed studies looking at adoption, social class and culture, social networks, life events, and familial factors. He first points out that while a genetically transmitted vulnerability to schizophrenia may be necessary for development of the illness, a disturbed rearing environment may also be necessary. Thus, the "at risk" children of schizophrenic mothers, when raised in a disturbed family environment, show a higher rate of psychotic illness than those at risk who are raised in normal adoptive family environments (Tienari et al. 1985).

A consistent finding in the literature of schizophrenia is the relationship of the illness to low socioeconomic status. The classic study was that of Hollingshead and Redlich (1958), who found that schizophrenia in the lowest social classes was nine times as frequent as in the upper classes. Part of this effect may be due to "downward drift": the tendency of preschizophrenic or schizophrenic individuals to drift into areas of social disorganization or poverty. Part may result from the effects of poverty itself (i.e., increased stress, limited opportunities, etc.), although few would argue that poverty causes schizophrenia (Liberman 1982). Interestingly, some data indicate a more benign course for schizophrenic patients in agrarian countries—ones we sometimes dismiss as "underdeveloped" (Strauss and Carpenter 1981). Perhaps such societies provide schizophrenic individuals with a less demanding and more supportive social system.

The role of stress in schizophrenia has been a source of ongoing controversy (McGlashan 1986). It is always difficult to know, for example, whether a so-called stressor preceded or resulted from the incipient psychotic episode: did the schizophrenic episode "flare up" because the patient lost his job, or did he lose his job because his boss detected the deterioration of incipient psychosis? These subtleties aside, there is reasonably good evidence that certain kinds of stressors increase the likelihood of relapse in schizophrenia. Families that show high levels of "expressed emotion" (EE) toward their schizophrenic members—for example, intense criticism, guilt induction, or intrusiveness—tend to precipitate relapses and rehospitalization (Leff and Vaughn 1981). Moreover, some data point to a correlation between onset or worsening of schizophrenia and the (antecedent) occurrence of major loss, death of a friend or relative, acute illness, or change of living situation, particularly if these events were unexpected (McGlashan 1986).

The "high EE" family studies remind one of earlier theories of schizophrenia that were based on notions of "faulty" family interaction. Thus, Lidz and his colleagues (1965) argued that schizophrenia arises out of continual covert and overt fighting between parents and the degree of "schism" or "skew" that results; in effect, children become pawns in the power games played by their parents and thereby become prone to psychosis. Fromm-Reichmann (1948) focused more specifically on the role of the "schizophrenogenic" mother, generally characterized as overprotective, hostile, cold, distant, and so forth (Arieti 1974). Bateson and colleagues (1956) advanced the "double-bind theory" of schizophrenia, arguing that inherently conflicting messages from significant figures in the child's life lead to helplessness, exasperation, and ultimately psychosis. This "damned if you do, damned if you don't" situation is summed up nicely in the example given by McNeil and Soreff (1987), in which "the double binding mother gives her son two neckties for his birthday. When he arrives at the breakfast table wearing one, she asks why he did not wear the other one" (p. 138). Bateson's formulation is actually more complex than this (Arieti 1974), involving a "tertiary negative injunction" that prohibits the child from escaping (e.g., the son must show up at the breakfast table wearing one of the two ties).

Arieti (1974) has criticized both Bateson's hypothesis and the notion of the "schizophrenogenic" mother. Most authorities today would argue that "family pathology" is, at most, one of many factors implicated in the etiology of schizophrenia, and that even when present, such pathology must fall on the "fertile ground" of abnormal biochemistry before schizophrenia arises.

Pitfalls in the Differential Diagnosis

Organic Conditions

Schizophrenia may be "mimicked" by a plethora of medical, neurological, and toxicological conditions. Let's consider the following vignette.

Vignette

Mitch was a 14-year-old male with, according to his parents, a 2-year history of "weird behavior." He was brought by them to the ER, where he expressed the delusion that "my guidance counselor has the FBI out looking for me." On physical examination, Mitch showed significant tremor and rigidity. A faint, greenish-brown ring was noted on slit-lamp examination of the cornea. Liver function tests were markedly elevated. A tentative diagnosis of Wilson's disease was made and later confirmed by decreased serum ceruloplasmin.

The many medical conditions that may present with "schizophreniform" features are summarized in Table 5–2. In general, the mental status and physical examinations are the key to differential diagnosis. Organically based psychoses are more likely than schizophrenia to be accompanied by visual hallucinations and impaired orientation, level of consciousness, and cognition. They are also more likely to be associated with neurological or other physical abnormalities, as well as abnormal laboratory findings. Of course, the old adage still applies: "The body can have as many diseases as it pleases." Someone may have schizophrenia and also suffer from anemia, thiamine deficiency, and Cushing's disease!

Functional Disorders

After the clinician has ruled out organic factors in the etiology of schizophreniform symptoms, a number of functional disorders must be considered, as listed in Table 5–3. With so many conditions in the differential diagnosis, where is the clinician to begin? The "decision tree" provided in Appendix B of DSM-III-R itself gets us off to a good start by emphasizing the following features: duration of psychotic symptoms; presence or absence of major depressive or manic symptoms and their temporal relationship to psychotic symptoms; and the presence or absence of hallucinations and bizarre behavior. To this list we would add, "presence or absence of life-long pattern of maladaptive behavior," in order to include the above-noted personality disorders. Let's see how, in clinical practice, some of these features point us toward a diagnosis.

Vignette

Mark, a 23-year-old white male with no previous psychiatric history, presented in the ER with symptoms of decreased sleep and racing

Table 5–2.   Medical conditions sometimes presenting with schizophreniform features

---

Neurological: head trauma, tumors, infarcts, CNS infection, dementia

Endocrine: hyper-/hypothyroidism, hyper-/hypoparathyroidism, pituitary, adrenal disorders

Metabolic: Cardiac, hepatic, renal, respiratory failure; Na^+/K^+ imbalance

Deficiencies: thiamine, pyridoxine, niacin, cobalamine

Intoxication-withdrawal: alcohol, barbiturate, amphetamines, PCP

Iatrogenic: antidepressants/anticholinergics, antihypertensives, L-dopa

---

Source. Extensively modified from McNeil and Soreff 1987.

thoughts, stating, "The spirit of Martin Luther King has infiltrated my metabolism." He also stated that God's voice was instructing him to "minister to the needs of all the world's peoples." Mark showed loud, pressured speech, loosening of associations, and occasional bizarre posturing. His affect was generally euphoric or irritable. Mark's older brother, who accompanied him to the ER, gave the following history. One month prior to evaluation, Mark began to talk of being "possessed by the spirit of black godliness," and claimed to be receiving "messages from the Imperator." At that time, however, Mark did not appear euphoric or irritable. His brother stated, in fact, that Mark was "quiet and calm, but with these weird ideas." Two weeks prior to evaluation, there was a dramatic shift in Mark's affect: he "got real loud and aggressive and stayed up the whole night singing." In addition to hearing God's voice, Mark also felt that his brother and mother were "warring in my head . . . trying to take over the respective hemispheres of my brain." Mark's family history was positive for "mood swings" in his uncle, who was taking lithium carbonate. Physical and laboratory evaluations were totally normal.

Table 5–3.   Psychiatric disorders with psychotic features

Schizoaffective disorder	Obsessive-compulsive disorder
Major depression with psychotic features	Personality disorders
Manic episode with psychotic features	Schizotypal Schizoid Borderline
Schizophreniform disorder	Paranoid
Delusional disorder	Histrionic
Brief reactive psychosis	Factitious disorders
Autistic disorder	Malingering
Mental retardation	Multiple personality disorder

Note. Cultural and/or religious beliefs may sometimes be misunderstood as "delusions."
Source. Extensively modified from American Psychiatric Association 1987; McNeil and Soreff 1987.

The first thing you may have noticed about Mark's clinical presentation is its polymorphous quality: it has features of both mania and schizophrenia. Indeed, a close inspection will show that at the time of his evaluation, Mark met criterion A for schizophrenia. He also showed—simultaneously—the classic symptoms of mania. The next thing you should have noticed is the "temporal uncoupling" of affective and psychotic features for the first 2 weeks of Mark's illness; that is, he experienced delusions and hallucinations in a state of relative euthymia. Finally, the mood syndrome (mania) made up a substantial part of the total duration of the psychosis (2 of the 4 weeks). Taken together, these features point to a diagnosis of schizoaffective disorder, bipolar (manic) type—a condition sometimes called "schizomania" (Levitt and Tsuang 1988).

Even though DSM-III-R provided fairly specific criteria for schizoaffective disorder, a good deal of confusion still surrounds this diagnosis (Levitt and Tsuang 1988). DSM-IV considers schizoaffective disorder to entail "an uninterrupted period of illness during which, at some time, there is either a major depressive episode, a manic episode, or a mixed episode concurrent with symptoms that meet criterion A for schizophrenia"; during the same period of illness, there must also be "delusions or hallucinatiions for at least 2 weeks in the absence of prominent mood symptoms" (American Psychiatric Association 1994, p. 292). The mood-episode symptoms must be present for "a substantial portion" of the total duration of the illness (active and residual phases). No doubt, these criteria will be modified as we refine our understanding of this disorder—if it is a single entity in the first place.

It appears that schizoaffective disorder (variously defined) is heterogeneous with respect to familial, genetic, clinical, and prognostic factors. Mendlewicz (1979), for example, compared family history profiles of schizoaffective patients with those of bipolar, unipolar, and schizophrenic patients. He found high "loading" for affective illness in first-degree relatives of schizoaffective patients, but also a higher-than-expected rate of schizophrenia in those relatives. Recent attempts at subtyping schizoaffective illness have focused on the distinction between "manic" and "depressive" types. It may also prove useful to distinguish patients in whom affective and psychotic episodes occur consecutively from those in whom they occur concurrently (Maj and

Perris 1985). We shall say more about schizoaffective disorder in our discussion of treatment directions and goals.

Continuing our discussion of differential diagnosis, let's consider another vignette, based on a case I recently evaluated.

Vignette

Luther was a 23-year-old black male who had moved from a southern state to the Northeast 3 years prior to evaluation. He had no psychiatric problems until 2 months prior to evaluation, at which time Luther began to experience intense anxiety surrounding "the people in the trees." He described these as "KKK types who drop down on you in the night," and stated that he heard these "tree people" discussing him in racially derogatory terms. Luther also reported several experiences of "seeing men in white hoods in my room." On examination, the patient showed intense anxiety, confusion, disorientation to day and date, and loosening of associations. Physical and laboratory testing were completely normal. An electroencephalogram in the emergency unit (to rule out organic brain syndrome) was also completely normal. There was no history of substance abuse, as confirmed by Luther's family. Family psychiatric history was negative, except for an aunt "who used to get real excited now and then." Premorbidly, Luther was described as "a shy boy, but always helpful and polite." He had completed high school and 1 year of college, after which, "he wanted to live at home." His behavior had been normal up until the current episode.

Luther's case presents us with another illness whose precise nature still eludes us: namely, schizophreniform disorder. In effect, this condition is a symptomatic "phenotype" of schizophrenia, with the distinction being mainly in the time course. Schizophreniform disorder meets criterion A of schizophrenia, does not fit the criteria for schizoaffective disorder or mood disorder with psychotic features, and has a duration of at least 1 month but less than 6 months. This criterion for duration includes the prodromal, active, and residual phases of the illness. Typically, schizophreniform disorder presents with more emotional turmoil, anxiety, confusion, and hallucinatory symptoms than does schizophrenia. Interestingly, the presence of intense affect, confusion, and disorientation bodes well for the patient, as does good premorbid and social functioning—thus, the DSM-IV designation "with good prognostic features." (Historically, many such patients would have been termed "good prognosis schizophrenics.")

What if our last patient, Luther, had moved to the Northeast just 2 weeks ago and had just been the victim of a racially motivated assault? What if he had presented with the same symptoms as described previously, except that they had begun 1 week prior to evaluation? The most likely diagnosis would be brief reactive psychosis. This condition generally begins after "one or more events that, singly or together, would be markedly stressful to almost anyone in similar circumstances in that person's culture" (American Psychiatric Association 1987, p. 205). A brief reactive psychosis may last for a few hours or up to a month, and there is full return to the premorbid level of functioning. (While "awaiting" the expected recovery, the diagnosis is qualified as "provisional.") We do not know much about the genetic and biochemical underpinnings of this condition. DSM-III-R noted that a variety of personality disorders (e.g., paranoid, borderline, or schizotypal) may predispose the individual to brief reactive psychosis.

Let's consider another vignette.

Vignette

A 42-year-old male sales clerk developed the delusion that a well-known television personality was "desperately in love" with him. In most respects, the patient appeared "normal." He was well dressed and polite, and showed no loosening of associations. He denied auditory or other hallucinations, and no Schneiderian symptoms could be elicited. The patient had never met the actress, but insisted that he "knew" she loved him because he had received a kind reply to one of his fan letters. Physical and laboratory studies were normal.

The man in question may bring to mind John Hinckley, the would-be assassin of former President Ronald Reagan and the would-be lover of movie star Jodie Foster. Our patient appears to meet the criteria for DSM-III-R delusional (paranoid) disorder, erotomanic type. This particular syndrome—historically associated with a condition described by Clerambault—is distinct from schizophrenia in the following respects: 1) the delusion lacks the bizarre quality of many schizophrenic delusions (e.g., "The CIA has planted a radio transmitter in my brain"); 2) there is little or no thought process disorder; 3) auditory or visual hallucinations are absent or minimal; 4) the patient's behavior is not odd or bizarre, except in the very circumscribed area of the delusion; and 5) social and occupational functioning are not usually severely impaired (unless, like Mr. Hinckley, the patient comes into conflict with the law). Familial and genetic data suggest that delusional (paranoid) disorder is distinct from schizophrenia (Kendler 1980). Most commonly, the delusion is persecutory in nature, but DSM-III-R also recognizes grandiose, jealous, and somatic subtypes.

The movie *Rain Man* (1988) focused attention on the syndrome of autism and, indirectly, on mental retardation. Both these conditions may sometimes be confused with schizophrenia. An important diagnostic clue is the age at onset. Both autistic disorder and mental retardation have their onset in infancy, childhood, or adolescence; for example, the autistic child usually gives evidence of dysfunction before age 3 years. Schizophrenia rarely has its onset in childhood.

Obsessive-compulsive disorder (OCD) may occasionally resemble schizophrenia, albeit superficially. The OCD patient's "rituals" (e.g., hand washing, checking doors, etc.) may appear "crazy" to the casual observer, but close analysis usually reveals that these behaviors are ego-alien and subject to the patient's reality-testing ability. Obsessive or ruminative thoughts may sometimes be hard to distinguish from auditory hallucinations, but here, too, differences may be discerned (Pies 1984). Let's consider the following vignette.

Vignette

A 30-year-old male complained of hearing "voices" and had been placed on Thorazine, 100 mg/day, by his physician. This sedated him but did not affect the "voices." The patient also exhibited a variety of peculiar rituals, including cleaning the seats of chairs before sitting down, "sterilizing" silverware by boiling it before use, and sleeping only on sheets that had "just been washed." On interview, the patient conceded that these behaviors "don't make a whole lot of sense" and added, "I know it sounds crazy, but I just can't help feeling that I'm going to pick up AIDS. I know they say you can't get it from seats and things, but I just can't help myself." The "voices" described by the patient were actually his own ruminative thoughts, usually involving the question "Why can't you be a nice clean boy?" Further exploration in psychotherapy revealed that this was what his mother used to say to him as a boy "whenever she wanted to embarrass me." Treatment with fluoxetine 20 mg/day plus psychotherapy led to substantial improvement.

Although the personality disorders are usually conceptualized as nonpsychotic in nature, a number of them may, from time to time, "cross over" into the psychotic realm. Moreover, the suspiciousness associated with paranoid personality disorder or the "odd beliefs" of schizotypal personality disorder may sometimes verge on the frankly delusional. DSM-III-R emphasized the role of "extreme stress" in precipitating transient psychotic episodes in such individuals. The differentiation of severe character pathology from schizophrenia rests on the absence of persistent delusions or hallucinations in the former. The degree of loosening of associations also tends to be greater in schizophrenia, though in the midst of a transient psychotic episode the individual with personality disorder may sound quite disorganized. It is evident that the "cross-sectional" symptom picture—that is, the symptoms at a given time—is not as helpful as the longitudinal course in making the diagnosis of schizophrenia.

In our discussion of the biopsychosocial model in Chapter 1, we hinted at some of the difficulties in distinguishing certain cultural beliefs from psychosis. This is nowhere more evident than in making the diagnosis of schizophrenia in an individual from, say, the Haitian or Puerto Rican cultures, in which some "normal" beliefs sound strikingly psychotic to the unaccustomed ear. Let's consider the following case vignette (adapted from Nandi et al. 1985).

Vignette

A 23-year-old Bengali (Indian) woman who had recently immigrated to the United States was brought to the ER by her American roommate. The patient had been having anxiety attacks for the 3 weeks prior to evaluation, characterized by frequent palpitation, trembling, dyspnea, and a choking sensation. Her roommate, however, was more concerned with what she described as "these weird gestures" the patient had been making over the past week and her "ranting about this Indian goddess." On examination, the patient did appear anxious and tearful, but was able to state in rather good English, "You would be upset too if people thought you were crazy." The patient was alert and fully oriented. Despite the language barrier, it was evident that the patient's thought processes were coherent.

She denied any ideas of influence or reference with respect to other people, but stated, "I believe the goddess Kali [believed to protect people from diseases] is angry with me. That is why I am choking and trembling." She explained that, in her village, Kali was worshipped at a regularly occurring festival. She believed that at the last such festival, just prior to her immigration, she had performed the ritual improperly. The "weird gestures" noted by her roommate were an attempt to placate the "angry" goddess. A diagnosis of panic disorder was established, based on the patient's personal and family history. Her condition responded well to low doses of alprazolam.

The case above demonstrates the necessity of considering cultural factors before jumping to the diagnosis of schizophrenia. Finally, let's consider the following vignette.

Vignette

A 34-year-old male was admitted to the impatient psychiatric unit on a court order "for assessment of competency to stand trial." The defendant had been arrested on a charge of "breaking and entering" and "aggravated assault." On interview, the patient stated that he had "heard a voice" telling him to break into a house and steal some money. When asked by the psychiatrist if he could ever resist this voice, the patient replied that he could not. He stated that the voice was "constant . . . like a constant droning in my head . . . it's been going on for months now." When asked what he did to make the voices go away, the patient looked surprised. After a brief pause, he stated, "Nothing makes them go away." When asked if the voices came from inside or outside his head, the patient replied, "I don't know . . . both." When asked what, specifically, the voice said to him, the patient replied, "It says, 'Break into a house and steal some money.'" No delusions associated with this voice could be elicited, and no ideas of influence, reference, and so forth were noted. The patient's behavior on the unit appeared normal, except when observed by staff. At such times, the patient would make convulsive movements of his arms or begin screaming.

I hope that you are ready to send this particular nonschizophrenic person off to stand trial and that you noted the classical features of malingered psychosis. Resnick (1988) has summarized these features as follows:

1. Claimed auditory hallucinations are not accompanied by a congruent delusion. (Eighty-eight percent of true auditory hallucinations are so accompanied.)
2. The "voices" can never be resisted. (Most schizophrenic individuals with command auditory hallucinations can resist acting on them.)
3. The auditory hallucinations are continuous. (True "voices" are usually intermittent.)
4. The patient claims to have no strategies for reducing the "voices." (At least in chronic schizophrenia, the patient has usually developed such strategies, such as listening to music, humming, exercising, and so forth.)
5. The content of the hallucination is stated by the patient in very dry, concrete language. (Usually, command auditory hallucinations are vulgar or highly charged emotionally—for example, "Kill the lousy bastard!")
6. The overall symptom picture and behavior of the patient do not comport with a diagnosis of schizophrenia (e.g., the patient interacts normally except when observed by staff).

Adjunctive Testing

Neuroendocrine Studies

Although it is probably premature to classify these as true "adjunctive" diagnostic tests, there are several intriguing leads in the neuroendocrinology of schizophrenia. Meltzer and colleagues (1984) have done seminal research on the relationship between growth hormone and limbic system dopaminergic activity. There is some evidence, for example, that certain schizophrenic patients show a blunted growth hormone response to the dopamine agonist apomorphine, and perhaps to GABA and norepinephrine as well (Monteleone et al. 1986; also see comments by Meltzer 1988). Interestingly, schizophrenic patients with smaller ventricles may show a greater growth hormone response to apomorphine than do those with larger ventricular-brain ratios (Losonczy et al. 1986), suggesting—once again—the biological heterogeneity of schizophrenia. Another promising area of investigation involves the endogenous tridecapeptide neurotensin (Nemeroff 1986). Several studies have shown a reduction in cerebrospinal fluid neurotensin concentration in drug-free schizophrenic patients who were compared with age- and sex-matched control subjects; interestingly, this finding does not seem to hold up in paranoid schizophrenia, again arguing for the heterogeneity of this disorder (Nemeroff 1986). Because neurotensin concentration appears to be normal in depressed patients, this test may someday prove useful in differential diagnosis. Finally, a variety of lipid-related abnormalities have been found in schizophrenia, though none has proved a reliable adjunctive test (Pies et al. 1992).

Electroencephalography and Related Techniques

Over the past two decades, electroencephalographic studies in schizophrenic patients have revealed an increased incidence of nonspecific abnormalities (Cummings 1985; Small 1983); however, the electroencephalogram (EEG) in general has low sensitivity and poor resolution in relation to the sort of subtle brain abnormalities we would expect in schizophrenia. Morihisa and his colleagues (1983) and Guenther and Breitling (1985) found brain electrical activity mapping

(BEAM) abnormalities in schizophrenic patients compared with control subjects. Schizophrenic patients may show increased delta activity over the entire cortical surface of the brain (Morihisa et al. 1983) or left-sided sensorimotor dysfunction during the performance of various coordination tasks (Guenther and Breitling 1985). Complementing this last finding are data from Jutai et al. (1984) on visual evoked potentials in schizophrenic patients and normal subjects. Schizophrenic patients showed abnormal cortical-subcortical interactions during the analysis of visual information. A more recent study of REM latencies by Zarcone et al. (1987) suggested that medication-free schizophrenic individuals may have abnormally low REM latencies when compared with normal control subjects. As we saw in our discussion of major depression (Chapter 4), however, this finding is not pathognomonic for schizophrenia. Finally, Flor-Henry (1983), in reviewing the abundant literature linking psychotic symptomatology with temporal lobe epilepsy, concluded that dominant lobe pathology is implicated in the schizophreniform psychoses of temporal lobe epilepsy. But aside from this neurophysiological "overlap," it is sometimes useful to obtain an EEG in those patients with "atypical" schizophrenia who fail to respond to antipsychotics or who manifest features suggestive of partial complex seizures (e.g., olfactory hallucinations or amnesic periods).

Imaging Techniques

In our discussion of the biological underpinnings of schizophrenia, we briefly discussed the literature on structural brain abnormalities, rCBF studies, and PET scanning. Now we delve into these areas in more detail in the belief that these techniques may serve as useful adjunctive tests, given the right clinical context.

A great deal of work has now appeared linking schizophrenia to various computed tomography (CT) scan abnormalities (Weinberger and Kleinman 1986). As a generalization, CT studies have shown that a proportion of schizophrenic individuals have enlarged cerebral ventricles compared with control subjects. However, a study by Farmer et al. (1987) pointed out the many inconsistencies in the CT data. Thus, there is a popular hypothesis stating, in essence, that schizophrenia can be subdivided into a familial form, characterized by normal cerebral ventricles, and a sporadic form, associated with enlarged ventricles. But in their study of 35 chronic schizophrenic patients, Farmer et al. found no correlation between ventricular-brain ratio (VBR) and family history of schizophrenia. Further, patients meeting Crow's type 1 description, contrary to expectation, were among those with the largest VBRs.

Let us concede, then, that subtyping of schizophrenia according to CT abnormalities has not proved feasible. Is the CT scan still useful in confirming a diagnosis of schizophrenia per se? Here the evidence is more encouraging. Weinberger and Kleinman (1986) examined 29 controlled studies of CT findings in schizophrenia and noted that all but 5 found larger lateral ventricles in schizophrenic subjects. Moreover, the two studies with the largest sample sizes affirmed this finding (Johnstone et al. 1981; Takahashi et al. 1981). Measurements of third ventricle size also strongly suggest abnormal enlargement in schizophrenia (Weinberger and Kleinman 1986). Of course, the meaning of these findings is still unclear, and their specificity is limited. Thus, enlarged ventricles are also seen in some patients with affective disorders (Pearlson et al. 1984). Nonetheless, in a "close call" case, the finding of enlarged ventricles—in the absence of another neurological or psychiatric disorder—would tend to increase one's confidence in the diagnosis of schizophrenia. More recently, magnetic resonance imaging (MRI) has yielded both new and confirmatory findings. Thus, Degreef et al. (1992), in an MRI study comparing first-episode schizophrenic patients with normal control subjects, found that the patients showed lateral ventricular enlargement early in the course of illness. Moreover, enlargement of the left temporal horn was most related to the positive symptoms of the disease, a finding that is consistent with many studies showing left-sided temporal lobe abnormalities in schizophrenia.

Another promising imaging technique is PET. Tamminga et al. (1992) have recently reviewed rCBF studies in schizophrenia, noting that schizophrenic patients frequently show frontal cortical and/or basal ganglia abnormalities. Frontal cortical dysfunction seems particularly common in patients with chronic symptoms while performing "frontal lobe" tasks (e.g., the Wisconsin Card Sort). Tamminga et al. (1992) also found limbic system abnormalities (e.g., hippocampus, anterior cingulate cortex) in a group of drug-free, psychotic schizophrenic patients who were tested by means of PET.

It is of great theoretical interest that increased glucose metabolism in the basal ganglia has recently been demonstrated in PET studies of chronic schizophrenic patients with and without antipsychotic medication (Wolkin et al. 1985; see Gur et al. 1987a, 1987b for review). Early et al. (1987) confirmed these findings, demonstrating an abnormally high blood flow in the left globus pallidus of never-medicated schizophrenic patients. We normally think of the globus pallidus and other regions of the basal ganglia in terms of "movement disorder" such as parkinsonian or antipsychotic-related extrapyramidal symptoms. But the plot has thickened substantially. For example, there is evidence (Mesulam 1985) that—in primates, at least—the globus pallidus is involved in species-specific sexual display patterns (Mac-Lean 1978). Moreover, a part of the globus pallidus may mediate saccadic eye movements, which—as we shall see—may also be abnormal in schizophrenia. No doubt the basal ganglia will prove an important focus of study over the next several years. PET scan abnormalities in this area of the brain may prove to be a revealing diagnostic study, although, at present, we can't really speak of this as a true adjunctive test for schizophrenia.

Combined Electroencephalographic/Imaging Techniques

A very promising approach has recently been advanced by McCarley and associates (1993), who combined recording of auditory P300 event-related potentials with MRI technology. In a study of 15 schizophrenic subjects, these workers found gray matter volume reductions in the left posterior superior temporal gyrus (STG) that were specifically associated with P300 amplitude reduction and asymmetry; these findings differed significantly from those seen in control subjects. McCarley et al. concluded that the STG may be "an anatomical region of great importance in schizophrenia" (p. 195).

Neuropsychological and Neuropsychiatric Testing

There is little question that schizophrenic patients show abnormalities on standard personality and projective tests (Meyer 1983). On scale 8 (schizophrenia) of the Minnesota Multiphasic Personality Inventory (MMPI), schizophrenic patients typically score above 70 T, and usually fall in the 75 to 90 T range as they move toward chronicity (Meyer 1983). Extremely high scores are more likely to indicate severe patterns within other diagnostic categories or else an attempt to exaggerate illness ("faking bad"). On the Wechsler Adult Intelligence Scale (WAIS), subtest scatter is common and the verbal scaled score is generally higher than the performance scaled score (Meyer 1983). Interestingly, schizophrenic patients tend to fail some of the "easier" items while succeeding on the "harder" ones. Scores tend to be higher on block design and digit symbol, but lower on arithmetic, picture arrangement, and comprehension. On the Rorschach, Ogdon (1977) noted several response patterns associated with psychosis in general and schizophrenia in particular (Meyer 1983), including poor quality and low number of human movement responses; poorly organized animal movement responses; responses dictated only by the color of the blot ("pure C" responses); and perseverating by seeing the same "thing" in several sequential ink blots. On the Thematic Apperception Test (TAT), schizophrenic patients are apt to tell rambling, confused, self-referential, or bizarre stories (Meyer 1983). Finally, what about the time-honored "proverbs test," often a part of our mental status examination? On the comprehension subtest of the WAIS, patients with paranoid schizophrenia occasionally score lower because they make "peculiar and overinclusive" proverb interpretations (Meyer 1983). Meyer also notes that "exotic" proverbs may be more useful in bringing out the paranoid schizophrenic patient's delusional material, since, when given common proverbs, the patient will intentionally give the "common" meaning and hold back the more bizarre ones. Patients with schizophreniform disorder or brief reactive psychosis tend to show more evidence of "emotional upset and turmoil" on testing than do schizophrenic patients (Meyer 1983). Thus, for example, on the MMPI, one is likely to see higher 8, 7, and F scales.

Several neuropsychiatric tests are proving useful in the diagnosis of schizophrenia and, indeed, may also be revealing the nature of the disorder itself (Flor-Henry 1983; Gur 1986). At least four types of studies have suggested abnormalities in schizophrenia: sensorimotor studies, visual field studies, dichotic listening, and psychophysiological measures of hemisphere activity (Gur 1986). Among the most consistent—and perhaps the most practical—findings to be extracted from this literature is that involving abnormal eye movements in schizophrenia (Cummings 1985; Holzman et al. 1974, 1977; Tomer et al. 1981). Testing of oculomotor pursuit movements in schizophrenia reveals that the usually smooth "following" movements are fragmented, or "saccadic." Moreover, schizophrenic patients tend to have occasional bursts of horizontal eye movements and alterations of blink rates, with decreased blinking in chronic schizophrenia and increased blinking in acute cases (Karson 1983; Stevens 1978). Interestingly, there is also evidence showing a preponderance of lateral eye movements to the right in schizophrenia (Gur 1978), suggesting—once again—abnormal left-hemisphere function (Flor-Henry 1983). Cummings (1985) cautions that abnormal eye movements have also been seen in patients with a variety of neurological disorders and even in some normal control subjects. Nevertheless, in making the diagnosis in a puzzling case, eye movement studies may prove helpful. It is particularly intriguing that in one study, individuals with schizotypal personality disorder showed impaired visual tracking of a moving object, compared with nonschizotypal subjects (Siever et al. 1984). If this finding is confirmed in subsequent studies, it could demonstrate that the visual-motor system is a "connecting link" in the chain of schizophrenic-like syndromes.

One of the more promising neuropsychiatric tests in the diagnosis of schizophrenia involves so-called dichotic listening. In effect, this entails the presentation of simultaneous, competing acoustic signals to both ears. The neuronal connections involved in this procedure are complex (Flor-Henry 1983). For our purposes, it will suffice to say that in normal "dextral" (right-handed) individuals, there is a right-ear superiority in the detection of dichotically presented stimuli. Because of trans-callosal pathways, right-ear activation leads to stimulation of the left hemisphere. A number of studies (Gruzelier and Hammond 1976; Wexler and Heninger 1979) have suggested more "right-ear errors" in schizophrenic (vs. normal) subjects, suggesting, yet again, left-hemisphere dysfunction. Interestingly, improvement in right-ear function seems to be related to improvement in clinical status.

Recently, Goldsamt et al. (1993) reviewed the neuropsychological correlates of schizophrenia. They concluded that schizophrenic patients "show significant impairment in neuropsychological functioning," depending on the subgroup of schizophrenia, and that this impairment is "primarily in abilities mediated by the frontal and temporal lobes" (pp. 155–156).

A summary of our (admittedly flawed) adjunctive tests is provided in Table 5–4.

Treatment Directions and Goals

Somatic Approaches

In reviewing this burgeoning area, Kane (1986) began by noting that antipsychotic drugs remain the mainstay of treatment. However, a variety of adjunctive agents are now available and may enhance the

Table 5–4.   Adjunctive tests in schizophrenia

Test/Procedure	Schizophrenia	Control
Neuroendocrine	Blunted GH response to various releasing factors	Normal response
EEG/BEAM	Nonspecific abnormalities or left-side dysfunction	Normal
Imaging	CT: Enlarged ventricles	Normal
	PET: Hypofrontality or hyperactive basal ganglia	Normal
Psychological	Abnormalities on Rorschach, WAIS, TAT	Normal
Neuropsychiatric	Abnormal pursuit eye testing movements; abnormal dichotic listening	Normal

Note. GH = growth hormone; EEG = electroencephalogram; BEAM = brain electrical activity mapping; CT = computed tomography; PET = positron-emission tomography; WAIS = Wechsler Adult Intelligence Scale; TAT = Thematic Apperception Test.
Source. Siever et al. 1984; Stevens 1978; Takahashi et al. 1981; Tamminga et al. 1992.

overall response of the schizophrenic patient (Kane 1986; Osser 1988). In the past 10 years, we have refined our knowledge of antipsychotics in a number of ways. First, we now know that "megadoses" of these agents are, by and large, not more effective than standard doses. Specifically, the use of antipsychotics in excess of 1,500 mg/day of chlorpromazine or its equivalent is no more effective than, say, 600 mg/day of chlorpromazine (Kane 1986; Neborsky et al. 1981). In terms of the most commonly prescribed antipsychotic, haloperidol, there is no good evidence that 60 or 70 mg/day works better in the average schizophrenic patient than does 10 to 15 mg/day. The now defunct idea of "loading" an acutely disturbed psychotic patient with huge doses of antipsychotic in order to achieve "rapid neuroleptization" has been replaced with a more moderate approach—for example, using 2 to 5 mg of haloperidol im every hour or two, up to around 15 to 20 mg in a 24-hour period (Anderson and Tesar 1991). Some clinicians also add a small amount of a benzo-diazepine (e.g., lorazepam 1 to 2 mg im) to the antipsychotic, but this strategy makes it harder to know "what is doing what" if the patient responds paradoxically.

Despite the recommendations above, there is always the "outlier" on the bell-shaped curve who will require unusually large doses of antipsychotic medication. This may be an individual with very rapid hepatic metabolism of oral medication (the "first-pass" effect) or, less commonly, poor oral absorption. Conversely, some patients will do better on lower-than-average doses. This leads us directly into the area of plasma levels of antipsychotic agents and the corollary concept of the "therapeutic window" (Kane 1986; Mavroides et al. 1984). In essence, there is now moderately good evidence suggesting that for haloperidol, an inverted U-shaped curve best describes clinical re-sponse versus plasma level; that is, patients respond best when the plasma level of haloperidol is (roughly) between 5 ng/ml and 20 ng/ml (Davis and Bresnahan 1987). A similar curve may apply to fluphenazine (Prolixin, etc.). Controversy exists as to the strength of these relationships, but I find it useful to obtain a plasma level of fluphenazine or haloperidol in cases of poor clinical response. If the resultant level is either markedly above or below the putative thera-peutic window, it may be worthwhile decreasing or increasing the dose (Davis and Bresnahan 1987). In the future, red blood cell levels of antipsychotic medications may prove a more accurate way of gauging dose-response relationships.

Although intramuscular dosing eliminates the "first pass" effect (hepatic extraction) seen with orally administered medication, the intramuscular route is not necessarily preferable for acutely psychotic patients. (For example, some patients find the oral route less threatening than "the needle.") Moreover, similar blood levels can be achieved with oral medication (concentrate) if given in doses equivalent to the intramuscular dose (Kane 1986). For haloperidol concentrate, twice the (desired) oral dose will produce the same total amount of drug available to the body over a 24-hour period as the corresponding intramuscular dose (i.e., 10 mg po will equal 5 mg im) (Schaffer 1982).

Clozapine (Clozaril)—mentioned at the beginning of this chapter as a genuine breakthrough in the treatment of schizophrenia— improves the overall level of functioning in about 45% to 60% of "refractory" schizophrenic patients. Negative features, such as apathy and withdrawal, are clearly responsive to clozapine. Sometimes, a period of 6 or more months is required before the patient responds fully, and dosages as high as 900 mg/day may be necessary; the usual dosage is roughly 250 to 500 mg/day (see Ayd 1989 for review).

Common side effects with clozapine include hypersalivation (sometimes responsive to anticholinergic agents), weight gain, tachycardia, postural hypotension, and a seizure incidence of about 3% to 5% per year with doses of 400 mg or higher. The most feared complication of clozapine treatment is agranulocytosis, which occurs in about 1.3% of patients over the course of a year, most commonly during the first 4 or 5 months of treatment. On the positive side, clozapine rarely causes extrapyramidal side effects, neuroleptic malignant syndrome, or tardive dyskinesia (TD)—in fact, TD may actually improve with clozapine treatment. Clozaril is beginning to find use in the treatment of schizoaffective and resistant bipolar patients (Suppes et al. 1992).

The benzisoxazole antipsychotic risperidone (Risperdal) was recently released for the treatment of psychotic disorders (Chouinard et al. 1993). At the optimal dose of 6 mg/day, risperidone rarely causes extrapyramidal side effects and may also reduce negative features of schizophrenia. Unlike clozapine, risperidone does not appear to cause agranulocytosis. Nevertheless, it remains to be seen whether risperidone will prove as useful as clozapine in the treatment of refractory schizophrenic patients.

Keep in mind that "schizophrenia" and "psychosis" are not synonymous and that management may differ in the case of, for example, drug-induced psychosis (see Chapter 10).

Before discussing non-neuroleptic medications, we should discuss that much-feared complication of antipsychotic use, tardive dyskinesia. The "true" prevalence of TD is not precisely known, with figures ranging from 0.5% to 50% of patients on long-term antipsychotic medication (Jeste and Wyatt 1982; Kane et al. 1984). The average prevalence across many studies is around 15% to 20% (Kane 1986). Looked at optimistically, this suggests that most patients on maintenance antipsychotics will not get TD. Furthermore, most cases of TD are relatively mild and nonprogressive, at least over 2- to 3-year follow-up (Gardos et al. 1983; Kane 1986). Unfortunately, some cases of TD are severe and even incapacitating—possibly correlated with increasing age (Kane 1986). Furthermore, TD is a major source of malpractice litigation against psychiatrists. As Thomas Gutheil (1988) puts it, "The tardive dyskinesia liability tidal wave is just beginning" (p. 447). Thus, for both compassionate and self-protective reasons, the psychiatrist must treat the issue of TD with the utmost caution and concern. The key concept to remember is informed consent, and this is an ongoing process, not a hastily signed "consent form" (Gutheil 1988). We still have no good treatment for TD, though many cases—particularly in younger persons—will remit with discontinuation of the antipsychotic (Levinson and Simpson 1987). The use of cholinomimetic agents such as Deanol; GABA agonists; or reserpine may sometimes be helpful (Mason and Granacher 1980).

Finally, as noted earlier, there is preliminary evidence that clozapine (Clozaril) may actually mitigate TD; in any event, clozapine virtually never produces TD.

Although the antipsychotic agents remain the principal somatic treatment for all the functional psychoses, a variety of auxilliary or "second line" treatments are emerging (Kane 1986; Osser 1988). Some studies show that the addition of lithium carbonate to antipsychotics can benefit some "schizoaffective" or treatment-resistant schizophrenic patients (Biederman et al. 1979; Carman et al. 1981). However, the combination of lithium and antipsychotic medication increases the risk of extrapyramidal symptoms, even when lithium levels are within the therapeutic range (Addonizio et al. 1988). Beta-blockers appear to reduce psychotic symptoms when added to antipsychotics, but this effect may be due to their efficacy in reducing akathisia (Lipinski et al. 1988) rather than to a "primary" antipsychotic action. Benzodiazepines have long been thought useful as adjunctive or even primary treatment for psychotic conditions, but the evidence for this is modest (Kane 1986; Osser 1988). Occasionally, the addition of lorazepam to an agitated schizophrenic patient's antipsychotic regimen may be useful (Osser 1988). More recently, the anticonvulsant carbamazepine has been found useful in a few cases of chronic schizophrenia and schizoaffective illness, but it also has the potential to lower plasma antipsychotic levels significantly (Osser 1988). We have already commented on the heterogeneity of schizoaffective disorder; understandably, this fact affects the choice of somatic treatment (Levitt and Tsuang 1988). There is modest evidence that the "schizomanic" individual may benefit from a combination of lithium and antipsychotic. Treatment is less clear for the depressed schizoaffective patient, but a tricyclic/antipsychotic regimen or ECT may be useful (Levitt and Tsuang 1988).

A number of promising medications for schizophrenia are "waiting in the wings" (Hollister 1994). Most of these agents have two pharmacological features in common: selective dopamine receptor blockade (e.g., corticolimbic receptors being more affected than receptors in the basal ganglia) and some form of serotonergic receptor blockade (Hollister 1994). Amperozide, zotepine, and melperone exemplify this type of agent. An intriguing agent called ondansetron appears to have some antipsychotic properties without producing direct dopamine receptor blockade; rather, it antagonizes the serotonin 5-HT3 receptor, which may then lead to decreased dopamine release. These and other agents may bring new hope to the treatment of schizophrenia in the coming years.

We should not conclude our section of somatic therapies without saying a word about ECT. Is this an effective treatment for schizophrenia? The evidence on this issue is sorely lacking (Kane 1986), but ECT may be transiently effective in some schizophrenic patients (Welch 1987). There is also some evidence showing that in a subgroup of young psychotic patients with a "schizophreniform" profile (acute onset, family history of affective illness, etc.), ECT may produce sustained improvement (Salzman 1980; Welch 1987). ECT is probably worth trying in a truly refractory schizophrenic patient (Osser 1988) who remains severely incapacitated.

Psychosocial Approaches

McGlashan (1986) has admirably reviewed the psychosocial treatment of schizophrenia (Table 5–5). This is an issue that tends to polarize psychotherapists, because it touches on two fundamental clinical questions: Does psychotherapy really work in schizophrenia, and what are its potential risks? Few psychiatrists today would claim that individual psychotherapy alone (i.e., without at least occasional use of antipsychotic medication) is effective in the treatment of schizophrenia. Indeed, a number of controlled outcome studies suggest that individual psychotherapy of the traditional "exploratory" type is not effective in schizophrenia (May and Simpson 1980). May and Simpson (1980) concluded that psychodynamically oriented individual psychotherapy has little or no value for schizophrenic patients who are sick enough to be in a hospital. Two caveats are in order, however. First, almost all the studies in this area have significant methodological flaws (e.g., the use of inexperienced therapists, poor definition of technique). Second, as McGlashan (1986) notes, the available literature "does *not* . . . test or call into question the importance of the individual relationship between doctor and patient. The individual clinician remains central to any treatment effort, if only to coordinate other treatment modalities and provide ongoing evaluation" (p. 108). Moreover, if done with carefully selected patients in a "nonclassical" manner, individual psychotherapy with schizophrenic patients can sometimes be helpful (Cancro 1983). Some general principles of psychosocial treatment, as described by McGlashan (1986), are outlined in Table 5–5. In my own experience, the best general approach to psychotherapy with schizophrenic patients is a friendly, matter-of-fact, reality-oriented one that minimizes exploration of "unconscious" material. On the other hand, dealing with here-and-now feelings of anger, demoralization, or anxiety is very important in maintaining the therapeutic alliance.

Recently, a good deal of evidence has pointed toward the usefulness of what might be termed "family educational therapy" in the treatment of schizophrenia. You may recall our mention of "high EE" families: those who expose their schizophrenic members to intense criticism, guilt induction, or intrusiveness (Leff and Vaughn 1981). Treatment may be directed not at showing families how they "caused" their loved one's schizophrenia (a dubious notion, certainly), but at informing them about schizophrenia—its nature, likely course, and exacerbating factors. In particular, families are taught the prodromal signs of relapse and the ways in which inappropriate emotional expres-

Table 5–5.   Psychosocial treatment of schizophrenia

Psychosocial treatment principles in schizophrenia

A broad, flexible approach is needed, emphasizing stress reduction, mobilization of resources, and reinforcement of healthy ego function.

The core of treatment is the clinical relationship and the empathic involvement of the clinician.

Treatment must be consistent and temporally open ended, and must offer continuity of caregivers.

Therapists need to be flexible, realistic, and respectful of the patient's autonomy and need for distance.

General treatment strategies

A thorough initial evaluation must be made to rule out other conditions.

The treatment should constantly be reassessed and recalibrated, taking into account the phase of illness and the target symptoms.

Treatments should be applied with graded increases in intensity and complexity, consistent with the patient's tolerance.

Psychosocial treatment should be integrated with appropriate pharmacotherapy.

Source. Extensively modified from McGlashan 1986, pp. 100–103.

sion may promote relapse (McGlashan 1986). On the other hand, placing excessively low expectations upon schizophrenic patients in order to "spare" them from "too much emotion" may be self-defeating, too. Thus, reduction of EE level may reduce active symptoms and rehospitalization, but also decrease performance, increase "negative" symptoms, and worsen chronicity (Harnett 1988; Wing and Brown 1970). Osser (1988) has summarized the topic nicely in stating that "reasonable pressure should be placed on patients, in a supportive and accepting environment, in order to determine what their maximum level of functioning can be. Then, it would seem humane to allow them the most comfortable environment consistent with their limitation" (p. 313). Finally, Harnett (1988), having reviewed the data, has suggested that antipsychotic medication may act synergistically with social therapies and that exposure to the latter without benefit of antipsychotic medication may do more harm than placebo treatment (Hogarty et al. 1974).

Integrated Case History

Mr. Snyder was a 26-year-old single male brought to the psychiatric ER by his mother. She reported that for the past 3 months Kurt, the patient, had been increasingly seclusive, sometimes remaining in his room for days at a time. His hygiene and diet had been very poor, such that (according to his mother) the patient "smells horrible . . . I don't think he's showered in two weeks . . . and he's probably lost 15 pounds in the last couple of months." At times, the patient would be heard "laughing or talking to himself" from within his room. In the past 2 days, he had barricaded himself inside his room by piling chairs behind his door. This prompted his mother and older brother to "break in through a window" and forcibly bring the patient in for assessment.

There was no previous psychiatric history, and, according to the patient's family, he had been well until approximately 1 year ago, when he "began to say and do strange things"—for example, he started saying that the neighbors were "poisoning our lawn with Agent Orange" and that "someone had been looking in his window at night." Six months prior to evaluation, the patient had been fired from his job as a salesman in a record store, because (according to his brother) "the customers were getting freaked out . . . every time they'd buy something, Kurt would start in with this 'poisoning' business."

Kurt had had a normal birth and developmental history, but by age 10 he seemed "a little different than the other boys . . . quiet and very serious . . . he was always sensitive to teasing and kind of kept to himself." His family life had been quite chaotic, with Kurt's father's having left the family when the patient was 9 years old. According to the patient's mother, Kurt's father "had a terrible temper . . . we used to fight all the time . . . he never hit Kurt, but he was always yelling." In the past few months, according to the patient's brother, Kurt had come under intense pressure from his mother to "pick himself up by his bootstraps and get himself a job."

On mental status examination, the patient was alert and oriented to month and year, but not the date. He appeared dishevelled and malodorous. His speech was halting, with many interruptions, during which the patient would glance to one side and smile. He would not comment on what, if anything, he was hearing or seeing during these interruptions. His affect was guarded and suspicious through most of the interview. His thought process showed several tangential responses as well as "thought blocking." The patient denied auditory or visual hallucinations, but said, "I do get information that your kind doesn't have access to." He would not comment on the matter of his neighbors "poisoning" the lawn, but did state, "There is a great deal of danger in the world . . . if you had any brains, you'd know I'm right about that."

Kurt was admitted involuntarily to the inpatient psychiatric unit. Physical examination and laboratory testing disclosed no abnormalities, except mild dehydration. An MRI of the brain showed "mild to moderate volume reduction in the left hippocampus and left superior temporal gyrus." A subsequent neurological evaluation showed "no focal findings" but "some impairment of smooth pursuit eye movements on testing of EOM [electroculomyography]."

Neuropsychiatric testing showed an elevated scale 8 on the MMPI as well as "subtest scatter" on the WAIS, with verbal IQ greater than performance IQ (92 vs. 78). On the TAT, Kurt produced "rambling, confused" stories, mainly involving harm to himself from "the night people." Proverb interpretation was described as "bizarre or idiosyncratic"; for example, "A rolling stone gathers no moss" was interpreted as "The Rolling Stones are finished. They can't even play backup anymore . . . Keith Richards [a member of the Rolling Stones] wants to hire me and then screw me over."

A provisional diagnosis of "schizophrenia, paranoid type" was made. Kurt was begun on thiothixene 4 mg/day, which was gradually increased to 15 mg/day. Benztropine (Cogentin) 1 mg/day was added because of mild parkinsonian side effects.

Kurt attended group therapy on the unit three times per week, during which a supportive, "reality-centered" approach was used, with minimal confrontation or interpretation of unconscious impulses. Kurt also met twice weekly with a psychiatric resident who knew she could work with him after discharge from the unit. The resident also took a supportive, here-and-now approach to therapy, while allowing Kurt to express some anger at his mother "for pushing me to get a job." The resident also met with Kurt's mother and brother, informing them of Kurt's diagnosis, the likely prognosis, and ways of minimizing the risk of relapse. They were taught some of the stressors that may precipitate relapse, and also the premonitory signs of psychotic decompensation (e.g., poor sleep, anxiety, depression, and suspiciousness). After 4 weeks on the unit, Kurt had improved significantly. His affect was brighter, and he no longer seemed preoccupied with paranoid themes. He was discharged on thiothixene 15 mg/day, with an outpatient appointment scheduled in 1 week.

Conclusion

What is the future of schizophrenia? We have suggested that this disorder is, in all likelihood, the final common pathway for a number of different etiologies. As we enter the era of DSM-IV, we can anticipate greater effort at separating schizophrenia into clinically relevant subtypes rather than merely descriptive ones. We can also anticipate great efforts to link these subtypes with objective "validators" such as human leukocyte antigen (HLA) locus, MRI findings, and electrophysiological data. Concurrently, we can expect a vigorous and continuing search for more specific and effective antipsychotic agents—particularly agents that do not lead to tardive dyskinesia or agranulocytosis. In the psychosocial realm, we will undoubtedly try to refine our understanding of "expressed emotion" and its role in developing the optimal milieu for schizophrenic patients—one that is neither overwhelmingly stimulating nor hopelessly stultifying. Finally, we can expect further efforts to disentangle schizophrenia from its nosologic cousins: schizoaffective disorder, delusional disorder, and schizotypal personality disorder.

References

Addonizio G, Roth SD, Stokes PE, et al: Increased extrapyramidal symptoms with addition of lithium to neuroleptics. J Nerv Ment Dis 176:682–685, 1988

Akbarian S, Bunney WE Jr, Potkin SG, et al: Altered distribution of nicotinamide-adenine dinucleotide phosphate–diaphorase cells in frontal lobe of schizophrenics implies disturbances of cortical development. Arch Gen Psychiatry 50:169–177, 1993a

Akbarian S, Viñuela A, Kim JJ, et al: Distorted distribution of nicotinamide-adenine dinucleotide phosphate-diaphorase neurons in temporal lobe of schizophrenics implies anomalous cortical development. Arch Gen Psychiatry 50:178–187, 1993b

American Psychiatric Association: Diagnostic and Statistical Manual of Mental Disorders, 3rd Edition, Revised. Washington, DC, American Psychiatric Association, 1987

American Psychiatric Association: Diagnostic and Statistical Manual of Mental Disorders, 4th Edition. Washington, DC, American Psychiatric Association, 1994

Anderson WH, Tesar G: The emergency room, in Massachusetts General Handbook of General Hospital Psychiatry, 3rd Edition. Edited by Cassem NH. St Louis, MO, Mosby Year Book, 1991, pp 445–464

Andreasen NC: Affective flattening and the criteria for schizophrenia. Am J Psychiatry 136:944–947, 1979

Arieti S: Interpretation of Schizophrenia, 2nd Edition. New York, Basic Books, 1974

Ayd F: Clozapine update: benefits and risks. International Drug Therapy Newsletter 24:37–39, 1989

Bateson G, Jackson DD, Haley J, et al: Toward a theory of schizophrenia. Behav Sci 1:251, 1956

Benjamin JD: A method for distinguishing and evaluating formal thinking disorders in schizophhrenia, Language and Thought in Schizophrenia: Collected Papers. Edited by Kasanin JS. New York, WW Norton, 1964, pp 65–90

Biederman J, Lerner Y, Belmaker RH: Combination of lithium carbonate and haloperidol in schizo-affective disorder: a controlled study. Arch Gen Psychiatry 36:327–333, 1979

Bloom FE: Advancing a neurodevelopmental origin for schizophrenia. Arch Gen Psychiatry 50:224–227, 1993

Buchsbaum MS, Ingvar DH, Kessler R, et al: Cerebral glucography with positron tomography: use in normal subjects and in patients with schizophrenia. Arch Gen Psychiatry 39:251–259, 1982

Cancro R: Individual psychotherapy in the treatment of chronic schizophrenic patients. Am J Psychother 37:493–501, 1983

Carman JS, Bigelow LB, Wyatt RJ: Lithium combined with neuroleptics in chronic schizophrenia and schizoaffective patients. J Clin Psychiatry 42:124–128, 1981

Chouinard G, Jones B, Remington G, et al: A Canadian multicenter placebo-controlled study of fixed doses of risperidone and haloperidol in the treatment of chronic schizophrenic patients. J Clin Psychopharmacol 13:25–40, 1993

Crow TJ: The biology of schizophrenia. Experientia 38:1275–1282, 1982

Crow TJ, Owen F, Cross AJ, et al: Letter to the editor. Lancet 1:36, 1978

Cummings JL: Clinical Neuropsychiatry. Orlando, FL, Grune & Stratton, 1985

Davis JM, Bresnahan DB: Psychopharmacology in clinical psychiatry, in American Psychiatric Association Annual Review, Vol 6. Edited by Hales RE, Frances AJ. Washington, DC, American Psychiatric Press, 1987, pp 159–187

Degreef G, Ashtari M, Bogerts B, et al: Volumes of ventricular system subdivisions measured from magnetic resonance images in first-episode schizophrenic patients. Arch Gen Psychiatry 49:531–537, 1992

Diethelm O, Heffernan TF: Felix Platter and psychiatry. Journal of the History of the Behavioral Sciences 1:10–23, 1965

Early TS, Reiman EM, Raichle ME, et al: Left globus pallidus abnormality in never-medicated patients with schizophrenia. Proc Natl Acad Sci U S A 84:561–563, 1987

Farde L, Nordström A-L, Wiesel F-A: Positron emission tomographic analysis of central D_1 and D_2 dopamine receptor occupancy in patients treated with classical neuroleptics and clozapine: relation to extrapyramidal side effects. Arch Gen Psychiatry 49:538–544, 1992

Farmer A, Jackson R, McGuffin P, et al: Cerebral ventricular enlargement in chronic schizophrenia: consistencies and contradictions. Br J Psychiatry 150:324–330, 1987

Flor-Henry P: Cerebral Basis of Psychopathology. Boston, MA, John Wright/PSG Publishing, 1983

Fromm-Reichmann F: Notes on the development of treatment of schizophrenics by psychoanalytic psychotherapy. Psychiatry 11:263–273, 1948

Gardos G, Perenyi A, Cole JO, et al: Tardive dyskinesia: changes after three years. J Clin Psychopharmacol 3:315–318, 1983

Golden CJ, Moses JA Jr, Zelazowski R, et al: Cerebral ventricular size and neuropsychological impairment in young chronic schizophrenics. Arch Gen Psychiatry 37:619–623, 1980

Goldsamt LA, Barros J, Schwartz BJ, et al: Neuropsychological correlates of schizophrenia. Psychiatric Annals 23:151–157, 1993

Gottesman II, Shields J: Schizophrenia: The Epigenetic Puzzle. Cambridge, UK, Cambridge University Press, 1982

Gruzelier JH, Hammond N: Schizophrenia: a dominant hemisphere temporal-limbic disorder? Research Communications in Psychology, Psychiatry and Behavior 1:33–72, 1976

Guenther W, Breitling D: Predominant sensorimotor area left hemisphere dysfunction in schizophrenia measured by brain electrical activity mapping. Biol Psychiatry 20:515–532, 1985

Gur RE: Left hemisphere dysfunction and left hemisphere overactivation in schizophrenia. J Abnorm Psychol 87:226–238, 1978

Gur RE: Cognitive aspects of schizophrenia, in American Psychiatric Association Annual Review, Vol 5. Edited by Frances AJ, Hales RE. Washington, DC, American Psychiatric Press, 1986, pp 68–77

Gur RE, Resnick SM, Alavi A, et al: Regional brain function in schizophrenia, I: a positron emission tomography study. Arch Gen Psychiatry 44:119–125, 1987a

Gur RE, Resnick SM, Gur RC, et al: Regional brain function in schizophrenia, II: repeated evaluation with positron emission tomography. Arch Gen Psychiatry 44:126–129, 1987b

Gutheil TG: Liability issues and malpractice prevention, in Handbook of Clinical Psychopharmacology. Edited by Tupin JP, Shader R, Harnett DS. Northvale, NJ, Jason Aronson, 1988, pp 439–454

Harnett DS: Psychotherapy and psychopharmacology, in Handbook of Clinical Psychopharmacology. Edited by Tupin JP, Shader R, Harnett DS. Northvale, NJ, Jason Aronson, 1988, pp 401–424

Heston LL: Psychiataric disorders in foster home reared children of schizophrenic mothers. Br J Psychiatry 112:819–825, 1966

Hogarty GE, Goldberg SC, Schooler NR, et al: Drug and sociotherapy in the aftercare of schizophrenic patients, III: adjustment of nonrelapsed patients. Arch Gen Psychiatry 31:609–618, 1974

Hollingshead AB, Redlich FC: Social Class and Mental Illness. New York, Wiley, 1958

Hollister LE: New psychotherapeutic drugs. J Clin Psychopharmacol 14:50–63, 1994

Holzman PS, Levy D: Smooth pursuit eye movements and functional psychosis: a review. Schizophr Bull 3:1415–1420, 1977

Holzman PS, Proctor LR, Levy DL, et al: Eye tracking dysfunctions in schizophrenic patients and their relatives. Arch Gen Psychiatry 31:143–151, 1974

Holzman PS, Kringlen E, Levy DL, et al: Abnormal-pursuit eye movements in schizophrenia: evidence for a genetic indicator. Arch Gen Psychiatry 34:802–805, 1977

Jackson SW: Melancholia and Depression. New Haven, CT, Yale University Press, 1986

Jeste DV, Wyatt RJ: Understanding and Treating Tardive Dyskinesia. New York, Guilford, 1982

Johnstone EC, Owens DGC, Crow TJ, et al: A CT study of 188 patients with schizophrenia, affective psychosis and neurotic illness, in Biological Psychiatry. Edited by Perris C, Struwe G, Jansson B. Amsterdam, Elsevier–North Holland, 1981, pp 237–240

Jutai JW, Gruzelier JH, Connolly JF, et al: Schizophrenia and spectral analysis of the visual evoked potential. Br J Psychiatry 145:496–501, 1984

Kane JM: Somatic therapy [of schizophrenia], in American Psychiatric Association Annual Review, Vol 5. Edited by Frances AJ, Hales RE. Washington, DC, American Psychiatric Press, 1986, pp 78–95

Kane JM, Woerner M, Lieberman JA, et al: The prevalence of tardive dyskinesia. Psychopharmacol Bull 21:136–139, 1984

Karson CN: Spontaneous eye-blink rates and dopaminergic systems. Brain 106:643–653, 1983

Kendler KS: The nosologic validity of paranoia (simple delusional disorder). Arch Gen Psychiatry 37:699–706, 1980

Kendler KS: Genetics of schizophrenia, in American Psychiatric Association Annual Review, Vol 5. Edited by Frances AJ, Hales RE. Washington, DC, American Psychiatric Press, 1986, pp 25–41

Kline NS, Li CH, Lehman HE, et al: Beta-endorphin induced changes in schizophrenic and depressed patients. Arch Gen Psychiatry 34:1111–1113, 1977

Kraepelin RM, Dementia Praecox and Paraphrenia (1907). Translated by Barclay RM, Roberts GM. New York, Robert E Krieger, 1971

Leff J, Vaughn C: The role of maintenancy therapy and relatives' expressed emotion in relapse of schizophrenia: a two-year follow-up. Br J Psychiatry 139:102–104, 1981

Lehmann HE: Schizophrenia: history, in Comprehensive Textbook of Psychiatry/III, 3rd Edition. Edited by Kaplan HI, Freedman AM, Sadock BJ. Baltimore, MD, Williams & Wilkins, 1980, pp 1104–1112

Levinson DF, Simpson GM: Antipsychotic drug side effects, in American Psychiatric Association Annual Review, Vol 6. Edited by Hales RE, Frances AJ. Washington, DC, American Psychiatric Press, 1987, pp 704–723

Levitt JJ, Tsuang MT: The heterogeneity of schizoaffective disorder: implications for treatment. Am J Psychiatry 145:926–936, 1988

Liberman RP: Social factors in the etiology of the schizophrenic disorders, in Psychiatry Update: The American Psychiatric Association Annual Review, Vol 1. Edited by Grinspoon L. Washington, DC, American Psychiatric Association, 1982, pp 97–112

Lidz T, Fleck S, Cornelison AR: Schizophrenia and the Family. New York, International Universities Press, 1965

Lipinski JF Jr, Keck PE Jr, et al: β-Adrenergic antagonists in psychosis: is improvement due to treatment of neuroleptic induced akathisia? J Clin Psychopharmacol 8:409–416, 1988

Losonczy MF, Song IS, Mohs RC, et al: Correlates of lateral ventricular size in chronic schizophrenia, I: behavior and treatment response measures. Am J Psychiatry 143:976–981, 1986

MacKay AVP, Bird O, Bird ED, et al: Dopamine receptors and schizophrenia: drug effect or illness? Lancet 2:915–916, 1980

MacLean PD: Effects of lesions of globus pallidus on species—typical display behavior of squirrel monkeys. Brain Res 149:175–196, 1978

Maj M, Perris C: An approach to the diagnosis and classification of schizoaffective disorders for research purposes. Acta Psychiatr Scand 72:405–413, 1985

Mason AS, Granacher RP: Clinical Handbook of Antipsychotic Drug Therapy. New York, Brunner/Mazel, 1980

Mavroides ML, Kanter DR, Hirschowitz J, et al: Clinical relevance of thiothixene plasma levels. J Clin Psychopharmacol 4:155–157, 1984

May P, Simpson GM: Schizophrenia: overview of treatment methods, in Comprehensive Textbook of Psychiatry/III, 3rd Edition, Vol 2. Edited by Kaplan HI, Freedman AM, Sadock BJ. Baltimore, MD, Williams & Wilkins, 1980, pp 1192–1217

McCarley RW, Shenton ME, O'Donnell BF, et al: Auditory P300 abnormalities and left posterior superior temporal gyrus volume reduction in schizophrenia. Arch Gen Psychiatry 50:190–197, 1993

McGlashan TH: Schizophrenia: psychosocial treatments and the role of psychosocial factors in its etiology and pathogenesis, in American Psychiatric Association Annual Review, Vol 5. Edited by Frances AJ, Hales RE. Washington, DC, American Psychiatric Press, 1986, pp 96–111

McNeil GN, Soreff SM: Psychosis, in Handbook of Psychiatric Differential Diagnosis. Edited by Soreff SM, McNeil GM. Littleton, MA, PSG Publishing, 1987, pp 127–163

Meltzer HY: Commentary, in 1988 Yearbook of Psychiatry and Applied Mental Health. Edited by Freedman DX, Lourie RS, Meltzer HY, et al. Chicago, IL, Year Book Medical, 1988, pp 50–51

Meltzer HY, Kolakowska, Fang VS, et al: Growth hormone and prolactin response to apomorphine in schiaophrenia and the major affective disorders: relation to duration of illness and depressive symptoms. Arch Gen Psychiatry 41:512–519, 1984

Mendlewicz J: Current genetic concepts on schizoaffective psychosis, in Genetic Aspects of Affective Illness. Edited by Mendlewicz J, Shopsin B. New York, SP Medical & Scientific Books, 1979, pp 93–101

Mesulam M-M: Principles of Behavioral Neurology. Philadelphia, PA, FA Davis, 1985

Meyer RG: The Clinician's Handbook. Boston, MA, Allyn & Bacon, 1983

Monteleone P, Maj M, Iovino M, et al: Growth hormone response to sodium valproate in chronic schizophrenia. Biol Psychiatry 21:588–594, 1986

Morihisa JM, Duff FH, Wyatt RJ: Brain electrical activity mapping (BEAM) in schizophrenia. Arch Gen Psychiatry 40:719–728, 1983

Nandi DN, Banerjee G, Bera S, et al: Contagious hysteria in a West Bengali village. Am J Psychother 34:247–252, 1985

Neborsky R, Janowsky D, Munson E, et al: Rapid treatment of acute psychotic symptoms with high and low dose haloperidol. Arch Gen Psychiatry 38:195–199, 1981

Nemeroff CB: The interaction of neurotensin with dopaminergic pathways in the central nervous system: basic neurobiology and implications for the pathogenesis and treatment of schizophrenia. Psychoneuroendocrinology 11:15–37, 1986

Ogdon D: Psychodiagnostics and Personality Assessment: A Handbook. Los Angeles, CA, Western Psychological Services, 1977

Osser D: Treatment-resistant problems, in Handbook of Clinical Psychopharmocology. Edited by Tupin JP, Shader RI, Harnett DS. Northvale, NJ, Jason Aronson, 1988, pp 269–328

Pandey RS, Gupta AK, Chaturvedi UC: Autoimmune model of schizophrenia with special reference to anti-brain antibodies. Biol Psychiatry 16:1123–1136, 1981

Pearlson GD, Garbacz DJ, Breakey WR, et al: Lateral ventricular enlargement associated with persistent unemployment and negative symptoms in both schizophrenia and bipolar affective disorder. Psychiatry Res 12:1–9, 1984

Pies R: Distinguishing obsessional from psychotic phenomenon. J Clin Psychopharmacol 4:345–347, 1984

Pies R, Renshaw P, Goff D, et al: Water-suppressed nuclear magnetic resonance spectroscopy of plasma from schizophrenics and normal controls: a preliminary report. Research Communications in Psychology, Psychiatry and Behavior 17:26–32, 1992

Resnick PJ: Diagnosis of malingered hallucinations: forensic issues. Audio-Digest Psychiatry [Audio-Digest Foundation] 17 (July 25), 1988

Salzman C: The use of ECT in the treatment of schizophrenia. Am J Psychiatry 137:1032–1041, 1980

Schaffer CB: Bioavailability of intramuscular vs oral haloperidol in schizophrenic patients. J Clin Psychopharmacol 2:274–277, 1982

Shenton ME, Kikinis R, Jolesz FA: Abnormalities of the left temporal lobe and thought disorder in schizophrenia. N Engl J Med 327:604–612, 1992

Siever LJ, Coursey RD, Alterman IS, et al: Impaired smooth pursuit eye movement: vulnerability marker for schizotypal personality disorder in a normal control population. Am J Psychiatry 141:1560–1565, 1984

Small JG: EEG in schizophrenia, in EEG and Evoked Potentials in Psychiatry and Behavioral Neurology. Edited by Hughes JR, Wilson WP. Boston, MA, Butterworths, 1983, pp 25–40

Stevens JR: Eye blink and schizophrenia: psychosis or tardive dyskinesia? Am J Psychiatry 135:223–226, 1978

Strauss JS, Carpenter WT: Schizophrenia. New York, Plenum, 1981

Suppes T, McElroy SL, Gilbert J, et al: Clozapine in the treatment of dysphoric mania. Biol Psychiatry 32:270–280, 1992

Takahashi R, Inaba Y, Inanga D, et al: CT scanning and the investigation of schizophrenia, in Biological Psychiatry. Edited by Perris C, Strewe G, Jansson B. Amsterdam, Elsevier–North Holland, 1981, pp 259–268

Tamminga CA, Thaker GK, Buchanan R, et al: Limbic system abnormalities identified in schizophrenia using positron emission tomography with fluorodeoxyglucose and neocortical alterations with deficit syndrome. Arch Gen Psychiatry 49:522–530, 1992

Terenius L, Wahlstrom A, Lindstrom L, et al: Increased levels of endorphins in chronic psychosis. Neurosci Lett 3:157–162, 1976

Tienari P, Sorri A, Lahti I, et al: The Finnish adoptive family study of schizophrenia. Yale Journal of Biology and Medicine 58:227–237, 1985

Tomer R, Mintz M, Levy A, et al: Smooth pursuit pattern in schizophrenic patients during cognitive task. Biol Psychiatry 16:131–144, 1981

Weinberger DR, Kleinman JE: Observations on the brain in schizophrenia, in American Psychiatric Association Annual Review, Vol 5. Edited by Frances AJ, Hales RE. Washington, DC, American Psychiatric Press, 1986, pp 42–67

Weinberger DR, Berman KF, Zec RF: Physiological dysfunction of dorsolateral prefrontal cortex in schizophrenia, I: regional cerebral blood flow (rCBF) evidence. Arch Gen Psychiatry 43:114–124, 1986

Welch CA: Electroconvulsive theapy in the general hospital, in Massachusetts General Hospital Handbook of General Hospital Psychiatry. Edited by

Hackett TP, Cassem NH. Littleton, MA, PSG Publishing, 1987, pp 269–280

Wexler B, Heninger GR: Alterations in cerebral laterality during acute psychotic illness. Arch Gen Psychiatry 36:278–284, 1979

Widen L, Blomgrist G, DePaulis T, et al: Studies of schizophrenia with positron CT. J Clin Neuropharmacol 7 (suppl 1):538–539, 1984

Wing JK, Brown GW: Institutionalism and Schizophrenia. Cambridge, UK, Cambridge University Press, 1970

Wolkin A, Jaegar J, Brodie J, et al: Persistence of cerebral metabolic abnormalities in chronic schizophrenia as determined by positron emission tomography. Am J Psychiatry 142:564–571, 1985

Zarcone VP, Benson KL, Berger PA: Abnormal rapid eye movement latencies in schizophrenia. Arch Gen Psychiatry 44:45–48, 1987

6

Anxiety Disorders

The natural role of twentieth-century man is anxiety.
Norman Mailer

It has been over 40 years since W. H. Auden's poem "The Age of Anxiety" appeared. As Rollo May points out, the four characters in the poem have in common "loneliness, the feeling of not being of value as persons, and the experience of not being able to love and be loved" (May 1977, p. 5). Some of the lines in Auden's poem are well worth a psychiatrist's time—for example, "the fears we know are of not knowing." One can understand this on the level of "society," in an age when any hour might bring nuclear cataclysm; or on the level of individual neurosis, as in the obsessive-compulsive person's need to check the same lock a hundred times a day. Of course, neither global nor personal anxiety is really unique to our time. In the Middle Ages, anxiety "took the form of excessive dread of death and pervasive fears of devils and sorcerers" (May 1977, p. 178). In Freud's time, as we will discuss later, anxiety asserted itself quite without assistance from impending nuclear destruction. Still, our age—in which the stable and familiar structures of church and family have been sorely tested—may be producing subtle variations on the manifestations of anxiety, such as certain forms of pathological narcissism (Lasch 1979).

Given all this, it's important to distinguish what is generally termed "normal" from "abnormal," or pathological, anxiety. Easier said than done. But a good start is made by May (1977) in the following passage from *The Meaning of Anxiety.*

205

Normal anxiety is that reaction which (1) is not disproportionate to the objective threat, (2) does not involve repression or other mechanisms of intrapsychic conflict, and, as a corollary to the second point, (3) does not require neurotic defense mechanisms for its management. It (4) can be confronted constructively on the level of conscious awareness or can be relieved if the objective situation is altered. (p. 209)

May goes on to define "neurotic anxiety" as essentially the reverse of the above; that is, it involves a disproportionate reaction, repression or other forms of intrapsychic conflict, and management by pathological mechanisms such as symptom formation or withdrawal. Neurotic anxiety, as May notes, "tends to paralyze the person, and thus does not make for constructive or creative activity" (p. 214). Parenthetically, we should note that without "normal" anxiety, a good deal of artistic inspiration would be nullified—witness Edvard Munch's (1863–1944) painting "The Scream," which in many ways epitomizes the Age of Anxiety. Finally, we should add that some authorities use the term "fear" to describe something quite close to May's concept of "normal anxiety" (Shader 1988).

Generalized Anxiety Disorder

The Central Concept

The DSM-III-R (American Psychiatric Association 1987) construct of generalized anxiety disorder (GAD) was at once admirably specific and frustratingly broad. In the changeover from DSM-III (American Psychiatric Association 1980) to DSM-III-R, attempts were made to narrow the scope of GAD; thus, the required duration was extended from 1 month to 6 months, and the symptom list was expanded. DSM-IV (American Psychiatric Association 1994) has reversed the second approach: it has actually reduced the list of possible symptoms in GAD from 18 to 6, mainly by cutting most of the symptoms of autonomic hyperarousal (palpitations, sweating, etc.). The effect of this may be to reduce the overlap between GAD and panic disorder.

"Exaggerated startle response" has been cut, thus sharpening the distinction between GAD and posttraumatic stress disorder (PTSD). The new criteria, unlike those of DSM-III-R, also require "significant distress or impairment in social, occupational, or other important areas of functioning" (American Psychiatric Association 1994, p. 436). Despite these refinements, if we consider the following vignette, we may come away with the impression of GAD as an exceedingly widespread, if not "normal," condition.

Vignette

Mr. Angst was a 40-year-old accountant who complained that for the past 7 months he had felt "incredibly uptight." The patient noted two problems that were bothering him: the concern that he would "screw up" at work, and the worry that his wife might be having an affair. After careful interview with both the patient and his wife, no objective evidence to substantiate either concern could be found. Mr. Angst conceded that his worries "are probably unrealistic." Nevertheless, he continued to experience muscle tension, restlessness and irritability, difficulty concentrating, a feeling of being "keyed up," difficulty performing simple calculations on the job, and occasional initial insomnia. Physical examination and laboratory testing (including thyroid function) were unremarkable. The patient's caffeine intake was moderate, and there was no history of amphetamine or other substance abuse. A diagnosis of GAD was made.

It would seem that there are many "Mr. Angsts" walking around and that few of them would be considered "mentally ill" in the colloquial sense. Indeed, some studies suggest that GAD is present in 2% to 5% of the general population; however, other studies suggest that many patients so diagnosed actually suffer from one of the other anxiety disorders (Kaplan and Sadock 1988). Only around a third of patients with GAD actually seek psychiatric help (Kaplan and Sadock 1988). Nevertheless, for individuals with the more severe forms of GAD, the condition can lead to social-vocational incapacity and—based on my own observation—to substance abuse as a form of self-medication. (In an epidemiological study of young adults, Christie et al. [1988] found a correlation between the presence of an anxiety disorder and later substance abuse disorder; however, this study did not sort out generalized from other types of anxiety.)

Historical Development of the Disorder

The historical concept of "generalized anxiety" is difficult to tease out from the more circumscribed phenomenon we shall come to describe as panic disorder. Indeed, one of the signal accomplishments of modern psychiatry is the clinical differentiation of these two disorders. (Also bound up with the notion of generalized anxiety is that of hypochondriasis, which we shall explore in Chapter 7 in our discussion of somatoform disorders.) Nevertheless, if one hunts a bit, descriptions of something approximating GAD may be found as far back as classical times. Consider this description of the anxiety of old age, as described by the poet Anacreon (6th century B.C.):

> My temples have turned grey, and my crown is white.
> Charming youth is no longer here, and my teeth are decayed.
> Of sweet life not much time is left.
> Therefore I often groan, shuddering at Tartarus [Hell]
> For the abyss of Hades is frightful, and the descent to it
> Grievous. And once you have gone down, there is no coming back.
> (Snell 1982, p. 64)

As Snell (1982) notes, the poet's "eyes are centered upon his helplessness; his 'will to life' sees itself hemmed in" (p. 64). We see the element of "apprehensive expectation" typical of GAD. The groaning and shuddering of the poet suggest the somatic component of his anxiety, though—it must be said—it is difficult to ignore the depressive quality of this description. But then, as we shall see, generalized anxiety and depression are often admixed.

Rollo May (1977) notes that until the coming of Freud, the problem of anxiety lay in the provinces or philosophy and religion. In particular, the philosophers Spinoza, Pascal, and Kierkegaard had much to say about what we might now consider "normal" or "existential" anxiety. Kierkegaard, for example, emphasized the role of "freedom" in generating anxiety in human beings. Freedom to choose one's life exposes the individual to all sorts of inner tensions. Kierkegaard also added a new twist to the concept of anxiety (or "dread"), perhaps anticipating later psychoanalytic theories of unconscious conflict. Kierkegaard spoke of anxiety as "a desire for what one dreads, a sympathetic antipathy . . . one fears, but what one fears, one desires" (Kierkegaard 1944, p. xii). If one thinks of the psychoanalytic concept of reaction formation, Kierkegaard's idea seems remarkably prescient, especially in considering obsessive-compulsive rituals. In effect, Kierkegaard paved the way for later "conflict" theories of anxiety.

If Freud had done nothing else but separate "anxiety neurosis" from the hodgepodge of symptoms known as "neurasthenia," he would have made a significant contribution to psychiatry (Freud 1895[1894]/1962). (Neurasthenia, a term popularized by the American G. M. Beard, included symptoms of exhaustion and depression admixed with many autonomic signs of anxiety.) But Freud did a great deal more. First, he recognized that anxiety could be distinguished from depression on the basis of the "motor manifestations" of anxiety (e.g., dyspnea and palpitations). Second, Freud appreciated that anxiety could be manifested either as a chronic state or as discrete attacks (Nemiah 1980a), although he used the term "anxiety neurosis" to encompass both forms of the disorder. Of course, Freud's preeminent contribution to the theory of anxiety involved the idea that anxiety is a signal to the ego that some unacceptable drive is pressing for awareness and discharge (Kaplan and Sadock 1988). As a signal, anxiety prompts the ego to engage one or more defense mechanisms. We shall discuss Freud's theory in more detail in our discussion of psychological factors.

The Biopsychosocial Perspective

Biological Factors

Most biological theories of GAD fall under the general rubric of sympathetic nervous system (SNS) overarousal. The James-Lange theory posited that subjective anxiety was actually a response to peripheral (sympathetic) phenomena such as tachycardia or dyspnea—in effect, that we "learn" we are anxious because we perceive that our bodies are overaroused. Most modern theories, however, posit that central nervous system (CNS) arousal precedes peripheral manifestations of anxiety, except when there is a specific peripheral cause such as pheochromocytoma (Kaplan and Sadock 1988).

But what is the biological nature of "overarousal"? With respect to GAD (as opposed to panic disorder), it must be admitted that little is known, though much is hypothesized. Furthermore, our theories about GAD are largely inferential, based on the (putative) mechanisms of anxiolytics. One often hears, for example, that anxiety entails some sort of "GABA deficiency," since benzodiazepine anxiolytics are GABA (gamma-aminobutyric acid) agonists. This is rather like reasoning that if whacking the TV set restores the picture, the television must have been suffering from a "whack deficiency." Nevertheless, we can learn important things about anxiety by understanding the mechanisms by which it is relieved (Dubovsky 1990). We now know that brain cells contain receptors for benzodiazepines and that benzodiazepines differ in their relative affinities for these receptors. Furthermore, there is a good correlation between the percentage of occupied benzodiazepine receptor sites in the brains of experimental animals and the pharmacological effects of the drug. We also have good evidence that the benzodiazepine receptor exists as part of a larger complex that includes a GABA$_A$ receptor. GABA is the main inhibitory neurotransmitter in the CNS; it "works" by allowing influx of chloride ions into the neuron, thus "hyperpolarizing" the cell and, in effect, making it harder to fire. When a benzodiazepine locks on to its receptor, it increases the affinity of the GABA receptor for GABA, thereby "amplifying" chloride ion influx. So far, we have not discovered a naturally occurring benzodiazepine agonist—that is, one that would explain why our neurons are built to handle anxiolytic compounds from pharmaceutical companies. However, there is a naturally occurring compund called diazepam binding inhibitor that acts as an "inverse agonist": it decreases GABA receptor affinity for GABA and actually provokes anxiety! Pathological anxiety may reflect, in part, hyperactivity of such an endogenous benzodiazepine inverse agonist (Dubovsky 1990). Alternatively, perhaps some of us are born a few hundred milligrams short of some as yet unidentified "endogenous tranquilizer," and go on to develop GAD. It would be nice if the story were this simple, but, of course, it isn't. The anxiolytic buspirone, for example, does not appear to operate via benzodiazepine mechanisms at all (Riblet et al. 1984); instead, buspirone may (just for starters) block presynaptic dopamine receptors. It is also a serotonergic ($5\text{-}HT_{1A}$) "partial agonist," which gives it some special properties. As we will see, serotonin seems to play a pivotal role in some forms of anxiety. Add to this the role of adenosine and calcium and you have some sense of how much—and how little—we know of the mechanisms underlying generalized anxiety. We shall say more about these complex issues when we address the biological underpinnings of panic disorder.

Psychological Factors

Let's consider the following vignette, drawn from a detailed family history, family interviews, and information obtained over the course of 2 years in the patient's psychoanalytically oriented therapy.

Vignette

Mark was a 37-year-old single male who presented with generalized anxiety. His principal symptoms were "muscle tension all the time," a feeling of being "on edge," tremulousness, occasional palpitations, and initial insomnia. These problems had been present "as long as I can remember." Physical and laboratory studies were entirely normal. Mark gave a history of "having problems being alone" as a child. At the age of 5, he began sleeping in his parents' bed because "I was just too scared to sleep in my room." This behavior began around the time of the birth of Mark's younger brother Mitchell. Mark recalled—and his mother confirmed—being "kinda upset" when Mitch was brought home from the hospital. "I felt like I had been dethroned," Mark acknowledged, and he teased Mitch constantly as they grew older. At age 7, Mark developed almost constant abdominal pains without organic etiology, forcing him to miss school frequently. His father berated him for this, saying, "Don't be such a sissy." His mother would "get real cold" whenever Mark missed school, but acceded to his wish to be around her during the day. On the days he did get to school, Mark would worry that his mother "wouldn't pick me up . . . would just leave me stranded there." At times, he believed she would die in a car accident. Interview with Mark's parents revealed a critical, patronizing style on the father's part and a quiet, withdrawn, aloof attitude in Mark's mother.

The above vignette brings together a number of strands from the psychoanalytic and object-relations literature (Fishman 1989; McDermott et al. 1989; Nemiah 1985a). Psychoanalytic theory, as McDermott et al. (1989) have nicely summarized, holds that

> "anxiety disorders are caused by unconscious conflicts related to the basic drives of sex and aggression. The roots of these conflicts are found in earlier parent, child, and sibling interactions and are often Oedipal in nature. . . . Under certain pathogenic conditions these conflicts can no longer get successfully repressed, and the symptoms of overt anxiety erupt. . . . a number of childhood anxieties are related to losses at increasing chronological (developmental) age: loss of the womb with birth, loss of breast with weaning, loss of stool in toilet training, threatened loss of genitals in castration anxiety, loss of mother in hostile interactions with her, and loss of the mother object to the competitor (father). (pp. 408–409)

In Mark's case, we can see how the arrival of his little brother may have precipitated a number of these dynamics and how his parents' critical or withholding style may have exacerbated them. This leads us into the object-relations view of anxiety, which emphasizes the importance of the "holding environment" (Winnicott 1958). In essence, the holding environment is the atmosphere of safety and affirmation created for the infant by the mothering figure. Defective "holding" leaves the child "with an anxious vulnerability to feeling unprotected and empty" (Fishman 1989, p. 2012). Chronic deprivation, in this view, also makes the child feel enraged at his or her parents. But because this rage is intolerable and guilt provoking, it may be "split off" in the manner we will discuss in Chapter 9 (see G. Adler 1985; Kernberg 1975, for further discussion). As Fishman (1989) notes, "The child splits his inner views of self and others into good and bad; he keeps the two categories of experience completely separate from each other so that rage-contaminated images will not obliterate the small pocket of good ones. This is the unconscious, defensive process labelled 'splitting'" (p. 2013).

But of course, the ego's defenses are not perfect; sometimes, the child—and later, the adult—becomes dimly aware of his rage. Often, this is precipitated by some perceived deprivation or loss. At such a time, anxiety (or depression) may result.

The capacity to bear anxiety is itself a major developmental achievement, and the child who did not receive sufficient "holding" may be ill-equipped to tolerate the stresses of adulthood, perhaps developing GAD or other traumatic "neuroses" (Fishman 1989).

It must be said that the psychoanalytic and object-relations theories of generalized anxiety are just that—theories. The empirical evidence, such as it is, comes mainly from direct observation of infants who have experienced various kinds of separation or deprivation (Mahler et al. 1975; Spitz 1965). Inferential evidence, of course, has been gleaned from countless psychoanalyses. In any given case of GAD, however, it is difficult to prove that the disorder evolved from the dynamics discussed above (Fisher and Greenberg 1977). Indeed, cognitively oriented therapists such as Albert Ellis (1962) and Aaron Beck (Beck and Emery 1985) would argue that generalized anxiety arises from a variety of self-defeating, deeply internalized ideas, such as "I must be loved by my parents or it is horrible!" As Ellis and Harper (1975) so colorfully put it, "Life holds innumerable pains in the neck for all of us; but true catastrophes . . . rarely happen. And 'terrors,' 'horrors,' and 'awfulnesses' arise from fictional demons . . . which we foolishly make up in our heads and cannot really define or validate" (p. 146).

Sociocultural Factors

Alfred Adler, who developed the concept of "inferiority feelings," also commented on the profoundly social roots of anxiety. He stated that "only that individual can go through life without anxiety who is conscious of belonging to the fellowship of man" (A. Adler 1927, p. 238). But it was Harry Stack Sullivan who most cogently argued that anxiety is an interpersonal phenomenon arising "out of the infant's apprehension of the disapproval of the significant persons in his interpersonal world" (May 1977). Clearly, if this is what is meant by the "social" roots of anxiety, we will have a hard time separating them from the object-relations views we have just discussed. Therefore, we shall take a somewhat more circumscribed look at sociocultural influences in the development of anxiety. Let's illustrate this approach with a brief clinical vignette.

Vignette

Nguyen was a single 19-year-old Vietnamese male who presented in the outpatient psychiatric clinic with complaints of stomach pains, "weakness in the lungs," difficulty falling asleep, nervousness, and muscle aches. Physical examination and laboratory studies 1 week earlier had been totally within normal limits. The immediate precipitant for Nguyen's evaluation was a violent altercation with his father, leading to Nguyen's arrest. When his father did not press charges, Nguyen was sent by the court for "counseling." His symptoms had actually begun 2 years earlier, when Nguyen and his grandmother left Vietnam and joined the rest of Nguyen's family in Boston. The family had left Vietnam 8 years earlier with two of Nguyen's siblings, leaving Nguyen in the care of his maternal grandmother. [This practice is common in Vietnamese culture; see Ganesan et al. 1989.] Nguyen had difficulty adjusting both to American culture and to his rather fractured family system. He and his grandmother moved in with the rest of the family but were rather isolated from them emotionally. Nguyen's brother and sister had been quite "Americanized," and they often made fun of Nguyen for his "weird Vietnamese ways." Nguyen's father criticized his son for the latter's difficulties in school, where his performance was deemed "inferior." Testing by the school psychologist strongly suggested "a specific learning disability, but anxiety interfering with performance cannot be ruled out." Nguyen's parents were very distraught over his academic difficulties and blamed him for many problems within the family. His father set extremely strict limits on Nguyen's social life, resulting in anger and resentment on Nguyen's part. During the week prior to evaluation, Nguyen had been "sleeping on the streets," having been "kicked out by my father."

Nguyen's case (based on the work of Ganesan et al. [1989]) draws together a number of sociocultural factors associated with GAD: namely, familial issues, stressful life events, refugee status, and homelessness. Anxiety disorders in adolescents, according to family systems theory, may result from pathological interactions within the family (McDermott et al. 1989). For example, when one family member is "scapegoated" by the others, he or she may develop symptoms of GAD. Thus, Nguyen became the focus of the family's anger and the "carrier" of the family's many difficulties. In addition to the numerous cultural problems faced by newly arrived immigrants, adolescent refugees may also face intergenerational conflict within their families (Ganesan et al. 1989). In Nguyen's case, there was also the difference in "exposure" to the American culture between him and his siblings.

Although the evidence is conflicting, there are data pointing to a correlation between GAD and recent life stressors. Blazer et al. (1987) found that men who reported many recent stressful events had a risk of GAD that was 8.5 times that of men reporting few such events; surprisingly, this correlation did not hold up for women. Koegel et al. (1988) found that homeless adults, when compared with "housed" control subjects, had a higher lifetime and current prevalence of GAD, based on DSM-III criteria. (Of course, this correlation leaves open the question of causality.) In Nguyen's case, recent homelessness appears to have exacerbated a more chronic GAD. Finally, Nguyen's possible learning disorder (LD) raises two possibilities. First, such a disability might contribute to the generalized anxiety Nguyen himself was feeling. But there is also some evidence that parents of LD children are more anxious and more preoccupied with "control" than are parents of non-LD children (Margalit and Heiman 1986). Margalit and Heiman (1986) found that parents of LD children expected more from their children and did not encourage free expression of feelings. One can only guess how the added challenge of an LD child would exacerbate the already considerable anxiety of an immigrant family.

In closing our discussion of the biopsychosocial perspective on GAD, it is worth reexamining Morton Reiser's (1975) hypothesis of the "vicious cycle" at work in anxiety disorders:

Neurovegetative and endocrine changes in response to psychosocial stress have been shown to affect higher mental processes such as cognition, and could in this way influence perception and evaluation of danger signals and anxiety proneness . . .

. . . sustained pressure from active psychological conflict, with weakening of defenses, might set into motion a cyclic reaction whereby psychological processes involved in evaluation of danger would become increasingly more primitive . . . as a consequence of the physiologic responses they evoke, and that the physiologic responses would become increasingly more vigorous as danger signals were evaluated with increasing alarm. (p. 495)

In short, anxiety begets anxiety that begets anxiety. A modified version of Reiser's scheme is shown in Figure 6–1.

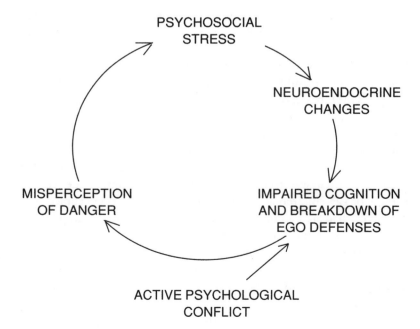

Figure 6–1. Psychosocial stress. *Source.* Extensively modified from Reiser 1975.

Pitfalls in the Differential Diagnosis

Organic Conditions

It is roughly accurate to say that GAD may be mimicked by *Harrison's Textbook of Medicine.* I mean, of course, that a multitude of organic disorders can present with symptoms of generalized anxiety. Before examining this daunting list, let's look at a clinical vignette.

Vignette

A 61-year-old widowed male with no prior psychiatric history presented with a 6-month history of feeling "nervous and jumpy . . . like I'm gonna crawl out of my skin." He related that 5 months earlier, his daughter and son-in-law had "kicked me out of their house." He had been forced to move into a small apartment in a housing project, which he described as "a real rat hole." Counseling at a senior citizen center had been helpful but had not eliminated the patient's anxiety. He complained of episodic headache, tremulousness, sweating, and recent weight loss. There was no complaint of dyspnea, tightness in the chest, tingling, numbness, depersonalization, or the fear of dying or "going crazy." Physical examination was normal except for blood pressure of 180/100 and minor hypertensive retinal changes. Measurement of urinary catecholamines confirmed a diagnosis of pheochromocytoma.

This vignette serves not only to introduce us to the differential diagnosis of GAD but also to warn us against the temptation of premature diagnostic closure. It would have been all to easy to have attributed this patient's anxiety to his recent eviction, even though the time course did not coincide precisely with his symptoms. Of course, the stress of being "kicked out" undoubtedly contributed to the patient's organically based anxiety.

Table 6–1 is only a partial list of the many organic disorders presenting with symptoms of generalized anxiety. Given this multitude of conditions, are there some general clues that might alert the clinician to an organic cause of generalized anxiety? Certainly, the onset of acute anxiety in an elderly individual ought to raise your level of suspicion—particularly when there is no previous psychiatric history. The presence of abnormal autonomic signs, although not pathognomonic, is also suggestive of organic factors. The medical review of systems, of course, is critical in uncovering an organic disorder. For example, a history of exercise intolerance may point to a cardiovascular origin of the patient's anxiety; weight loss and heat intolerance to hyperthyroidism; and excess thirst and urination to diabetes and its possible insulin-related hypoglycemic reactions (McNeil 1987). This last point should remind you how important the medication history is in differential diagnosis: a patient taking theophylline for asthma or

Table 6–1.   Organic causes of generalized anxiety

Cardiopulmonary	Transient ischemic attacks
Angina pectoris	Ménière's disease
Arrhythmias	
Congestive heart failure	**Metabolic**
Acute asthma	Hepatic failure
Pulmonary embolus	Hypokalemia
Mitral valve prolapse	Hypoxia
Pneumothorax	Acidoses (e.g., lactic acidosis)
Endocrine	**Drug-related**
Hyperthyroidism	Sympathomimetics (ephedrine, terbutaline)
Hypoglycemia	
Pheochromocytoma	Xanthine derivatives (caffeine, aminophylline)
Hypoparathyroidism	
Carcinoid syndrome	Thyroid preparations
	Insulin (via hypoglycemia)
Neurological	Psychotropics (e.g., fluoxetine, tricyclics)
Degenerative diseases (Alzheimer's, Huntington's)	
	Sedative withdrawal (alcohol, benzodiazepines)
Partial complex (temporal lobe) seizures	

Source.   Extensively modified from McNeil 1987.

"diet pills" for "lack of energy" is certainly a candidate for organically based generalized anxiety. Finally, substance abuse and its accompanying withdrawal symptoms should always be assessed in taking a history from an anxious patient.

Before leaving the organic causes of generalized anxiety, let's examine a vignette with immediate relevance to clinical psychiatry.

Vignette

A 47-year-old female presented with marked psychomotor retardation, depression, and hypersomnia (up to 16 hours per day). Her psychiatrist considered prescribing a monoamine oxidase inhibitor (MAOI), but the patient would not agree to the dietary limitations. Fluoxetine 20 mg/day was prescribed, with modest improvement over the subsequent 3 weeks. Increases in fluoxetine dosage up to 80 mg/day had no further benefit. The psychiatrist decided to "potentiate" the serotonergic action of fluoxetine with the more noradrenergic action of desipramine, which was begun at 150 mg qhs. Within 5 days, the patient complained of feeling "like I'm crawling out of my skin," jittery, shaky, and sweaty. Serum level of desipramine was 460 ng/ml, considerably higher than the putative therapeutic range. Gradual discontinuation of the desipramine resulted in a return to the patient's postfluoxetine baseline.

We should state at the outset that the combination of fluoxetine and desipramine has not been rigorously evaluated and is not presented here as an example of correct practice. Rather, we see in this vignette an example of "iatrogenic" anxiety. In the first place, fluoxetine alone may cause agitation and tremor (Stark and Hardison 1985), as may desipramine early in the course of treatment. Moreover, fluoxetine may elevate plasma levels of tricyclics, leading to a variety of toxic side effects (Vaughan 1988).

Functional Disorders

The "nonorganic" psychiatric disorders that may be confused with GAD are summarized in Table 6–2. To appreciate this differential diagnosis, let's consider the following vignette.

Vignette

Mr. Gemisch was a 34-year-old (English-speaking) German immigrant who presented with what he called "depression." He reported having felt this way for the past 7 months, during which time he had been promoted to a rather high level in an engineering firm. He described initial insomnia, poor appetite with no associated weight loss, constant worry about losing his job (without any real evidence of risk), and vague ruminations about his health. These symptoms had led him to increase his usual alcohol consumption from "one glass of wine per week to two or three glasses per day." Mr. Gemisch also complained of feeling "cold and clammy" and tremulous and of having occasional trouble swallowing. He denied constipation, decreased libido, or diurnal mood variation. He admitted to recent suicidal ideation, with a plan to "shoot myself if I don't get better-." He was admitted to the inpatient unit with a diagnosis of "agitated depression." A sleep electroencephalogram (EEG) showed a slightly reduced REM latency of about 75 minutes.

This vignette raises one of the most difficult questions in psychiatric differential diagnosis: the teasing out of anxiety from depressive disorders. Note that, despite the tempting chief complaint, Mr. Gemisch lacks many of the classic neurovegetative features of major depressive episode (i.e., weight loss, midcycle insomnia, decreased libido, constipation, and diurnal variation of mood). Moreover, his autonomic complaints (cold, clammy sensation and trouble swallowing) are more suggestive of anxiety disorder. His sleep EEG—a topic we will consider further under the subsection on adjunctive

Table 6–2.   Differential diagnosis of generalized anxiety disorder

Adjustment disorder with anxious mood	Depressive disorders
	Mania
Schizophrenia and related disorders	Somatoform disorders
Other anxiety disorders	Dissociative disorders

Source. Extensively modified from McNeil 1987.

testing—is also more consistent with anxiety and hyperarousal than with major depression (Uhde et al. 1984). Of course, the more we learn about anxiety and depression, the more we appreciate the common ground between them. Breier et al. (1985) have reviewed the data linking noradrenergic dysfunction to both depression and anxiety. These authors note the familial relationship between panic and depression—a topic we will explore later in this chapter. Although the symptomatic distinction between GAD and major depression is not as sharp as that between panic disorder and major depression (Breier et al. 1985; Dubovsky 1990; Roth et al. 1972), there are some clinically useful clues, as summarized in Table 6–3.

Let's now consider further the differential diagnosis of GAD using another vignette.

Vignette

Jim was a 22-year-old male who presented with a chief complaint of "feeling rotten . . . anxious, down, like my mind is going." For the past 2 years, Jim had been experiencing intermittent bouts of what he called "everything bending . . . like I'm in a dream." These bouts

Table 6–3. Differential diagnosis of generalized anxiety disorder (GAD) and major depression

	GAD	Major depression
Early awakening	Sometimes	Often
Suicidal ideas	Sometimes	Often
Psychomotor slowing	Uncommon	Common
Loss of interest	Sometimes	Often
Hopelessness	Uncommon	Common
Worthlessness	Uncommon	Common
Weight loss	Sometimes	Often
Decreased libido	Sometimes	Often

Source. Extensively modified from McNeil 1987.

would usually last hours, but sometimes days. They were characterized by a sense that "I'm outside by body, looking down on the
whole scene." The edges of tables, chairs, and other objects would
become "wavy" and indistinct. This was usually accompanied by
mild dizziness, but not by palpitations, dyspnea, tingling, or numbness. In between bouts, Jim reported feeling "on edge . . . waiting
for the thing to happen." There was no history of substance abuse
prior to onset of these symptoms, but Jim admitted that for the past
month he had been drinking "just to get rid of the feelings." An
EEG and other physical investigations were normal.

You have probably made the diagnosis of depersonalization disorder in Jim's case—one of the dissociative disorders we will discuss
later. As you can see, signs and symptoms of generalized or panic-type
anxiety may be present. Depersonalization can usually be distinguished from GAD by careful attention to alterations of sensory
awareness and "sense of reality." However, depersonalization as a
symptom may sometimes be present in other anxiety disorders, in
which case the additional diagnosis of depersonalization disorder is
not made. By the way, substance abuse may be either a precipitant or
a consequence of depersonalization. This is also true with respect to
GAD-type symptoms, although the rules of DSM-IV would prohibit
the diagnosis of GAD if a known organic factor initiates or maintains
the symptoms.

In Table 6–2 we noted that GAD may be confused with a number
of other functional psychiatric disorders, including adjustment disorder with anxious mood, schizophrenia and related psychotic disorders,
mania, and somatoform disorders. Because these conditions are discussed in detail in other chapters, we will present one vignette and
then summarize the features that distinguish these disorders from
GAD.

Vignette

Ms. Citamos was a 44-year-old divorced female who had emigrated
from Greece 2 months ago. She presented with a chief complaint
that "I am nervous around people all the time because of my odor.
The gas from my body comes out backwards." She explained that

ever since her coming to the United States, "my bowel gas comes out my mouth" and that people were systematically avoiding her for this reason. The patient expressed no other unusual beliefs, ideas of influence, thought insertion, and so forth. She denied auditory or visual hallucinations. Despite some minor problems with English, there was no thought process disorder. Affect seemed anxious and slightly depressed. There was a recent history of unusual eating habits (e.g., avoiding "any foods with meaty odors") but no loss of appetite or weight loss. The patient complained of initial insomnia but no midcycle or early morning awakening. She also complained of feeling "tightened" and "all wound up and fearful." She denied sudden attacks of anxiety, dyspnea, paresthesia, or fear of dying. With respect to her chief complaint, the patient remained adamant in her belief that "bowel gas" was escaping from her mouth, despite numerous physical examinations, a normal GI series, and the repeated reassurance of friends and family that she exhibited no unusual odors.

Although Ms. Citamos has some features of GAD—feeling nervous, wound up, fearful, and so forth—her presentation is actually consistent with delusional (paranoid) disorder, somatic type. The key here is the fixed, inflexible nature of the somatic preoccupation. As we shall see, patients with social phobia also present with anxious concerns about being scrutinized by others but lack the very specific somatic delusional material presented in this case.

Aside from other anxiety disorders, which will be discussed in the remaining sections of this chapter, a number of functional disorders may present with prominent anxiety. Table 6–4 summarizes the features that help distinguish these functional disorders from GAD:

Adjunctive Testing

Perhaps because of its more dramatic nature, panic disorder has inspired far more biological research than has GAD. Thus, the neuroendocrine, polysomnographic, and brain-imaging data on GAD are sparse.

Table 6–4. Differential diagnosis of functional disorders and generalized anxiety disorder (GAD)

	GAD	Adjustment disorder[a]	Schizophrenia	Mania[b]	Somatoform disorder	Dissociative disorder
Duration	>6 mo	<6 mo	>6 mo	Varies	Chronic	Varies
Precipitant	+/-	++++	+/-	++	+ (conversion)	+++
Affect	Anxious	Anxious	Flat, inappropiate	Irritable, euphoric	Depressed, anxious	Varies
Thought process	Normal	NL	+ disorder	+ disorder	NL	NL
Bodily preoccupations	+	+/-	+	-	++++	+
Disturbed integration of memory/ consciousness	-	-	++	-	-	+++

Note. −, usually absent; +/−, may or may not be present; +, present to a small degree/likelihood; ++, present to a moderate degree/ likelihood; +++, present to a considerable degree/likelihood; ++++, present to an extreme degree/likelihood.
[a]With anxious features. [b]Manic phase of bipolar disorder.

Neuroendocrine Studies

Thus far, no specific neuroendocrine abnormality has been linked with GAD. Avery et al. (1985) examined dexamethasone suppression test (DST) response in patients with GAD, panic disorder, and primary affective disorder. No difference in DST nonsuppression was found among patients with major depression, panic disorder, and panic disorder with agoraphobia. But somewhat surprisingly, patients with GAD showed higher rates of DST nonsuppression than did patients with major depression. It remains to be seen whether this finding will be borne out in larger studies or will prove useful in the differential diagnosis of GAD. Cowley et al. (1988) examined lactate response in patients with "pure" GAD (i.e., no history of panic attacks), patients with panic disorder, and normal control subjects. GAD patients had a significantly lower rate of full-blown panic attacks than did panic disorder patients, but had more than did control subjects. Furthermore, GAD patients had a higher-than-normal degree of anxiety and physical symptoms (without actual "terror") in response to lactate infusion. While these limited data suggest a biological differentiation of GAD from panic disorder, the utility of lactate infusion for purposes of diagnosing GAD remains to be determined.

Sleep Studies

You may recall our patient Mr. Gemisch, who suffered from a mixture of anxious and depressive symptoms and who showed normal REM latency. Although the data are few, it appears that most patients with GAD (vs. patients with major depression) will have normal REM latencies (Akiskal and Lemmi 1987; Sitaram et al. 1984). This also seems to be true of the patients with so-called anxious depression who often get called "atypically depressed" (Akiskal and Lemmi 1987). If this finding is borne out in further, large-scale studies, REM latency may prove useful in the differential diagnosis of GAD, depression, and "mixed" states.

Imaging Techniques

At the time of this writing, specialized imaging techniques would rarely be utilized in making the diagnosis of GAD. However, because anxiety is so pervasive—and because it may be seen in a variety of organic brain syndromes (Cummings 1985)—imaging techniques may sometimes be useful and appropriate. For example, the "anxious" elderly patient with deficits in short-term memory probably merits a computed tomography (CT) scan. Moreover, the future may bring more specific techniques with greater utility in diagnosing a variety of anxiety disorders (see sections on panic disorder and obsessive-compulsive disorder). Interestingly, Reiman et al. (1989) found that normal volunteers had significant blood flow increases confined to the same bilateral regions of the temporal lobes when anticipating painful electric shock. In a positron-emission tomography (PET) study of GAD patients treated with benzodiazepines, Buchsbaum et al. (1987) found decreased glucose metabolic rate in the visual cortex (eyes open) and increased rate in the basal ganglia and thalamus. It remains to be seen whether the work of Reiman et al. or Buchsbaum et al. proves useful in the clinical diagnosis of GAD. At this time, their techniques must be called investigational.

Psychological Testing

If you imagine our prototypical GAD patient to be an individual with a somewhat depressive, histrionic, and obsessive overlay, you will easily understand the profile on the Minnesota Multiphasic Personality Inventory (MMPI) associated with this disorder. Typically, the GAD patient shows elevated 2, 3, and 7 scales. Given our previous discussion of the overlap between anxiety and depressive disorders, it is not surprising that scale 2—the depression scale—is elevated. Scale 3 (hysteria) is tapping ego-alien anxiety and agitation. Scale 7 (psychasthenia) measures some of the obsessional features of the GAD patient, as well as general physical complaints (Meyer 1983). Chronic autonomic hyperactivity is reflected by the elevated scale 9 score (hypomania), and you will recall that "mania" was listed in our differential diagnosis of GAD. If the individual is beginning to fear loss of control, a rise on scale 8 (schizophrenia) is likely. A high F scale is also common. probably indicating general psychopathology (Meyer 1983). On the revised Wechsler Adult Intelligence Scale (WAIS-R), the GAD patient's level of tension may lower the digit span and arithmetic scores within the verbal scaled scores. Object assembly may also be impaired (Meyer 1983).

Treatment Directions and Goals

If our biopsychosocial approach to GAD has any merit, we might expect it to be reflected in the treatment of GAD—and, indeed, this is so.

Somatic Approaches

A variety of pharmacological agents are now available for the intermittent or chronic treatment of GAD. The mainstay of treatment for many years has been the benzodiazepines (Shader 1988). Because of the risk of dependency and even physical addiction associated with these agents, caution must be exercised; the use of benzodiazepines in patients with a history of alcohol abuse, for example, is rarely indicated. Nevertheless, for the average GAD patient, short-term use of these agents is both effective and safe. Chronic use is generally discouraged in the literature, but some GAD patients may require benzodiazepine therapy for months or even years, after attempts to treat them with other somatic and nonsomatic means (see below) have failed. An American Psychiatric Association task force (American Psychiatric Association 1989) emphasized the need for frequent reassessment of the severity of the patient's anxiety, with appropriate decreases in dose or discontinuation of the benzodiazepine. Shader (1988) has summarized some of the important pharmacokinetic and pharmacodynamic principles of benzodiazepine treatment. Primarily, you should keep in mind that short- and intermediate-half-life agents without active metabolites (e.g., oxazepam and lorazepam) may be preferable in elderly patients or in those patients with compromised hepatic function. However, withdrawal from shorter-acting agents may be more severe, especially in the case of alprazolam (Shader 1988). Conversely, long-half-life agents with long-lasting, active metabolites (e.g., diazepam and chlordiazepoxide) may cause some elderly or hepatically impaired patients to feel groggy or "hung over," at least in the initial stages of treatment. Withdrawal from such agents, however, appears to be less severe. Obviously, discontinuation of the shorter-acting agents requires more time (sometimes many weeks) and closer monitoring.

A variety of nonbenzodiazepine agents may be useful in the treatment of GAD. Some, such as the tricyclics, have been around a long time and have been underutilized. Newer agents such as buspirone may be useful in patients with a history of drug abuse, because buspirone appears to be nonaddictive. However, buspirone is not useful in acute situational anxiety, because its onset of action is 1 to 2 weeks. Moreover, buspirone may not be especially effective in patients who have been "spoiled" by recent benzodiazepine use (Dubovsky 1990). Another class of agents, the beta-blockers, is finding increasing use in a variety of anxiety disorders, but the role of beta-blockers in the treatment of GAD is not yet clear. Moreover, some of the beta-blockers can cause hypotension, depression, or exacerbation of asthma.

Occasionally, a brief course of an antihistamine such as diphenhydramine may be useful in mild situational anxiety. However, these agents probably lose their (marginal) effectiveness quite soon and may cause confusion in many elderly patients.

Finally, when generalized anxiety is accompanied by features of "atypical depression" (see Chapter 4), a monoamine oxidase inhibitor (MAOI) may be helpful.

Psychotherapeutic Approaches

Behavioral approaches to GAD have focused on the somatic component of the disorder (e.g., muscle tension or tremulousness). Wilson (1989) concluded that "overall, treatment of GAD with biofeedback and relaxation procedures has yielded distinctly modest results" (p. 2034). However, treatments featuring a combination of relaxation training and some form of cognitive restructuring have shown positive effects (Wilson 1989; Woodward and Jones 1989).

The psychoanalytically oriented approach to GAD harks back to our discussion of deficient "object constancy" (see discussion of psychological factors in the biopsychosocial perspective on GAD earlier in this chapter). The interventions that prove helpful, according to psychoanalytically oriented therapists (Fishman 1989), are those that enhance object constancy in the context of a "corrective emotional experience" (to borrow Franz Alexander's term). Fishman (1989) has summarized the treatment of a 40-year-old lawyer with severe, chronic anxiety and multiple somatic complaints. The patient had experienced his mother as "a devastating presence" who attacked him whenever she felt threatened:

> First, the therapist demonstrated a consistent willingness and ability to help the patient before his anxiety reached unbearable proportions. At times, all that was required was mentioning that the therapist understood how flooded and pained the patient was. These frequent exchanges gradually convinced the patient that the angry and provocative feelings he experienced would not only not be met in kind but also could be tempered by the therapist's understanding. Eventually, the patient was able to modulate his anxiety so that he could elaborate on his fantasies without becoming flooded. He was able to work through a variety of conflicts at the basis of his impoverished sense of self. (p. 2015)

Other psychotherapeutic approaches to GAD have been advocated, with little evidence that one is superior to another. Rogerian (client-centered) therapy, emphasizing empathy and warmth, may prove helpful. On the other hand, Beck (1976) advocates a rigorous cognitive-behavioral approach, arguing that "anxiety neurosis" is essentially a "thinking disorder" in which the patient repetitively alarms himself or herself with irrational or unrealistic cognitions. Therapy is directed as substituting more realistic cognitions and adaptive behaviors for the old ones.

Finally, we should note Salzman's astute comment (American Psychiatric Association 1989) that "judicious use of benzodiazepines . . . may actually allow psychotherapy, behavioral therapy, or psychoanalytic work to proceed more efficiently and productively with the ultimate goal of further reduction in anxiety without drugs" (p. 2044).

Panic Disorder and Agoraphobia

The Central Concept

Vignette

Ms. Shpilkes was a 26-year-old single female who was brought to the emergency room by her sister, who stated, "She's just been staying in the house now for weeks . . . I can't get her to come out. She just sits and watches TV and lately she's started drinking. When I ask her what's wrong, she just says she feels like crawling out of her skin and that she's sure she's gonna die." The patient herself appeared thin, pale, and tremulous. Physical examination was notable for tachycardia and a fine resting tremor. Alcohol was detectable on her breath, but the patient was not grossly intoxicated. Ms. Shpilkes gave a history of "feeling like I'm going crazy with fear" dating back to her late teens. She described her anxiety as—at first—coming in "spikes . . . like attacks that would last a few minutes," but added, "Later it got so I was expecting an attack to come at any time. All I would do is sit around and wait. So even when I wasn't having an attack, I was still nervous. I figured it was safer being inside than out, so I kinda stopped going places. I once had an attack in the supermarket and thought I was going to die—not just physically, but of embarrassment. Everybody looked at me like I was crazy and I wondered if I was. I still wonder!"

As our vignette suggests, the attacks in panic disorder (PD) usually last minutes, or occasionally hours. At least at first, the attacks are often "spontaneous"—that is, they do not appear to be precipitated by any obvious external stressor (as in simple phobia). (Some patients do identify "internal" or intrapsychic stressors—for example, "I had a thought of my husband dying and suddenly I felt the attack coming on.") Later in the course of the disorder, the attacks may become associated with, or precipitated by, certain anxiety-provoking situations (e.g., getting stuck in a crowded tunnel while driving). DSM-IV uses the terms "unexpected (uncued)," "situationally bound (cued)," and "situationally predisposed" to describe the spectrum of "endogenicity" seen in this disorder.

True panic attacks almost always begin with a 10-minute (or shorter) period of rapidly increasing symptoms; attacks described as building more slowly (e.g., over an hour or two) should be regarded as atypical or arising from some other cause. The symptoms of the attack itself include four or more of the following: shortness of breath, dizziness, palpitations, trembling, sweating, choking, nausea, depersonalization/derealization, paresthesias, hot flashes, chest pain or tightness, fear of dying, and fear of going crazy.

As our section heading suggests, PD and agoraphobia are closely related. Agoraphobia typically involves anxiety about being outside the home, particularly in situations from which escape might be difficult. Although the exact relationship is controversial, most cases of PD show some symptoms of agoraphobia, and many cases of agoraphobia appear to follow the onset of PD. However, as Weissman (1988) has shown through several epidemiological studies, many subjects with agoraphobia have no symptoms of PD. The most popular hypothesis relating PD to agoraphobia holds that the latter develops in response to the "embarrassment" of having an attack in public or to the fear that escape from such a setting will be impossible.

Panic disorder is anything but benign. More recently, Markowitz et al. (1989) demonstrated that PD is associated with "pervasive social and health consequences similar to or greater than those associated with major depression" (p. 984). These include alcohol and other drug abuse, impaired social and marital functioning, increased use of health services, and—rather surprisingly—an increased likelihood of suicide attempts.

Historical Development of the Disorder

The history of PD is intimately connected with that of "hypochondriasis," "hysteria," and "melancholia" (see Jackson 1986 for discussion). As early as 1764, Robert Whytt described a kind of "nervous" disorder in which the patient might experience "an uneasy, though not painful sensation about the stomach, attended with low spirits, anxiety, and sometimes great timidity . . . palpitations, or trembling of the heart . . . and a sense of suffocation . . . strange persuasions of their labouring under diseases of which they are quite free; and imagining their complaints to be as dangerous as they find trouble-some" (Whytt 1768, pp. 530–532). Whytt also noted that such patients may complain of flushing and chills, a variable pulse, giddiness, and occasional disturbances of sight, sound, or smell (Jackson 1986). As we will see in our look at the differential diagnosis of PD, Whytt may have been dealing with a rather heterogeneous group, including PD patients, "hypochondriacs," depressed patients, and perhaps even some patients suffering from complex partial seizures.

By 1889, Janet had described most of the features we associate with PD, though in the case of his patient the attacks may have occurred in response to a variety of stimuli rather than "spontaneously." Janet described the patient—a woman of 39—as experiencing tightness in her throat, a desire to cry, a feeling of suffocation and labored breathing, trembling, palpitations, and diaphoresis. These symptoms sometimes occurred in response to such apparently trivial precipitants as her children sniffling (Janet and Raymond 1898).

We have already mentioned Freud's insightful separation of "anxiety neurosis" and "neurasthenia," and his observation that anxiety may be manifested either as a chronic state or as discrete attacks (Nemiah 1980a). It is this latter observation that led, much later, to the separation of GAD from PD—a distinction first recognized officially in DSM-III.

The Biopsychosocial Perspective

Biological Factors

We are just beginning to understand the biology of PD, and the research continues apace. In considering some of the theories that follow, you should keep in mind that PD, like schizophrenia and depression, may be a heterogeneous condition. Why, for example, do certain "provocative tests" for PD provoke attacks in some PD patients but not in others? With this caveat in mind, we can examine some of the leading biological hypotheses (Shear and Fyer 1988).

Central noradrenergic activation. Clinical observation has long suggested that panic symptoms are related to surges in SNS activity—

the venerable "fight or flight" response. Pharmacological studies show that agents which increase noradrenaline release are anxiogenic, whereas those that decrease firing of noradrenergic neurons are anxiolytic. Thus, yohimbine, which boosts noradrenergic function, may provoke panic attacks in some PD patients (more so than in control subjects). Conversely, clonidine, which inhibits noradrenergic function, may block yohimbine-induced panic attacks (Uhde et al. 1984). The locus coeruleus, a noradrenergic center in the midbrain, may be intimately involved in the production of panic attacks.

Peripheral autonomic hyperactivity. Some patients with panic-like symptoms appear to have heightened sensitivity to (peripheral) beta-receptor agonists such as isoproterenol. These patients may get relief of their panic symptoms with beta-blockers such as propranolol. This fact has led to the logical notion that PD is a result of peripheral beta-receptor hypersensitivity. Appealing as this model is, it has not been borne out by recent research (Shear and Fyer 1988). Moreover, most PD patients get decidedly unspectacular results with propranolol or other beta-blockers.

Respiratory dysfunction. You may recall the old saw that "breathing into a paper bag" is a good way to stop a panic attack. This may be true for some "panicky" patients, but the same maneuver may actually induce a panic attack in others. This observation led to various theories implicating carbon dioxide in the etiology of PD. Thus, Gorman et al. (1986) and Klein (1991) have suggested that PD patients may have a hypersensitive, CO_2-responsive "suffocation alarm mechanism." The commonly observed hyperventilation of the anxious or PD patient is, on this view, an attempt to maintain low levels of CO_2, thus circumventing the alarm mechanism. Another related hypothesis (Carr and Sheehan 1984) is that CO_2 decreases the pH in brain stem neurons, in turn stimulating central chemoreceptors and triggering panic in susceptible individuals. Finally, in an attempt to integrate biological and psychological mechanisms, Griez and van den Hout (1986) have suggested that patients panic with CO_2 inhalation because of their cognitive response to the (normally subclinical) somatic sensations induced by the CO_2. Most normal individuals will experience some somatic anxiety upon inhaling 35% CO_2, but not everyone will have a panic attack; it may be the cognitive-phobic quality of the PD patient's cognitions that actually brings on the attack (e.g., "Oh, my God! I'm gonna have a heart attack!").

But as Klein (1993) astutely observes, panic attacks can occur during relaxation and deepening non-REM sleep, despite the lack of danger cues or (presumably) irrational cognitions. Klein's recent review provides an integrated hypothesis of panic, the suffocation response, and specific evolutionary mechanisms. Klein summarizes the hypothesis in the following way:

> [A] physiologic misinterpretation by a suffocation monitor misfires an evolved suffocation alarm system. This produces sudden respiratory distress followed swiftly by a brief hyperventilation, panic, and the urge to flee. Carbon dioxide sensitivity is seen as due to the deranged suffocation alarm monitor. (p. 306)

We will discuss the matter of cognitions in more detail in our discussion of psychological factors.

Metabolic imbalance.   Nearly 40 years ago, Cohen and White (1951) discovered that patients with panic-like symptoms developed higher postexercise blood lactate levels than did normal control subjects. Later, Pitts and McClure (1967) made the seminal discovery that "anxiety neurotics," unlike normal control subjects, often experienced panic attacks in response to sodium lactate infusion. This led to a number of theories implicating "lactate hypersensitivity" in PD, none of which has been borne out completely. (It is important to note that roughly a third of PD patients do not show a "panic" response to lactate infusion, which suggests, as you might expect, the probable heterogeneity of this disorder.)

Psychological Factors

As an introduction to this area, let's consider the following vignette.

Vignette

Ms. Trennung was a 34-year-old married lawyer who presented with a 3-month history of "anxiety attacks" characterized by palpitations, shaking, paresthesias, and "the feeling that I'm choking to death." She had been feeling well in all respects until just after her husband of 12 years had announced that he would be filing for divorce. Her first response had been "shocked disbelief," followed by angry threats to "drag him through the courts until he drops." A few days later, the attacks began. The patient was a highly accomplished professional with no psychiatric history other than what she described as "school phobia" at age 5. She characterized this as "a horrible feeling that I would never see my mother again once she left me at school. I used to get diarrhea and feel dizzy as soon as she left the building."

This vignette brings together two strands in the psychological fabric of PD: the concept of separation anxiety and the notion of symbolic representation (Barlow 1988). The empirical research on PD strongly suggests that panic attacks in agoraphobic patients may well be an adult expression of the panic some children demonstrate upon separation from their mothers (Gittelman and Klein 1973). Psychoanalytic theory has incorporated this finding into the larger context of unconscious infantile needs and their adult counterparts.

Specifically, as Barlow (1988) notes,

adult panic would be conceived as a response to cues that have been learned or associated with earlier fundamental innate psychological and biological threats to the organism. Thus, mental imagery involving symbolic representations of very frightening early themes such as castration, separation, or parental disapproval may be sufficient to trigger panic attacks. (p. 20)

In our vignette, the obvious "trigger" was the imminent threat of divorce. In a middle-aged widowed female patient I have treated, the frequency of the patient's panic attacks increased dramatically after she learned that one of her cats had feline leukemia, showing clearly that "separation" is a uniquely personal construct.

The psychoanalytic understanding of PD is by no means alone in the marketplace of ideas; nor is it incompatible with superficially "competing" theories. The cognitive model of PD, as Barlow (1988) puts it, "assumes that the sharp spiral into panic is due to catastrophic misinterpretations of otherwise normal bodily sensations" (p. 11)—which was already intimated in our discussion of Griez and van den Hout's (1986) work.

Conditioning theory also contributes to our understanding of PD and, perhaps, of various phobic disorders as well (as will be discussed in our section on phobias). Briefly stated, conditioning theory views PD as a conditioned response to internal cues—so-called interoceptive stimuli. In one experiment, the colon of a dog was slightly stimulated at the same time that an electric shock was administered. Subsequently, the dog began to evince signs of anxiety during the natural passage of feces (Barlow 1988). Is it possible that the PD patient is similarly conditioned? The mechanism might be as follows: Initially, an interoceptive cue such as tachycardia might accompany a panic attack. A strong association is then formed between the tachycardia and the panic attack. A subsequent episode of "innocent" tachycardia acts as the trigger that sets off panic attacks, in what conditioning theorists might call a "learned alarm" (Barlow 1988).

It should be evident that a panic attack could also become "paired" with an external cue, such as a mother's dropping off her child at school. Through the process of "stimulus generalization," a much later separation—for example, the departure of one's spouse—might also trigger a panic attack. And if the panicky patient also happens to "catastrophize" by thinking "I'm having a heart attack!," we have the consummate psychoanalytic-cognitive-behavioral grand slam!

Social Factors

It is almost impossible to separate so-called psychological from social factors in any straightforward way; our psychology, after all, is largely the product of our object relations (i.e., our internalized social connections). Nevertheless, it is convenient here to examine what are commonly called "psychosocial stressors."

There is a persuasive research literature suggesting that "negative life events" often precede a patient's first panic attack or agoraphobia (Barlow 1988). For example, Roth (1959) found that 96% of a sample of 135 agoraphobic individuals reported some kind of "stress" preceding the onset of their disorder. The most common antecedent stressors were bereavement, illness or acute danger, and disruption of family or domestic relations. These stressors were seen less frequently in Roth's control patients, who were characterized as "neurotic." More recently, Roy-Byrne et al. (1986) partially replicated Roth's findings in a study of PD patients and healthy control subjects. Nevertheless, there appears to be no simple cause-and-effect relationship between stressful events and panic attacks or onset of PD. For example, many people experience severe life stressors without developing panic attacks. As Barlow (1988) noted, "The initial panic is most likely mediated by biological and/or cognitive variables such as stress-related noradrenergic . . . activity or information processing mechanisms" (p. 18) rather than by a simple stressful event. Recently, Shear et al. (1993) proposed a model in which the panic response results from an interaction between inborn neurophysiological irritability and psychological vulnerability, with the latter involving dependency/independence conflicts and disturbed object relations. According to this model, a significant life stressor falling on such "fertile soil" is likely to set off a panic attack.

Because demographic, ethnic, and cultural factors also enter into the social part of our model, we should touch on these matters as they relate to PD. One large-scale study of PD showed higher rates in women, in persons ages 25 to 44, and in separated and divorced persons. (The increased rate in women may be due partly to cultural factors that preferentially permit women to express, and seek help for, anxiety.) There appeared to be no consistent relationship with race or education (Weissman 1988). However, a study of panic attacks in three communities found higher rates among those persons with low education (Von Korff et al. 1985). (Panic "attacks," of course, are not necessarily equivalent to panic disorder.)

In Chapter 1, we discussed the ataque as a manifestation of stress and anxiety in Puerto Rican culture. We mention it now because the ataque appears to be a culturally sanctioned "cry for help" in the face of severe stress (Schlesinger and Devore 1980). Although the ataque takes various forms (e.g., tearing off clothing in public, twitching, screaming, falling into a stuporous state), it may superficially resemble a panic attack and may mistakenly lead to the diagnosis of PD.

Pitfalls in the Differential Diagnosis

Panic Disorder With or Without Agoraphobia

Organic factors. We have already discussed the "medical" differential diagnosis of GAD, and virtually the same considerations apply to the diagnosis of PD. Raj and Sheehan (1987) have thoroughly discussed this topic, and their main points bear repeating. They point out that "panic attacks" are part of the clinical picture in several medical conditions, notably thyroid disease, hypoglycemia, and pheochromocytoma. However, these authors believe that careful physical examination and history taking can all but exclude these conditions, without the need for sophisticated "screening" tests. The approach described by Raj and Sheehan (with testing being done when history or physical examination warrants it) is summarized in Table 6–5.

In addition to the above, Raj and Sheehan note that pheochromocytoma patients experience less frequent and less severe attacks than do "true" PD patients, and that somatic components of anxiety predominate over "psychic" ones in pheochromocytoma. Also, patients with pheochromocytoma rarely go on to develop agoraphobia (Starkman et al. 1985).

Raj and Sheehan clearly emphasize the importance of history and physical examination. They recommend, in addition, the following routine screening for patients presenting with panic attacks: CBC, urinalysis, renal and hepatic studies, and serum calcium and phosphorous levels. They do not advise routine thyroid function tests absent "positive" findings on history or physical; neither do they advise routine fasting blood sugar (FBS) or urine for catecholamines. Not all authorities would agree with this "cost-effective" approach. Thus, Stein and Uhde (1988)—even after finding no differences in thyroid function between 26 PD patients and 26 normal control subjects—stated that "these findings by no means obviate the need for thyroid screening in the clinical evaluation or patients presenting with panic attacks" (p. 746). In clinical practice, thyroid functions are often part of a panel of tests that includes those recommended by Raj and Sheehan, thus rendering the controversy moot. In my own practice, I order thyroid function tests on all patients presenting with panic attacks, particularly when history and physical examination are suggestive of thyroid dysfunction, or when response to standard treatment is poor.

Table 6–5. Differential diagnosis of medical disorder and panic disorder

Medical disorder	Clinical history	Physical examination	Tests
Thyroid disorder	Increased appetite, weight loss; heat intolerance; neck and chest irradiation; ^{131}I treatment; thyroidectomy	Ophthalmopathy; goiter; fine tremor; warm, moist skin	T_3, T_4 TSH
Hypoglycemia	Postprandial anxiety attacks; panic attacks with hunger; gastric surgery; insulin use; family history of adenomas	Tachycardia; warm, moist skin (if symptomatic)	FBS (if < 40, do GTT)
Pheochromo-cytoma	Familial pheochromo-cytoma; neurofibro-matosis; panic attacks accompanied by headache, sweating, and flushing; GI pain; cholelithiasis; weight loss	Hypertension (sustained or episodic); postural tachycardia and/or hypotension; café au lait spots	Urine for VMA, normeta-nephrine (24-hour)

Note. TSH = thyroid-stimulating hormone; FBS = fasting blood sugar; GTT = glucose tolerance test; VMA = vanillylmandelic acid; GI = gastrointestinal.
Source. Adapted from Raj and Sheehan 1987.

Raj and Sheehan also discuss mitral valve prolapse (MVP) and temporal lobe epilepsy as two conditions that may be associated with panic-type symptoms. However, the relationship between PD and MVP remains murky, and it is by no means clear that the latter "causes" panic attacks. Although it is worth "listening for" MVP— you may detect the classic midsystolic click and/or late systolic murmur—the implications of this condition in PD are not clear (Jacob and Turner 1988). It appears that patients with panic attacks and MVP do not differ from those with panic alone with regard to family history of PD or response to treatment (Gorman et al. 1981). However, because MVP may have long-term health consequences such as cardiac arrhythmias, it is appropriate to order echocardiography in suspected cases. Parenthetically, DSM-III-R permitted the diagnosis of PD in the presence of MVP. DSM-IV specifies that in PD without agoraphobia, "the panic attacks are not due to the direct physiological effects of a substance . . . or a general medical condition (e.g., hyperthyroidism)" (American Psychiatric Association 1994, p. 402). It may be difficult, in some cases, to establish whether a medical condition is having a "direct" effect.

Partial complex seizures (temporal lobe epilepsy) can present with symptoms similar to panic attacks (Volkow et al. 1986), an especially interesting finding in light of some recent regional cerebral blood flow studies (see subsection on adjunctive testing in PD). Both PD and temporal lobe epilepsy are paroxysmal disorders that occur without any obvious precipitants. Both may be accompanied by intense feelings of anxiety and "unreality" or depersonalization. Autonomic symptoms such as diaphoresis, flushing, hyperventilation, and tachycardia may also be present in both (Raj and Sheehan 1987). However, partial complex seizures—unlike PD—typically show automatisms (such as picking at one's clothing), a markedly altered level of consciousness, and amnesia for events occurring during the seizure. Visual and olfactory hallucinations—often seen in temporal lobe epilepsy— would be most unusual in PD.

Functional psychiatric disorders.   Panic disorder may present with symptoms suggesting one or more psychiatric disorder and vice versa. Let's consider the following case.

Vignette

A 19-year-old female presented in the ER with a complaint of "severe anxiety attacks." She gave a 3-month history of episodic anxiety characterized by sudden onset of tingling, numbness, dyspnea, and "a feeling that I'm going to die." Typically, these attacks lasted for an hour or two and usually were precipitated by "visions." When pressed to describe this last symptom, the patient became tearful and agitated. She then stated that "the whole thing started after this guy fooled around with me." She went on to describe how a man she had dated had forced her to have sex with him approximately 3 months before the onset of symptoms. The "visions" the patient described were essentially "flashbacks" of the rape and involved no delusional elaboration. Psychiatric and family history, as well as cardiac examination, were unremarkable.

You have probably deduced that the patient is actually suffering from PTSD, which we will discuss in detail at the end of this chapter. For now, keep in mind that panic-type symptoms may occur in PTSD and many other disorders. An important point in this vignette is that, strictly speaking, the patient's attacks were not "spontaneous" (as is typically the case in panic disorder). Rather, they were usually precipitated by an internal stimulus—the "flashback." Of course, it is often difficult to rule out the presence of such "mental" precipitations in PD, as we have already discussed. Other psychiatric diagnoses that may be confused with PD are listed in the Table 6–6, along with a few discriminating features.

The occurrence of panic attacks in the context of major depression poses some interesting diagnostic, prognostic, and treatment problems. First of all, unlike DSM-III, DSM-IV permits the concurrent diagnosis of major depression and PD. Moreover, there is evidence suggesting that this co-occurrence has important implications. Thus, Van Valkenburg et al. (1984) found that patients with major depression and panic had significantly more chronic depression, more family history of alcoholism, and poorer response to treatment than did patients with "pure" depression.

We noted earlier in this chapter that sedative withdrawal may produce symptoms of generalized anxiety (also see Chapter 10). In the differential diagnosis of PD, the issue of substance abuse and dependence is also extremely important (Jacob and Turner 1988). (We are considering this topic under "functional psychiatric disorders" because substance abuse and dependence disorders are listed on Axis I.) Let's examine the following vignette.

Vignette

A 42-year-old male presented to the outpatient psychiatric clinic complaining of "panic attacks" over the past 5 years. The attacks

Table 6–6.   Differential diagnosis of panic disorder (PD) and other psychiatric disorders

Condition	Differences vis-à-vis panic disorder
Other anxiety disorders	See discussion in text.
Hypochondriasis	Anxiety concerning heart or heartbeat in hypochondriasis is generalized, accompanied by belief of "serious illness," not by discrete attacks.
Somatization disorder	Shortness of breath, palpitations, dizziness, and anxiety in somatization disorder are part of larger symptom complex including body pain, and conversion symptoms (blindness, aphonia). SD is almost always in females. PD without agoraphobia is equally prevalent in males and females.
Depersonalization disorder	"Out of body" experience and feeling of "unreality" in DD are not accompanied by massive autonomic signs and symptoms (dyspnea, choking, sweating, etc.). Dizziness and sensory anesthesia may be seen in DD.
Avoidant personality disorder	Anxiety in APD focuses on social discomfort and fear of evaluation or disapproval; the APD individual has few close friends (which may be true in some PD/agoraphobic patients, but PD patients per se maintain friendships). There is prominent rejection-sensitivity in APD (cf. social phobia).

tended to occur in the morning and were characterized by tremor, palpitations, "funny feelings in my skin," and "seeing weird things." The patient requested medication for relief of these symptoms. Further interview revealed a history of heavy alcohol abuse for the preceding 6 years, usually characterized by consumption in the late evening. The patient had used alprazolam "off and on" over the years to relieve his attacks, but found that this had ceased to help in the past year.

What's going on in this case? Frankly, it's difficult to sort out the various components of the patient's anxiety. That his "panic attacks" usually occur in the morning—after a drinking bout—suggest that withdrawal from the alcohol is the primary cause. The apparent visual and tactile hallucinations (formication) suggest full-blown delirium tremens (DTs). It is also possible that the patient is withdrawing from alprazolam, whose short half-life (10 to 15 hours) and "triazolo" structure make withdrawal particularly severe. The picture may be more complex, however. Panic attacks are found frequently in alcoholic individuals and, in around 40%, may precede the excessive drinking (Jacob and Turner 1988). Many patients who experience panic attacks report using alcohol as a form of self-medication. It is possible that subsequent alcohol withdrawal predisposes them to anxiety or panic attacks. Bottom line: Have a high degree of suspicion for alcohol or substance abuse in patients complaining of "panic attacks," particularly when they are evasive or defensive about their drinking and drug history.

Agoraphobia

Agoraphobia without panic disorder is rare in clinical samples, but it may be more common in the general population (American Psychiatric Association 1987; Weissman 1988). The differential diagnosis of agoraphobia per se includes a rather motley crew of disorders: major depression, schizophrenia, paranoid disorder, social phobia, obsessive-compulsive disorder, and avoidant, paranoid, and dependent personality disorders (McNeil 1987). What do these conditions have in common? Essentially, any of them can lead to an avoidant, "housebound" state, but for widely differing reasons.

Vignette

An unemployed 47-year-old single male refused to leave his apartment beginning 1 month prior to evaluation. His brother reported that the patient "sent out" for food, or had it delivered to him, and that he was living off "welfare checks." His brother became so concerned that he had the police enter the patient's apartment and bring him into the ER. Upon evaluation, the patient stated that he was terrified of leaving his apartment because of the "attacks," which he described as intense feelings of terror accompanied by palpitations, sweating, and dyspnea. When asked if anything brought on the attacks, the patient replied, "Of course. It's the damn airplanes. Every time I go outside and a plane flies over, it bombards me with gamma radiation. Then I get the attack." He denied that the attacks ever occurred spontaneously or in the absence of the airplanes. The patient manifested no thought process disorder or hallucinations in any modality. His thought content showed no delusional material beyond the idea of influence surrounding airplanes. Until 6 months prior to evaluation, he had worked successfully as an engineering consultant.

As you can see, all who are housebound are not agoraphobic. This patient appears to fit the criteria for delusional (paranoid) disorder (see Chapter 5), and his "panic attacks" are directly related to his circumscribed delusional belief. The following questions, directed to the patient, may help you reach or exclude a diagnosis of agoraphobia (Greist and Jefferson 1988):

1. Are there specific situations or places you avoid? [The agoraphobic patient will often avoid crowded stores, open spaces, traveling on a bus or train, etc.]
2. What do you feel would happen if you would end up in one of those places or situations? [The agoraphobic will describe fear of having a panic attack, dying, of "going crazy," or of being humiliated in public because of a panic attack.]
3. Do you think your fears are realistic or a little exaggerated? [The agoraphobic patient has intact reality testing and usually recognizes the fears as exaggerated or "silly." In contrast, the schizo-

phrenic or paranoid individual will often have a rigidly held delusional belief justifying the fear.]

4. If you must face the frightening situation or place, how do you handle it? [Agoraphobic individuals will usually describe anticipatory anxiety and the use of "phobic partners" to accompany them outside the home. Some will also give a history of alcohol or substance abuse as a means to decrease anxiety.]

5. Have you ever noticed that your anxiety lessens if you "ride out" the frightening situation or are prevented from leaving it? [Many agoraphobic individuals will describe a reduction in anxiety in such fortuitous "exposure therapy" situations.]

Adjunctive Testing

Because most clinical cases of agoraphobia are associated with PD, we will focus mainly on the latter.

Neuroendocrine Studies

In their review of this topic, Shear and Fyer (1988) concluded that "the result of the neurotransmitter and neurohumoral studies to date do not clearly support any specific hypothesis of panic vulnerability" (p. 37). Nor is there any single neuroendocrine test that enables one to "diagnose" PD. There is some preliminary evidence that patients with spontaneous panic attacks have lower urinary epinephrine levels than do normal subjects. Moreover, plasma levels of prolactin are elevated at the height of most attacks and are correlated with severity of the attacks (Cameron et al. 1987). This finding, if replicated sufficiently, could be useful in distinguishing PD patients from malingerers (who, in my experience, are sometimes seeking alprazolam).

Perhaps the closest we have come to a biochemical test for PD is the sodium lactate infusion test, mentioned earlier. Some investigators have reported a 70% incidence of lactate-induced panic in PD patients compared with a negligible incidence in normal control subjects (Shear and Fyer 1988). However, other studies have failed to support this finding (Gaffney et al. 1988). Interestingly, successful treatment of PD with tricyclics significantly decreases the frequency of lactate-provoked panic attacks (Ortiz et al. 1985). On the whole, when the diagnosis is unclear, lactate infusion is a reasonable test to obtain. It remains to be seen whether other provocative tests (e.g., using carbon dioxide, caffeine, or yohimbine) will prove more useful than lactate infusion in diagnosing PD.

Sleep Studies

You may recall that REM latency (i.e., the time between sleep onset and first REM period) is often decreased in many patients with major depressive episodes (Kupfer et al. 1988). In contrast, patients with various anxiety disorders appear to have REM latencies similar to those of normal control subjects (Sitaram et al. 1984). Panic disorder patients as a group also seem to have normal REM latencies, although the number of such patients studied by means of sleep EEG is quite small and the data sometimes contradictory (Mellman and Uhde 1989). Interestingly, the subgroup of PD patients with so-called sleep panic attacks may have increased REM latency, compared with PD patients who do not have sleep panic attacks and with normal control subjects (Mellman and Uhde 1989). This suggests a biological discontinuity between nocturnal panic attacks and major depression. However, Paul (1988) has presented important data suggesting a biological affinity between anxiety and depressive disorders in general. PD patients in the Mellman and Uhde study also tended to show increased sleep latency (i.e., time needed to fall asleep), decreased sleep time, and decreased sleep efficiency.

Imaging Techniques

Imaging techniques constitute an exciting and burgeoning area of research that may soon provide objective diagnostic evidence of PD. Using PET, Reiman et al. (1986) demonstrated abnormal asymmetry of parahippocampal blood flow in lactate-vulnerable PD patients, compared with PD patients who do not panic with lactate and with control subjects. Stewart et al. (1988) found that panic attacks appear to be accompanied by a significant increase in regional cerebral blood flow in the right occipital region. Moreover, lactate infusion produced a 20% to 23% increase in whole-brain blood flow in normal control subjects and PD patients who did not panic with lactate; in contrast, PD patients who panicked with lactate infusion had only a 2.2% increase in whole-brain blood flow. These data suggest biological heterogeneity in PD patients but require replication before becoming clinically useful.

Psychological Testing

Although traditional assessment instruments may be useful in the diagnosis of PD—the MMPI, for example, often shows elevation of the 7, 3, 1, and 4 scales (Meyer 1983)—a variety of "structured interview schedules" may be more useful (Jacob and Turner 1988). The Anxiety Disorders Interview Schedule (ADIS; DiNardo et al. 1983), for example, is designed specifically to differentiate among the anxiety disorders. The ADIS also incorporates the Hamilton Anxiety and Depression Rating Scales, making it possible to quantify the anxious and depressive components of the patient's condition.

As we have seen, panic anxiety is multidimensional, having behavioral, somatic, and cognitive components. To address these dimensions, a number of testing instruments have been developed (Jacob and Turner 1988). For example, Chambless et al. (1984) have developed the Body Sensations Questionnaire (BSQ) and the Agoraphobic Cognitions Questionnaire (ACQ), which together provide a good symptomatic description of panic/agoraphobia.

Finally, we should mention some adjunctive tests that are waiting in the wings and that someday may prove clinically useful. Because heart rate can increase by up to 35 to 40 beats per minute during a panic attack, attempts have been made to utilize ambulatory cardiac monitoring in the diagnosis of PD (Jacob and Turner 1988). However, the sensitivity and specificity of heart rate as a measure of panic are low; only around 58% of panic attacks show characteristic heart rate changes, and only around 30% of tachycardia episodes are accompanied by a subjective sense of panic (Taylor et al. 1986). Other techniques, such as measurement of skin conductance, are not yet clinically feasible.

Treatment Directions and Goals

In approaching the PD patient, you will be aiming at short-term relief of "catastrophic" symptoms and long-term modification of anticipatory anxiety and agoraphobia. You will need to understand any dynamic issues that "fuel" the patient's panic attacks without assuming that "there must be some unconscious issue" behind the disorder. You will need to help the patient in very direct cognitive-behavioral ways so that he or she regains a sense of personal control. Finally, you will need to educate the patient about the course of PD and the long-term risk-benefit ratio of treatment.

Somatic Approaches

There are three "old reliables" in the pharmacotherapy of PD: high-potency benzodiazepines, tricyclic antidepressants, and MAOIs. There is also a coterie of promising "contenders" whose value has yet to be established (e.g., calcium channel blockers, beta-blockers, clonidine, and a variety of nontricyclic antidepressants).

Among the high-potency benzodiazepines, alprazolam appears to have fallen out of favor, with clonazepam rushing in to fill the void. This stems from three difficulties with alprazolam: its relatively short therapeutic action in preventing panic attacks, its tendency to promote dependence and withdrawal, and its relatively high potential of abuse (Fyer and Sandberg 1988). Alprazolam-induced mania and paradoxical agitation or disinhibition are also potential problems. Clonazepam—in doses ranging from 0.5 to 9.0 mg/day—appears to be a better alternative. It usually reduces the periods of "breakthrough" panic associated with alprazolam and appears less likely to promote dependence, severe withdrawal, or abuse than does alprazolam; however, controlled studies are needed to confirm this clinical impression (Fyer and Sandberg 1988). (By the way, be very cautious in taking a patient off alprazolam; an "ordinary" nontriazolo benzodiazepine, such as diazepam, may not "cover" all the withdrawal symptoms associated with sudden discontinuation of alprazolam.)

Among the tricyclics, imipramine is the most studied, if not the most effective, treatment; there are at least six double-blind, placebo-controlled studies establishing its efficacy in PD (Fyer and Sandberg 1988). Although effective treatment of PD may require 150 to 200 mg/day of imipramine, it is best to start out with very low doses and move up gradually—for example, 10 mg at hs, with increases at a rate of 10 mg every 2 days or so (Fyer and Sandberg 1988). Such caution is due to the fact that PD patients are notoriously sensitive to tricyclic side effects, especially the "jitters." It is important to warn patients of this side effect and to advise them that it usually subsides with time. (Some practitioners will "cover" the patient with a benzodiazepine in low doses during the first week or two of treatment [e.g., clonazepam 0.25 mg po bid], but this approach runs the risk of inducing additional side effects.) Although other tricyclics such as desipramine and nortriptyline may also be effective in PD, they have not been studied as extensively as imipramine. Of great interest is the recent study by Mavissakalian and Perel (1992) showing that PD patients treated acutely with imipramine gained protection against relapse if they were maintained on half-dosage imipramine (i.e., one-half the acute dosage) for an additional year.

The new antiobsessional drug clomipramine also appears effective, but PD patients appear peculiarly sensitive to clomipramine and may do best on relatively low doses (25 to 50 mg/day), at least initially (Grunhaus et al. 1984).

Last among the "old reliables" are the MAOIs—phenelzine, tranylcypromine, and isocarboxazid—though phenelzine (Nardil) is by far the best studied (Fyer and Sandberg 1988). The use of an MAOI, of course, presupposes that the patient is willing and able to comply with the tyramine-free diet. Although this diet is less stringent than in years past, it still requires a certain amount of "healthy" obsessiveness. Phenelzine is usually begun at 15 mg q A.M. for 3 days, followed by 30 mg q A.M. for 4 days, with increases as tolerated up to about 60 to 90 mg/day. Because insomnia is a common side effect, a benzodiazepine or trazodone (25 to 50 mg) may be necessary before bed. I have begun giving patients on MAOIs a couple of tablets of nifedipine (10 mg) to use sublingually, in case of the so-called cheese reaction to tyramine (Clary and Schweizer 1987).

Several recent studies have shown fluoxetine to be effective in the treatment of panic attacks, including attacks associated with PTSD

(Gorman et al. 1987; Nagy et al. 1993). However, some PD patients may be very sensitive to the energizing effects of fluoxetine and thus may require extremely low doses (2 to 5 mg/day) in the early phases of treatment. The role of other selective serotonin reuptake inhibitors (SSRIs) in PD has yet to be clarified.

A variety of other agents have been used to treat PD, with mixed results (Fyer and Sandberg 1988). In general, the beta-blockers have not been especially effective for panic per se, although they may reduce the "background" anxiety of the PD patient. The new anxiolytic buspirone also seems relatively ineffective in PD (Sheehan et al. 1990). Other agents such as clonidine and calcium channel blockers show some promise but remain second- or third-line treatments.

Psychosocial Approaches

Much of the supporting evidence in the area of psychosocial approaches to treatment of PD is anecdotal, and it is still not clear what form of psychotherapy is best for this disorder (Greist and Jefferson 1988). The psychoanalytic literature—contrary to most theorizing in the 1980s—often views agoraphobia as the "primary" illness in patients with panic attacks and agoraphobia (Fishman 1989). Great importance is attached to the "self-fragmentation" associated with failures of "early holding and affirmation" (Fishman 1989). The therapist examines and explores the feelings of emptiness and impoverished self-esteem that are thought to underlie panic-agoraphobic symptoms. Latent feelings of dependency on others (for love, protection, etc.) are also examined. Fishman (1989) gives a vignette, excerpted below, that nicely summarizes the psychoanalytic view of the PD patient:

> Mr. G. adamantly avoided any awareness of his need of and vulnerability to women because of the repeated devastation he had experienced from his mother. He, like all other panic patients, feared most an even greater fear: to be in a self-fragmenting terror. The major cost of his vigilance against this danger was a skittish manner of relating. He could not bear to receive any serious feedback from his girlfriend. (p. 2017)

A direct or premature therapeutic assault on the patient's core "neediness" may only intensify the patient's resistance. Rather, the therapist initially tries to empathize with the patient's ambivalent dependence on others. Later, the therapist tries to link current difficulties to childhood problems in order to deepen the patient's awareness of his or her dependent traits, which may become manifest in the transference. Eventually, these, too, may be "worked through" with the patient.

The psychodynamic approach to PD has not been validated by well-controlled studies, nor is it necessarily incompatible with other approaches. Cognitive-behavioral approaches are receiving increasing study and appear to benefit many PD/agoraphobic patients (Craske 1988). The basic procedure for treating agoraphobia entails repeated exposure to situations that are feared and/or avoided and that have become associated with panic attacks—a technique known as in vivo exposure (Craske 1988). Direct treatment of panic has also been attempted, using "interoceptive exposure." This entails the repeated induction of autonomic effects associated with panic (e.g., rapid heart beat), with a resultant "desensitization" to these internal stimuli after a few weeks. "Cognitive reattribution" (Beck and Emery 1985) may also be useful, in which the PD patient is taught to interpret bodily sensations more realistically. For example, instead of thinking "I am going to die!" in response to a rapid heartbeat, the patient is taught to think "This is just a panic attack. I've gotten through these before and I'll get through this one." Such cognitive strategies may be combined with various relaxation techniques aimed at reducing hyperventilation and muscle tension (Craske 1988). Adjunctive medication may enhance outcome.

Integrated Case History

Ms. Temblor, a 24-year-old single woman with no prior psychiatric history, presented for evaluation with the chief complaint that "I'm too scared to leave the house . . . I feel like I'm gonna die or really lose it." Her mother had accompanied the patient to the psychiatrist's office, noting, "I take her everywhere she goes." The patient gave a history of "nerve attacks" over the preceding 6 months, characterized by shortness of breath, palpitations, sweating, choking sensation, and a fear of dying or "going crazy." Typically, the attacks would come on "out of the blue," build rapidly to a crescendo, and dissipate in about an hour. The patient was experiencing as many as four attacks per week. Sometimes, the attacks seemed to be precipitated by the thought that "I'm gonna be alone like this for the rest of my life." When asked to explain this remark, the patient related that the attacks had started shortly after she had broken up with her boyfriend of 2 years.

Since the breakup, she had been living alone in the apartment they once had shared. The patient's mother added, "She used to be like this when I took her to kindergarten . . . I couldn't get her to let go of my dress . . . she'd even throw up, she was so nervous." The patient's mother had suffered from similar attacks when she was in her 30s, but "they just seemed to go away." The patient gave no history of significant depression, guilt, weight loss, or sleep disturbance, but described "always worrying that I'm gonna have another attack." She had been largely confined to her house for the past 3 months, venturing out only when accompanied by her mother.

Mental status examination was unremarkable, except for significant cognitive distortions regarding her "attacks"—for example, "I always think I'm gonna have a heart attack . . . or that maybe I'm schizo or something . . . sometimes I feel like the only way to end this is to jump out the window."

Medical history was noncontributory, except for significant caffeine use (5 cups of coffee per day) and occasional episodes of "my heart skipping a beat" for several years preceding onset of frank panic attacks. A subsequent physical examination revealed "midsystolic click/murmur suggestive of mitral valve prolapse [MVP]," which was confirmed on echocardiogram.

Psychological testing revealed elevation of scales 7, 3, 1, and 4 on the MMPI and a score of 30 on the Hamilton Anxiety Rating Scale.

The diagnosis after assessment was "panic disorder with agoraphobia, possibly complicated by mitral valve prolapse." The case formulation also noted "possible childhood separation anxiety (school phobia) and recent loss of significant other" as psychodynamic factors to be explored.

The patient was begun on imipramine, 25 mg at hs, with the warning that "this may make you feel a little jittery during the first week or so." She was able to tolerate gradual increases over the following 3 weeks, up to 150 mg/day. Beta-blockers were considered for her MVP, but a cardiac consultation advised "waiting to see how she does on the imipramine," noting that "sometimes mitral valve prolapse will actually disappear with treatment of the panic disorder." The patient was advised to reduce and eventually eliminate caffeine. She also entered a cognitive-behavioral form of therapy that emphasized correction of her cognitive distortions, desensitization to interoceptive stimuli (palpitations, dyspnea, etc.), and "graded exposure" aimed at getting her out of the house. After moderate improvement in the patient's symptoms and development of sufficient rapport, her therapist began exploring some of the dynamic factors contributing to the PD. Particular attention was given to the patient's long-standing fear of "being abandoned" and to the impact of her recent breakup. The connection between separation anxiety and onset of panic attacks was clarified and worked through over the subsequent 2 months. Three months after initial intake, the patient was markedly improved, experiencing only one or two attacks per month.

Social Phobia and Specific (Simple) Phobia

Although some recent data suggest that social and simple phobias may have distinct familial patterns (Fyer et al. 1990), we will consider them together because of their historical and symptomatic associations. (For example, both disorders are often associated with situationally bound panic attacks.) In DSM-IV, the term "specific phobia" replaces "simple phobia," but there have been few major changes in criteria from DSM-III-R.

The Central Concept

Let's approach phobic disorders by considering a patient who has features of both specific and social phobia.

Vignette

Mr. Kleinhans was a 42-year-old professional horse breeder who presented with the complaint that "I can't stand being in crowded rooms." The problem had begun about 3 years ago, seemingly following (by some weeks) an embarrassing episode during a lecture that Mr. K. had given. In the course of addressing a group of colleagues in an extremely crowded hotel conference room, Mr. K. noted laughter from the back of the room. Fearing that the laughter was directed at him, he became flustered, stumbled in his presentation, and experienced a choking sensation associated with profuse sweating. He was unable to complete his talk and left the meeting feeling "humiliated and panicky." Ever since that event, Mr. K. has been unable to sit in a crowded room without fearing that people were "looking at me funny," or experiencing dyspnea and profuse sweating. Over time, Mr. K. also felt panicky entering any sort of conference room, even when no one else was present and he was not required to speak. Mr. K. did not experience spontaneous panic attacks and knew "intellectually" that "people probably aren't laughing at me." He did, however, describe himself as "a sensitive person all my life . . . even in grade school, I used to fear the teacher more than the other kids did."

This vignette brings out the key features of both social phobia and specific (simple) phobia and shows how sometimes they may be confused with panic disorder. In social phobia, there is a persistent fear of situations in which the individual may face the scrutiny or criticism of others. Exposure to the feared situation usually produces an anxiety response characterized by panic-like symptoms. Anticipatory anxiety is common (e.g., prior to a public-speaking engagement). In specific phobia, there is a persistent fear of some "circumscribed stimulus" (other than social situations), with resultant anxiety and avoidance. Classic examples include claustrophobia (fear of closed spaces), animal phobias, and fear of germs or contamination (mysophobia). (We are using the word "fear" more or less synonymously with "anxiety" in this discussion, as is done in DSM-IV.) In both social phobia and simple phobia, there is marked interference with the individual's occupational or social functioning, and/or marked distress about having the fear. (In dynamic terms, the condition is "ego-alien.") In both conditions, the individual retains reality testing (i.e., understands that the fear is excessive or unreasonable).

Historical Development of the Disorders

The history of phobic disorders is intimately bound up with Freud's theories concerning "the transformation of undischarged sexual energy" (Nemiah 1980c, 1985c), repression, and symbolization. We will say more of this below. But we cannot avoid mentioning Freud's famous case of Little Hans, the 5-year-old boy who developed a phobia of horses. The dynamics of the case have been beautifully summarized by John Nemiah (1980c), as follows:

> [Little Hans's] naturally occurring oedipal libidinal strivings for his mother and his rivalrous aggression toward his father were repressed as forces unacceptable to his developing ego. Unable to find an outlet for discharge because of repression, the drives were partially transformed into anxiety. At the same time, some of the aggressive energy was projected outward onto the little boy's father. . . . it was still difficult, however, for Little Hans to find relief from his painful anxiety, since the father who provoked it was constantly present. . . . to find relief, he needed . . . the displacement of the anxiety related to his father onto horses, objects that in Little Hans's experiences had been associatively linked with his conflict and could, therefore, act in a symbolic way as the carrier of the anxiety. Since horses could be avoided, Hans could escape from anxiety. (p. 1496)

You may find the psychoanalytic formulation a bit contorted, but it has had an incontestable and profound influence on our formulation and treatment of phobias. As we shall see, such dynamic mechanisms are not incompatible with other causal factors.

The Biopsychosocial Perspective

Biological Factors

There have been few investigations of biological factors in social and specific phobic disorders. From the standpoint of genetics, a study by

Fyer et al. (1990) showed a significantly higher risk for simple phobia among first-degree relatives of simple phobic probands compared with first-degree relatives of normal control subjects. Female relatives were more likely to be affected than male relatives. Significant between-group differences were not found for risk of other anxiety disorders, including social phobia. These results—though preliminary—suggest at least a familial, if not a genetic, factor in simple phobia. Similar findings on social phobia were recently reported by Fyer et al. (1993). These authors found that relatives of social phobia probands have a significantly higher risk for social phobia, but not for other anxiety disorders, including simple phobia.

The biology of phobic disorders remains obscure, but some hints derived from treatment outcome are emerging (Liebowitz et al. 1988). We do know that during a performance of the feared activity (e.g., public speaking), the social phobic patient will show an increase in heart rate from around 75 to 130, and a doubling of adrenaline levels. The individual becomes distracted by the rapid heartbeat, trembling, sweating, and so forth, and wonders if others are perceiving these symptoms (Liebowitz et al. 1992). The individual's mental processes become fuzzy, resulting in poor performance (which would be expected to reinforce the initial anxiety). Liebowitz et al. (1992) have hypothesized that the social phobia per se (not necessarily these acute autonomic changes) may be related to CNS dopamine dys-regulation, because the social phobic patient responds to MAOIs, which boost dopamine (see discussion of somatic approaches to the treatment of social phobia). However, MAOIs boost other biogenic amines as well; moreover, it is usually hazardous to infer biochemical etiology from pharmacological response.

Psychological Factors

We have already alluded to the psychoanalytic formulation of phobic disorders. Despite much controversy over Freud's views, our modern understanding of social and simple phobias is influenced by psycho-analytic theory. In Freud's later formulation of phobias, anxiety was not the *result* of repression (see Nemiah's summary of the Little Hans case presented earlier in this section) but the *cause* of repression; that is, anxiety prompts the ego to employ repression as a defense against an unacceptable impulse, one that is generally sexual in nature. This is the concept of "signal anxiety": anxiety "signals" the ego to employ repression as a defense. This may be only partially successful, however, and "auxiliary" defenses such as symbolization and displacement may be called upon and may be manifested as phobic symptoms. The diagram in Figure 6–2 depicts this scheme. Recent modifications of Freud's model include other forms of anxiety besides that associated with "castration" or "oedipal level" anxiety. Thus, pregenital sexual impulses, aggressive impulses, and—perhaps most important—separation anxiety may all "alert" the ego to activate phobic defenses. Obviously, it is difficult to obtain empirical evidence in support of these intrapsychic mechanisms; however, as a heuristic model, the scheme presented in Figure 6–2 may be helpful to the therapist. Moreover, if you decide to treat the patient with a psychodynamically oriented form of therapy, this scheme may be crucial to your handling of the case.

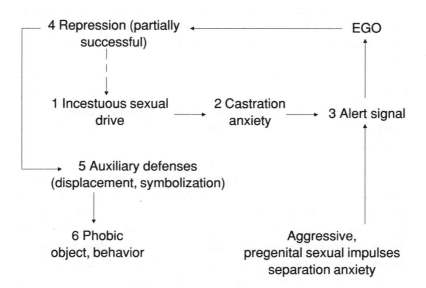

Figure 6–2. Psychodynamic model of phobia.

The psychodynamic model of phobia has been challenged by alternative theories (see discussion of social factors in panic disorder earlier in this chapter). J. B. Watson and Rayner (1920), for example, introduced the concept of phobia as a conditioned response. They presented the case of "Little Albert," who developed a phobia of rats and rabbits after having been exposed repetitively to a loud noise in the presence of these animals. This model may partially explain the development of certain simple phobias, such as fear of snakes. More recently, operant conditioning theory has attempted to explain the persistence of phobic avoidance, even in the absence of any apparent external reinforcement. On this view, anxiety is seen as a drive that motivates the patient to avoid the source of the anxiety. Such avoidant behaviors (e.g., staying away from public-speaking engagements) are maintained because they result in reduced anxiety.

Social Factors

With respect to simple phobias, a variety of interpersonal, cultural, and social factors appear to be at work. Of course, as always, it is difficult (and a bit artificial) to separate such factors from the "psychology" of the individual—yesterday's interpersonal contact may be today's "internal object." It is interesting that many otherwise "phobic" individuals can function in the company of a so-called phobic companion. What does this mean? Is the phobia itself—for example, the fear of crossing bridges—the result of some kind of separation anxiety that is mitigated by the phobic companion? Or does the companion function merely to "calm down" the phobic individual in the phobic situation? The particular type of simple phobia may suggest different interpersonal dynamics. Most animal phobias seem to begin in childhood— perhaps during the oedipal period (Marks and Gelder 1966). In contrast, most circumscribed phobias of heights, driving, closed spaces, and air travel seem to begin most frequently in the fourth decade (American Psychiatric Association 1987). Could it be that the phobic "animal" is symbolically related to the child's father or mother, as suggested by the case of Little Hans? In contrast, could phobias of later onset have a symbolic connection to nonparental "significant others" (e.g., one's spouse or lover)? We do not have the answers to these questions. However, there is evidence that simple phobias may be maintained (not necessarily caused) by interpersonal factors. As P. Friedman and Goldstein (1974) have noted,

> In some cases, secondary gains from a relationship of dependence on others—e.g., in the case of phobias which restrict the individual's locomotion—may contribute to the persistence of phobias whose origin is due to other factors. It is of interest to note in this connection that . . . dependence is a frequent characteristic of phobic patients . . . the phobic need for dependence on others may also have a strongly hostile underlying quality. (p. 125)

Cultural factors may also affect the development of simple phobias. For example, Burnam et al. (1987) showed that Mexican-American women ages 40 years or older had a significantly higher rate of current phobia than non-Hispanic white women in the same age group. However, this study lumped all phobias under one category and thus may have included agoraphobic individuals among simple and social phobic individuals. The authors also pointed out that socioeconomic factors (not controlled for in the study) rather than ethnicity may have contributed to this difference. In a study of psychiatric disorders in Puerto Rico, Canino et al. (1987) found a prevalence of social and simple phobia similar to that in "Anglo" populations. However, this study showed higher lifetime and 6-month prevalences of social and simple phobia in urban areas than were found in rural areas of Puerto Rico. The reasons for this difference are not clear, though one might speculate on the role of urban stressors in precipitating phobic symptoms.

It may seem redundant to speak of "social factors" in social phobia. Nevertheless, it is reasonable to ask what interpersonal, cultural, and socioeconomic factors may be correlated with this persistent fear of scrutiny by others. Liebowitz (1990) has hypothesized that social phobia encompasses two subtypes: discrete social phobia, as exemplified by simple public-speaking anxiety; and generalized social phobia, as characterized by widespread social avoidance affecting many aspects of the phobic individual's life. Liebowitz further suggests that social phobic individuals in general share with some "atypical depressive" individuals a marked rejection sensitivity. Indeed, if we conceive of rejection sensitivity as the underlying disorder, we can posit an "avoidant" pathway leading to social phobia and a "depressive" pathway leading to atypical depression (and especially the syndrome Liebowitz and his colleagues have called "hysteroid dysphoria"). Liebowitz—drawing on the work of Jerome Kagan—also believes that "shyness" and "submissiveness" as part of an individual's inborn temperament play a role in social phobia. While Liebowitz's ideas are intriguing, one must also ask whether they actually explain social phobia or merely break it down into its constituent parts—rejection sensitivity, shyness, submissiveness, and so forth. Perhaps more useful is Liebowitz's suggestion that separation anxiety plays a role in the development of some social phobias, thus bringing this condition into the "fold" of panic disorder and agoraphobia. Indeed, as we shall see, the differential diagnosis of these conditions is often complex.

Pitfalls in the Differential Diagnosis

Social Phobia

Vignette

Mr. Schreber was a 45-year-old engineer referred for psychiatric evaluation by his minister, who believed that the patient had "a social phobia." The patient himself gave a 3-year history of avoiding social gatherings of any kind. He had even given up going to his neighborhood church, where he had once been an active participant in many church functions. When asked about his reluctance to socialize, the patient gave this explanation: "Well, it's hard to explain, Doctor. I get embarrassed around people and a little scared. I don't think I trust them. You see, Doctor, I find that people are always, well . . . staring at my crotch. Especially men. It's like they don't really believe I'm a man or something . . . like they have to check me out to make sure. Sometimes it feels like they are burning a hole in my pants with their eyes." The patient showed no thought process disorder and gave no history of auditory hallucinations. There were no delusional ideas except as already noted. The patient described his premorbid and childhood history as unremarkable, "except that I've always kind of shied away from people and felt a little different."

If you feel that we're missing important data in this case, you're right. But so far, Mr. Schreber sounds suspiciously like his namesake, Daniel Paul Schreber, who was the focus of Freud's study of paranoid psychosis. Indeed, our Mr. Schreber has the hallmarks of someone with DSM-IV delusional disorder—probably of the persecutory type. Freud posited an underlying homosexual dynamic in paranoia that seems evident in our vignette. This is not commonly seen in "pure" social phobia, nor is loss of reality testing. Also, note the age at onset in our Mr. Schreber's case (i.e., age 42). This later age at onset is fairly typical of delusional disorder. In contrast, social phobia usually has its onset around puberty and rarely presents de novo after age 30 (Goldman 1988).

Marked anxiety in and avoidance of social situations may occur in a wide range of psychiatric disorders (Figure 6–2). As a general rule, the "reason" for the patient's avoidance in these other disorders clearly differs from that given in true social phobia. For example, the socially avoidant individual with a primary major depressive disorder may say, "I just don't feel like being around anybody. I don't have the energy or interest." (Severely depressed individuals, of course, may not have the energy to make such a long statement!) Avoidant personality disorder poses some sticky diagnostic issues and may actually coexist with social phobia. In avoidant personality disorder, the avoidance of social contact tends to be more pervasive than in social phobia; that is, the avoidant individual often has no close friends and rarely enters into meaningful relationships. In contrast, the social phobic individual may be fairly successful, personable, and well liked, but is unable to "perform" in specific social settings (e.g., speaking in public).

Social phobia may also be confused, or may "overlap" with, several other anxiety disorders (Table 6–7), as discussed later in this chapter.

Specific (Simple) Phobia

Ordinarily, the diagnosis of specific phobia is not likely to involve a complex set of conditions for exclusion. Goldman (1988) points out that some "flying phobia" is not truly a "fear of flying" (or of airplanes) but a form of agoraphobia; that is, the individual fears confinement in the plane's cabin without means of escape. In schizophrenia, certain objects or situations may be avoided, but the patient does not recognize the irrational nature of the anxiety. In obsessive-compulsive disorder, as we shall see, certain stimuli may be avoided, but such avoidance occurs in the context of a recurrent, ego-alien idea, impulse, or behavior. To appreciate this distinction, let's consider the following.

Vignette

A 37-year-old male presented in psychotherapy with the chief complaint of "germ phobia." He insisted on cleaning off the chair in the therapist's office several times before sitting down. He often felt the need to wear rubber gloves when shopping "in order to keep from contaminating everything." He acknowledged that this might be an irrational fear, but stated, "I can't stop myself from thinking this way." On further exploration in therapy, the patient revealed a long history—preceding the "germ phobia"—of recurrent, intrusive

Table 6–7.   Differential diagnosis of social phobia

Diagnosis	Clues to differential
Simple phobia	Phobic stimulus is not a social situation involving possibility of humiliation.
Panic disorder with agoraphobia	Origin of condition is often characterized by spontaneous panic in nonsocial context.
Obsessive-compulsive disorder	Avoidance of social situation is based on intrusive ego-alien idea (e.g., contamination by others' clothing); reality testing is intact.
Posttraumatic stress disorder	Avoidance is based on generalized numbing or detachment or on the effort to avoid reexperiencing the original trauma.
Schizophrenia/ delusional disorder	A delusional idea underlies the avoidance (e.g., in schizophrenia: hallucinations, thought process disorder, abnormal affect, etc.).
Avoidant personality disorder	See discussion in text.

thoughts involving the idea of defecating in his pants. He had no recent history of actually soiling his pants, though, as a child, he had been severely punished for having done so while walking home from school. He recalled his father's laughing at him for this and his mother's calling him "a filthy little boy." At around age 20, the patient began experiencing the recurrent, ego-alien thought "Don't mess your pants," or "You've messed your pants." This roughly coincided with his first sexual involvement with a woman he had met at college. Subsequently, he developed a ritualistic habit of checking his underpants throughout the day and of cleaning any chair he would sit on. The patient explained these behaviors by stating, "It's not really that I'm afraid of picking up germs, so much as I am of spreading them." However, he had recently begun ruminating about the possibility that others might be soiling their pants and thus contaminating him.

Although phobic features are present in this case, the presence of intrusive, ego-alien ideas involving defecation *preceding* the "germ phobia" suggests an obsessive-compulsive disorder.

Adjunctive Testing

Neuroendocrine Studies

Because we don't know the pathophysiology of social or simple phobias, it will come as no surprise that we don't know the neuroendocrinology of these disorders, either. It may be significant, however, that the lactate infusion test seems to produce different results in social phobic versus panic disorder patients. Thus, Liebowitz et al. (1985) found that lactate infusion produced panic attacks in 10 of 20 patients with panic disorder compared with only 1 of 15 patients with social phobia, suggesting, to these authors, a different pathophysiology in the two disorders.

Imaging Techniques

Imaging techniques are an area of investigation that is still in its infancy with respect to specific and social phobia. A study by Mountz et al.

(1989) showed no differences in regional cerebral blood flow between patients with "animal phobia" and normal control subjects. It remains to be seen what social phobic patients or patients with specific phobias will show on PET and other imaging techniques.

Psychological Testing

Standard tests such as the MMPI are not strikingly abnormal in social and simple phobic patients (Meyer 1983). Social phobic individuals may show a mildly elevated F scale, reflecting their concern about obtaining help, and a modestly lowered 9 scale, reflecting decreased "outgoingness" (Meyer 1983). Simple phobic individuals may also show a moderately elevated F scale, as well as minor elevations on scales 2, 3, and 7, reflecting depression and rumination.

More useful, perhaps, than such standard tests are structured interview questionnaires that help "dissect" social phobia from other anxiety disorders (Reich et al. 1988). The specific symptoms reported more commonly in panic disorder patients than in social phobic patients are palpitations, chest pain, tinnitus, blurred vision, headaches, and fear of dying. Social phobic patients are more likely than panic disorder patients to report dry mouth (Reich et al. 1988).

Treatment Directions and Goals

Social Phobia

Somatic approaches.   Liebowitz and colleagues (1988, 1990) have suggested that the more discrete form of social phobia (e.g., public-speaking anxiety) may respond to small doses of propranolol (10 to 20 mg 1 to 2 hours before performance). It appears that the more generalized form of social phobia responds quite well to the MAOI phenelzine, although it may take up to 8 weeks before response is seen. Interestingly, the efficacy of MAOIs does not seem related to the patient's degree of depression but may relate directly to what Liebowitz et al. (1988) have called "interpersonal hypersensitivity." (Phenelzine may not be effective for discrete performance anxiety, however.) Benzodiazepines (notably alprazolam and clonazepam) may also be helpful in treating social phobia, but the risk of dependence must be borne in mind (Ontiveros and Fontaine 1990). It is probably too early to say whether tricyclics are effective in either type of social phobia, but Liebowitz (1990) doubts that they are.

Psychosocial approaches. The psychoanalytic literature does not deal with social phobia as a discrete disorder, but rather as part of a constellation of character traits (Fishman 1989). A psychoanalytic approach may be useful if, for example, social phobia is embedded in a narcissistic character disturbance. Thus, Fishman (1989) describes a patient presenting with social phobic symptoms in whom

> the core issue was the patient's difficulty experiencing adequate self-valuation in everyday life. Psychotherapy in this instance proved to be of considerable benefit by helping the patient to recognize his basic lack of confidence, his need for exaggerated reparative responses from others, and his poorly contained vengeance when these responses were not forthcoming. Simple behavioral paradigms could not encompass the relevant center of the difficulty. (p. 2023)

Fishman also notes that social phobic symptoms may be based on a classic "neurotic conflict"; for example, a young man avoids parties because he fears his own sexual impulses (which, simultaneously, he wishes to express). In such cases, psychoanalytically oriented therapy may be helpful.

On the other hand, growing evidence suggests that a cognitive-behavioral approach may suffice for many patients with social phobia (Liebowitz 1990; Wilson 1989). Treatment may involve in vivo exposure to the feared situation, progressive relaxation techniques, rational self-talk, and social skills training. Liebowitz (1990) believes that group therapy focusing on the irrational cognitions that undermine self confidence (e.g., "I'm stupid. I have nothing to contribute") may be most effective. Role playing and rehearsal in such groups may also be helpful. Apparently, group therapy of this sort may be of benefit in both the discrete and generalized forms of social phobia.

Specific Phobia

Somatic approaches.   The literature is sparse with respect to the pharmacotherapy of DSM-III-R simple phobia. Nemiah (1980c) states that chlordiazepoxide and diazepam "are both effective aids to the patient in his struggle with the phobic situation," but there appear to be few reliable studies in this area. It makes clinical sense to consider using a benzodiazepine when a patient must face a phobic situation for a brief period of time (e.g., when a patient with "airplane phobia" must take a plane). The role of tricyclics and MAOIs remains to be defined.

Psychosocial approaches.   Fishman (1989) has noted that the psychoanalytic literature does not separate panic from simple phobic anxiety, adding that "both types of anxiety disorders often involve similar underlying conflicts and personality deformations" (p. 2019). Fishman discusses a case of "elevator phobia" that stemmed from the patient's underlying fears of abandonment and intimacy. Therapy involved the interpretation of these unconscious issues, including their manifestations in the transference. Fishman notes, however, that "if a phobic symptom can be treated in isolation by . . . behavioral techniques, it should be" (p. 2019). Indeed, the cognitive-behavioral treatment of simple phobic disorders is gaining increasing prominence. Goldman (1988) has noted that "spider phobia" can often be alleviated in a single 2-hour session using in vivo exposure. Similarly, patients with flying phobia can be treated in one or two flights in a small plane, in which they are exposed repeatedly to phobic stimuli such as takeoffs and landings. Using such behavioral methods, around 80% of patients with simple phobias will improve (Ost 1989). Incidentally, Walder et al. (1987) have shown that "fear of flying" is not a unitary phenomenon but may involve more discrete fears of being enclosed, crashing, becoming airsick, and so forth.

Finally, hypnosis, self-hypnosis, biofeedback, and related procedures may be integrated into both the psychodynamic and the behavioral approaches to phobic disorders (Frankel and Orne 1989).

Obsessive-Compulsive Disorder

The Central Concept

Once thought to be a rare condition, obsessive-compulsive disorder (OCD) is now known to afflict as many as 2% to 3% of individuals in the United States—more than 4 million people (Jenike 1989). Let's look at a typical case involving both obsessions and compulsions.

Vignette

Mr. Tobor, a 35-year-old computer programmer, presented with a 10-year history of what he described as "feeling like my thoughts are taking over my whole life." He suffered from the recurrent thought that he had neglected some vital step in developing a computer program for his company and that this resulted in the spread of a computer "virus" that would "shut down all the important computer systems in the country." These thoughts, which had waxed and waned over the years, had been exacerbated recently when reports of such a "virus" made national headlines. Mr. Tobor stated, "Intellectually, I know I didn't do anything wrong at all. But I can't get the stupid thought out of my head. What's really bad is that I keep going back to the office two or three times a night, checking and double-checking to make sure I haven't screwed up the program. It's nuts, I know, but if I don't go back and check, I can't sit still—I climb the walls at home and can't fall asleep." Mr. Tobor described significant feelings of anxiety and depression following the recent exacerbation of these intrusive thoughts and actions. He had increased his consumption of alcohol in recent months, "just to calm myself down." As a result of his need to "check back at the office," Mr. Tobor was unable to socialize and had recently broken off a brief relationship with a young woman "who thought I was a real nut case."

Mr. Tobor's case is fairly typical for OCD. He experienced recurrent, intrusive, illogical thoughts that he recognized as his own, and not "broadcast" to him from some external source. He felt compelled to act in order to neutralize these thoughts, and when unable to do so, he would experience intense discomfort. Nonetheless, he derived no real pleasure from the performance of his ritualized "checking" behavior. His social life had suffered as a consequence. In some cases of extreme OCD, the individual is virtually paralyzed. I recently examined a young woman whose obsessive processing of her own thoughts—in an attempt to say precisely the right thing—resulted in a kind of obsessional mutism: she would move her mouth spasmodically but could enunciate no words.

Insel (1990) describes four clinical subtypes of OCD, characterized by varying obsessions, compulsions, degrees of "resistance" to symptoms, and associated features. Most common are patients who have contamination obsessions and "washing" compulsions. These patients show moderate resistance and a good deal of avoidant behavior; for example, they will avoid public rest rooms, doorknobs, hand shaking, and so forth. The next subtype includes patients with "obsessional doubt," as typified by our Mr. Tobor. These patients generally show "checking" compulsions, intense resistance, and high degrees of guilt. (Many describe a very strict religious upbringing.) Third are those with so-called pure obsessions (e.g., intrusive urges or thoughts of a sexual or aggressive nature). Compulsions are often absent, or, if present, they are on a "cognitive" level (i.e., having counterthoughts to neutralize the obsessions). These patients are often very secretive about their upsetting thoughts or urges. Insel (1990) describes patients with "primary obsessional slowness": those who may spend 3 or 4 hours a day on a simple activity like shaving. Curiously, these patients show little resistance to their habits and little anxiety. (One wonders if such patients have features in common with passive-aggressive personality disorder, which, in DSM-IV, is included under the NOS [not otherwise specified] heading.) Finally, DSM-IV uses the specifier "poor insight type" for the OCD patient who, "for most of the time during the current episode, . . . does not recognize that the obsessions and compulsions are excessive or unreasonable (American Psychiatric Association 1994, p. 423).

Historical Development of the Disorder

The physician and clergyman Richard Napier (1559–1634) (see Jackson 1986 for discussion) left us a vivid description of a woman with an "obsessive-compulsive preoccupation of delusional proportions":

> Extreme melancholy, possessing her for a long time, with fear; and sorely tempted not to touch anything for fear that then she shall be tempted to wash her clothes, even upon her back. Is tortured until . . . she be forced to wash her clothes, be them never so good and new. Will not suffer her husband, child, nor any of the household to have any new clothes until they wash them for fear the dust of them will fall upon her. Dareth not go to the church for treading on the ground, fearing lest any dust should fall upon them. (Mac-Donald 1981, p. 154)

It is hard to tell from Napier's description whether this patient was actually psychotically depressed, or whether she suffered from severe OCD with phobic features. As we saw in our earlier case of apparent "germ phobia," it is often hard to disentangle obsessive-compulsive from phobic symptomatology. Indeed, by the latter part of the 19th century, George M. Beard (1839–1883) had lumped obsessive-compulsive and phobic states, along with other anxious-depressive conditions, under the rubric of "neurasthenia," which was conceptualized as "a want of nervous force." Even Freud, in his early formulations, failed to differentiate between phobic and obsessive-compulsive phenomena—that distinction came in his later psychodynamic schema (Nemiah 1980b, 1980c). Some modern writers still include phobias in the clinical syndrome of OCD, while others consider that phobic and obsessive-compulsive phenomena lie along a continuum (Nemiah 1980b, 1980c). And, as Napier's case suggests, there is also controversy as to the demarcation between OCD and psychotic disorders (Pies 1984). We shall say more of this in our subsection on differential diagnosis.

It is of interest that German clinicians of the 19th century viewed obsessive-compulsive pathology as essentially a disorder of cognition, foreshadowing, in some ways, the work of Beck, Ellis, and other "cognitive" therapists. Westphal, for example, believed that the core of OCD (or what he called *Vorstellung*) was the emergence of irrational thoughts (Insel 1990). He recognized that OCD patients knew that their obsessions were senseless, and used the term "abortive insanity" to describe OCD. Westphal also observed that, unlike patients with "true" insanity, the OCD patient would get worse rather than better when put into an asylum (Insel 1990).

The Biopsychosocial Perspective

Biological Factors

The biology of OCD is not completely understood, but we are coming closer. First, there is good evidence that familial and probably genetic factors are involved (Jenike 1989). Family members of OCD patients have a higher prevalence of OCD (and of anxiety and affective disorders) than do controls. Indeed, 20% of the nuclear family members have overt OCD, and another 15% have a subclinical form of the disorder. Isolated case reports indicate a higher concordance for OCD in monozygotic than in dizygotic twins, but rigorous studies are lacking.

PET scan studies suggest abnormalities in the frontal lobes and basal ganglia of patients with OCD compared with depressed and healthy control subjects (Baxter et al. 1987, 1992). Specifically, several PET scan studies have shown evidence of "hypermetabolism" in orbitofrontal regions of OCD patients (Swedo et al. 1992). Volumetric CT scan studies suggest bilateral decreased caudate volumes in OCD patients compared with normal control subjects (Luxenberg et al. 1988).

What might such findings mean in the larger context of neuropsychiatric disorders? It is intriguing that around 20% of patients with OCD have tics, and that around 25% of patients with Tourette's disorder—a tic disorder—will develop obsessive-compulsive features (Jagger et al. 1982; Lishman 1987). Is it possible that basal ganglia dysfunction may result in two (or more) forms of "stereotypy," involving repetitive thoughts and rituals in the case of OCD and repetitive vocal and facial tics in the case of Tourette's disorder? We are just beginning to clarify these issues.

There is now growing evidence that OCD involves some kind of dysregulation in serotonergic function. We shall see later, in our discussion of treatment directions and goals, that a variety of "pro-serotonin" agents are effective in the treatment of OCD. A recent study by Swedo et al. (1992) examined PET scans in 10 adults with OCD, before and after pharmacotherapy. These authors found that among patients treated with clomipramine ($n = 8$) and fluoxetine ($n = 2$), decreases in right orbitofrontal metabolism were directly correlated with improvement of OCD symptoms. This finding suggests that initial hypermetabolism in orbitofrontal regions of OCD patients may actually be "corrected" by serotonergic agents.

Other basic research confirms the role of serotonin (5-hydroxy-tryptamine [5-HT]) but also raises some questions and seeming paradoxes. For example, Zohar et al. (1987) tested the effects of the direct-acting 5-HT agonist *m*-chlorophenylpiperazine (m-CPP) in OCD patients and healthy control subjects. These authors found that m-CPP caused a transient but marked exacerbation of obsessive and compulsive symptoms in the patients but not in the control subjects. Because m-CPP acts by stimulating postsynaptic 5-HT receptors, these findings suggest that OCD is due to increased serotonergic activity, which is seemingly in opposition to the clinical findings using drugs such as clomipramine. However, Meltzer (1989) has suggested that m-CPP may stimulate 5-HT autoreceptors, which would decrease 5-HT synthesis and release. Recently, Lucey et al. (1993) found evidence of cholinergic supersensitivity in OCD.

Finally, there is some intriguing but preliminary evidence implicating hormonal factors in OCD (Rasmussen and Eisen 1990). Thus, it is not uncommon to see OCD symptoms in late pregnancy or following childbirth. About 60% of female OCD patients report that their symptoms worsen around their menstrual period. Interestingly, there has been at least one report that anti-androgen therapy in males improves OCD symptoms (Casas et al. 1986).

Psychological Factors

Insel (1990) has nicely summarized the classic, psychoanalytic formulation of OCD, as represented in Table 6–8.

The psychoanalytic view holds that as obsessive-compulsive personality defenses [see Chapter 9] break down, obsessive-compulsive symptoms may emerge; for example, checking rituals, hand washing, etc. Both the obsessive-compulsive personality structure and the "neurosis" are seen as disorders of "control"; that is, the sufferer is one who constantly struggles for intrapsychic and interpersonal control (Insel 1990).

A variation of this view is expressed in the formulation of MacKinnon and Michels (1971), who see the obsessive individual as involved in a conflict between obedience and defiance, leading to a continual alternation between fear and rage. Although the psychoanalytic view has been helpful in a heuristic way, there is little empirical evidence that OCD is associated with premorbid obsessive-compulsive personality traits. Nor is there good evidence linking OCD with "trauma" during the anal phase, though this has been described clinically (Fenichel 1945).

Having issued these disclaimers, we can still acknowledge that the psychoanalytic formulation may enrich our understanding of *some* patients with OCD (Nemiah 1985b). In particular, we can understand how a mother who compulsively kisses her screaming, hyperactive infant may be utilizing reaction formation (i.e., unconsciously transforming her anger into affection). We can also understand how the individual who compulsively washes his or her hands may actually harbor the unconscious wish to "soil." The hand-washing ritual may represent both a reaction formation and an "undoing" of the underlying (unacceptable) impulse. If you are impressed with my use of the "may" in this paragraph, you will also appreciate that none of these psychodynamic factors has proved fundamental in the etiology of OCD, nor do any of them necessarily generate useful treatment strategies. Then again, such hypotheses at least provide the therapist

Table 6–8.　Psychoanalytic concepts of "obsessional neurosis"

1. Continuum with obsessive-compulsive personality traits

2. Anal-sadistic id material

3. **Defenses:** denial, repression, regression, reaction formation, isolation, undoing, magical thinking, intellectualization

4. **Causes:** Constitutional excess of anal-sadistic tendencies or defenses; precocious ego development; rigid superego; trauma during anal stage

Source. Adapted from Insel 1990.

with a tiny island of conceptual order in the midst of this rather mysterious disorder.

Learning theory has quite different things to tell us about OCD and may explain things more parsimoniously than does the psycho-analytic view. For example, how does it come about that an individual will obsess over the matter of "contamination" and subsequently develop a ritual to relieve the anxiety associated with the obsession? A behavioral model might hold that a random, neutral thought such as "I have dirt on my hands" somehow becomes "paired" with an (unconditioned) anxiety-provoking stimulus—let's say, an automobile accident. The next time the thought occurs—say, after gardening—the individual again experiences extreme anxiety but has no idea why. Soon, a conditioned anxiety response is established, such that each time the person has the thought "I have dirt on my hands," anxiety ensues. According to the behavioral model, the individual may fortu-itously discover that hand washing (or some other behavior) reduces this anxiety. The act of hand washing is reinforced and perpetuated by this reduction in anxiety, and a compulsion is born.

Sociocultural Factors

Meth (1974) has suggested that "in cultures which regulate their members' daily life by strict rules, obsessive-compulsive neuroses seem to be infrequent, as if the need for this particular defense mechanism had been satisfied by the compulsiveness of the culture . . . [and con-versely] it is more common in societies which allow greater freedom of choice" (p. 733). This is an interesting claim, and it may be correct, but it cannot be inferred from the epidemiological data available thus far. Indeed, the prevalence of OCD seems quite consistent across a wide spectrum of cultures, including the United States, Taiwan, Germany, and Canada (Rasmussen and Eisen 1992).

Stressful life events have not been clearly linked with the onset of OCD, at least in adolescents (Rapoport et al. 1981). Nevertheless, some of the case histories reported by Rapoport et al. (1981) strongly suggest a precipitating stressor. One 14-year-old boy's symptoms may have been precipitated by the death of his father. Another boy of the same age seemed to develop washing, dressing, and checking rituals quite acutely, after observing his pregnant mother faint. A 14-year-old girl developed OCD symptoms at age 11, apparently after watching a movie about (the alleged ax-murderer) Lizzie Borden. Although Rapoport et al. found such recollections "unconvincing," it seems plausible that precipitating stressors may play a role in individuals who are biologically and psychologically predisposed to OCD.

Pitfalls in the Differential Diagnosis

Although classic OCD is often unmistakable in its presentation, the mere report of repetitive, stereotyped thoughts or behaviors suggests a wide range of underlying disorders. Let's look at an illustrative vignette.

Vignette

Mr. Taeper was a 35-year-old engineer who carried a diagnosis of chronic paranoid schizophrenia. The patient had been able to function quite well on an outpatient basis for many years, although his social life was extremely restricted. He had been maintained on thiothixene 20 mg/day without evidence of hallucinations or overt delusions, though he remained chronically suspicious and litigious. Two months prior to evaluation, Mr. Taeper reported to his psychiatrist that "I have the idea over and over again these days. It comes to me night and day, and even in my dreams. The same thought, over and over: that I am about to invent a perpetual motion machine." Because the patient seemed otherwise "intact" and coherent, his psychiatrist concluded that he had developed an "obsession." The patient was begun on the antiobsessional drug clomipramine 25 mg bid. Within 1 week, the patient reported the belief that his psychiatrist was poisoning him and that "the voice of Satan" was commanding him to "perform ritual ablutions."

The differential diagnosis of OCD does include the psychotic disorders, and sometimes the correct "call" is difficult (Pies 1984). This is particularly true of the patient with the "poor insight type" of OCD. In the case presented, our psychiatrist made two critical errors: failing to recognize the ego-syntonic quality of the patient's initial recurrent thought, and failing to "reality-test" the supposed obsession. By definition, obsessions are ego-alien, at least initially. The patient typically fights to get rid of the recurrent thought. In Mr. Taeper's case, the grandiose nature of the idea (i.e., inventing a perpetual motion machine) was gratifying, and he did not report any wish to rid himself of the idea. Moreover, close questioning would have revealed the "fixed" quality of the idea: Mr. Taeper truly believed, against all logic, that he was about to invent a perpetual motion machine. The worsening in his condition after initiation of clomipramine is not surprising; such worsening is often seen when a psychotic person is started on a tricyclic.

The differential diagnosis of OCD also includes the following conditions: 1) major depressive episode with "obsessive brooding"; 2) other anxiety disorders, in which rumination is common; 3) Tourette's disorder, in which "mental coprolalia" may be present (sudden, intrusive, senseless thoughts of obscene words that are not "fought" or suppressed); 4) various impulse control disorders such as kleptomania, pathological gambling, or trichotillomania; 5) eating disorders such as bulimia or anorexia nervosa in which rituals are common; and 6) idiosyncratic rituals/habits that fall short of OCD criteria.

The severely depressed individual may "brood" about being guilty, worthless, and so forth, in a manner that may suggest a genuine obsession. But typically, the depressed individual doesn't regard these thoughts as senseless or even necessarily inaccurate. For example, I recall an extremely depressed elderly accountant who brooded constantly over a $20 error he had made while preparing a relative's income tax return. Believing that this was an egregious failure on his part, he did not regard the intrusive thoughts as irrational, although he did express the hope that he would be rid of them eventually. (Psychodynamically, he may well have been punishing himself with these recurrent thoughts as a means of "atoning" for his "sin.")

Tourette's disorder usually begins by age 7 and almost always before age 14. Thus, it differs from OCD, which more typically begins in adolescence or early adulthood (American Psychiatric Association 1987). Moreover, the Tourette's patient usually shows multiple motor or vocal "tics," such as grunts, sniffs, or coughs, which are not common in most OCD patients. Unlike the OCD patient, the

Tourette's patient does not make strenuous efforts to "fight" the intrusive thought or motor movement. Nonetheless, these conditions may share biological and genetic factors; for example, OCD appears to be more common in first-degree relatives of Tourette's patients than in the general population.

In impulse control disorders such as pathological gambling or kleptomania, there is a "compulsive" quality to the person's life (e.g., feeling "driven," "powerless," and so forth). But unlike OCD patients, the patient with an impulse disorder derives pleasure from the specific behavior (e.g., stealing). According to DSM-III-R, "the act is ego-syntonic in that it is consonant with the immediate conscious wish of the individual" (American Psychiatric Association 1987, p. 321). However, guilt or self-reproach may follow the act or the resulting adverse consequences. Of note, there is a high incidence of trichotillomania in families having one or more members with OCD (Rapoport 1990).

In bulimia nervosa or anorexia nervosa, the patient may show peculiar preoccupations and/or rituals (e.g., constantly thinking about food, cutting it up into tiny pieces, hoarding it, etc.). However, the patient often has a near-delusional rationale for these rituals, relating either to the fear of gaining weight or to a markedly disturbed body image. For example, the anorexic individual may believe that cutting her food into tiny pieces reduces the risk of gaining weight. A true OCD patient would generally acknowledge the "senselessness" behind such an activity. Despite such theoretical distinctions from OCD, Rapoport (1990) notes that 15% of adult women with OCD had anorexia in adolescence. Furthermore, the anorexic individual sometimes merits the concurrent diagnosis of OCD, as, for example, when there is an ego-alien hand-washing compulsion present.

Many people have idiosyncratic habits, such as cracking their knuckles or whistling the same tune over and over. There are also a great many culturally sanctioned rituals (such as "crossing" oneself or "knocking on wood") that do not qualify as OCD. These habits and rituals typically do not distress the individual, occupy only a small amount of time each day, and do not significantly compromise social or occupational functioning.

Finally, we should note some of the organic disorders with which OCD may be associated, including epilepsy, Sydenham's chorea, frontal lobe or basal ganglia lesions, and postencephalitic Parkinson's disease (Rapoport 1990).

It is of great interest that only 26% of adolescents with OCD have no other Axis I disorder (Rapoport 1990; Swedo et al. 1989); around 25% have major depression, and many more have some other anxiety disorder. Learning disorders may also be associated with OCD. Thus, while differential diagnosis is a useful exercise, you should be sure to entertain that ever-present possibility, comorbidity.

Adjunctive Testing

Neuroendocrine Studies

There are no known consistent neuroendocrine abnormalities in OCD, but some lines of research suggest that OCD patients may resemble patients with major depression in some neuroendocrine functions. Thus, Siever et al. (1983) measured growth hormone response to clonidine administration in nine nondepressed patients with OCD. The OCD patients, when compared with control subjects, showed significantly decreased growth hormone response—similar to the response seen in many depressed patients. Also, baseline plasma norepinephrine levels were significantly greater in patients than in control subjects. Insel et al. (1982) found abnormal DST results in 6 of 16 patients with primary OCD, again suggesting a biochemical link between OCD and depression. However, this was not confirmed by Lieberman et al. (1985), who found no abnormal DST results in 18 OCD patients (vs. 37% abnormal sets of results in patients with major depression). It may be that supervening depressive features and/or the timing of the test determine the outcome of the DST in patients with OCD. Finally, Gorman et al. (1985) showed that patients with OCD react similarly to normal control subjects when infused with sodium lactate (see discussion of panic disorder).

Sleep Studies

There is limited evidence showing reduced REM latency in OCD, once again suggesting an affinity with major depression.

Imaging Techniques

Baxter et al. (1988), using PET, compared 10 nondepressed OCD patients with 10 normal control subjects. The OCD patients showed significantly elevated metabolic rates in the whole cerebral hemispheres, heads of the caudate nuclei, and orbital gyri. This group of investigators has also found high absolute glucose metabolic values for these brain regions in OCD patients compared with patients with unipolar major depression (Baxter et al. 1987). An interesting complementary study by Luxenberg et al. (1988) examined neuroanatomic abnormalities in OCD using quantitative X-ray CT. Ten males with severe OCD were compared with 10 healthy male control subjects. Caudate nucleus volume in the OCD patients was significantly less than that seen in the control subjects, once again supporting the hypothesis that the basal ganglia are involved in OCD (see discussion of biological factors earlier in this section).

Psychological Testing

On the MMPI, OCD patients often show the 2-7-8 high point combination. This pattern "reflects people who are self-analytic and inclined toward catastrophic expectations and a sense of hopelessness" (Meyer 1983, p. 122). We should note that while scale 7 originally denoted "psychasthenia," it is now felt to be more related to psychological turmoil and obsessive-compulsive traits (Newmark 1985). On the WAIS-R, an overall higher IQ is seen in OCD than in other disorders, with especially good performance seen on vocabulary, similarities, and comprehension subtests. However, the OCD patient's difficulty in changing mental "set" can sometimes reduce performance on similarities (Meyer 1983). On the Rorschach, there are usually few color responses but a high number of W (entire blot) and/or Dd (uncommon detail) responses. There is a high F+% and many "edge details." OCD patients "like to criticize the blots . . . and may express concern about the symmetry of the cards" (Meyer 1983, p. 123). On the Thematic Apperception Test (TAT), pedantic wording and an emphasis on details are common.

A number of rating scales for OCD have been developed. For example, the Yale-Brown Obsessive Compulsive Scale (YBOCS;

Goodman et al. 1989) rates 10 criteria of symptom severity and "patient control" over obsessions and compulsions.

Treatment Directions and Goals

Somatic Approaches

Greist (1990b) has reviewed the pharmacotherapy of OCD. There are essentially two main classes of pharmacotherapeutic agents: anxiolytics and antidepressants. In general, benzodiazepines are unreliably effective, although some open studies have reported success with alprazolam, clonazepam, diazepam, and oxazepam (Greist 1990b). The commonly used tricyclics have also been rather unimpressive in the treatment of OCD. However, several studies have shown clearly that the tricyclic agent clomipramine, which recently became available in the United States, is superior to placebo in the treatment of OCD. The largest study (DeVeaugh-Geiss et al. 1989) involved 519 patients at 21 sites in the United States. Fifty-eight percent of patients treated with clomipramine improved significantly, compared with only 3% on placebo. Unfortunately, clomipramine may produce troublesome side effects, even in relatively low doses (e.g., sedation, dry mouth, and sexual dysfunction). (A patient of mine experienced delayed ejaculation on only 25 mg clomipramine per day.) On occasion, I have found imipramine to be of modest effectiveness in OCD. There is growing evidence indicating that fluoxetine—and probably other SSRIs—may be nearly as effective as clomipramine (Jenike et al. 1989). (Fluvoxamine, a SSRI, has recently been approved by the FDA for use in OCD.) Lithium, which also boosts serotonergic function, may be useful as an adjunctive agent in OCD—for example, when combined with clomipramine—but is not especially effective when used alone (Rasmussen 1984).

Although antipsychotic agents are generally not indicated for OCD, there is preliminary evidence that they may be helpful in OCD patients with comorbid schizotypal personality disorder (McDougle et al. 1990). Bear in mind, of course, the risk of tardive dyskinesia in such cases. We should also note that none of the pharmacotherapies discussed has demonstrated ongoing efficacy once the medication is stopped.

Finally, there may be a role for so-called psychosurgery (e.g., leucotomy) in extremely refractory cases of OCD. Reportedly, over 80% of patients respond favorable to such surgery (Greist 1990b).

Psychosocial Approaches

John Nemiah (1985b), in discussing the psychotherapy of OCD, makes the telling observation that "it is possible . . . to effect a complete disappearance of compulsive behavior in some patients by the simple device of informing them that the doctor will assume complete responsibility for anything that may happen as a result of their impulses. . . . unfortunately, the improvement usually lasts for only a few hours" (p. 916).

Indeed, it is difficult to demonstrate the lasting effectiveness of psychodynamically oriented therapy in the treatment of OCD (Nemiah 1985b), although the literature abounds with anecdotal reports of benefit. While a psychodynamic understanding of OCD may be useful in the therapist's formulation of the case, it is not clear that a psychodynamic form of treatment is especially helpful; indeed, in my experience, delving into putative unconscious mechanisms may be the "nidus" for further rumination. Thus, behavior therapy is considered by many as the treatment of choice (Greist 1990a). "Exposure" and "response prevention" are the main behavioral treatments. Patients are asked to make contact with or to imagine their anxiety or ritual-provoking stimuli. For example, a patient obsessed with being "contaminated by germs" might be instructed to touch a toilet seat (exposure). The patient is also instructed to forgo the usual ritual associated with exposure—in this case, for example, hand washing. (You can undoubtedly see how this disorder and its treatment overlap with various phobic disorders and their treatment.) As you can imagine, such a procedure might itself evoke anxiety, and approximately 25% of patients will not comply with this approach (Foa et al. 1985). Those who can comply often show lasting gains—perhaps more so than when pharmacotherapy alone is used and then discontinued.

Obsessional thoughts not associated with rituals may be more refractory to treatment. One technique, called "saturation," requires the patient to focus exclusively on the obsessional thought for 10 to

15 minutes. This seems to result, paradoxically, in diminished attention to the obsessional thought (Nemiah 1985b). Thought stopping—a technique in which the patient learns to interrupt obsessional thoughts by hearing the word "Stop!"—may also be helpful in mild cases.

Posttraumatic Stress Disorder and Acute Stress Disorder

The Central Concept

Posttraumatic stress disorder and its more acute "cousin," acute stress disorder, develop after a susceptible individual is exposed to a particularly distressing event or set of events. In DSM-III-R, the nature of the trauma was conceptualized as one "outside the range of usual human experience and that would be markedly distressing to almost anyone" (American Psychiatric Association 1987, p. 250). DSM-IV has dropped the "beyond the pale" requirement but has narrowed down the kinds of trauma that "count" for PTSD. Specifically, the person has "experienced, witnessed, or been confronted with an event or events that involved actual or threatened death or serious injury, or a threat to the physical integrity of self or others" (American Psychiatric Association 1994, p. 427). DSM-IV also stipulates that the person's response to the event "involved intense fear, helplessness, or horror" (p. 428). The new criteria would permit, say, a victim of sexual assault to claim PTSD, but not someone whose business had gone down the drain, however "traumatic" that may have been. The new category, acute stress disorder, is quite similar to PTSD symptomatically but lasts only 2 days to 4 weeks; PTSD symptoms, by definition, must be present for more than 1 month.

Although combat experience is probably the most common etiological trauma in men, PTSD may follow rape, assault, terrorism, serious injury of a family member, natural disaster, and many other traumata. It appears to be equally prevalent in men and women, affecting around 1% of the general population (Goldman 1988). The diagnosis of PTSD requires substantial disruption of psychosocial functioning, as is demonstrated in the following vignette.

Vignette

Kevin was a 22-year-old male who had been assaulted by a gang of youths after he had "wandered onto their turf." Although his physical injuries were minor, Kevin began to experience severe symptoms of anxiety and depression within a few days after the trauma. He reported "waking up in a cold sweat" from nightmares of the incident, and the persistent fear that "someone might come into my apartment through the window." Although Kevin was able to "reality-test" this idea, it was nevertheless terrifying to him. Even during the day, Kevin experienced "flashbacks" of the assault; for example, he would see the face of one of the youths who had held a knife to his throat. At such times, Kevin would "break into a sweat" and experience trouble breathing. The flashbacks were often precipitated by driving by the street on which the assault occurred. Kevin described a "spaced out" feeling that overcame him during the flashbacks, stating, "It's like I'm right back there getting jumped again . . . I can practically feel that guy's breath against my face." Over the ensuing month, Kevin learned to avoid passing by the street, but the flashbacks would occur in other contexts (e.g., upon seeing someone who resembled one of the assailants). Kevin became withdrawn and isolated, spending most days inside his apartment. He had to quit his job as a short-order cook. Despite the attempts of friends and family to help him "cheer up," Kevin became progressively estranged from others, and he "kind of dried up inside . . . just numb." He lost interest in most of his usual hobbies, grew irritable with others, and had trouble concentrating. His appetite was poor, and he described "this clawing feeling in the pit of my stomach" that appeared without obvious reason. Kevin became startled by loud noises, and he found himself constantly glancing over his shoulder while walking on the street. Two months after the assault, Kevin's symptoms had not abated.

Kevin's history is fairly typical of the "acute" form of PTSD, in which symptoms are present less than 3 months. In the "delayed onset" form, symptoms begin at least 6 months after the trauma, though avoidance symptoms have usually been present during this hiatus. It is not yet clear whether important psychodynamic differences distinguish these subtypes (C. G. Watson et al. 1988). Horowitz

(1985) has pointed out that the response to trauma often occurs in phases. Thus, the immediate response to disaster is usually an "outcry" for help. There follows a "denial phase" in which the individual may feel "dazed" or "numb," sometimes showing selective amnesia for the trauma. Soon, an "intrusive phase" ensues in which the trauma victim may experience startle reactions, flashbacks, insomnia, and autonomic hyperactivity. Ideally, a process of "working through" allows the victim to "complete" the phases of trauma. When this process is blocked, severe disability may follow (Horowitz 1985). We will say more about "working through" when we discuss the treatment of PTSD.

Historical Development of the Disorder

Posttraumatic stress disorder, in one form or another, has been recognized for over a century (Andreasen 1980). In the late 19th century, Oppenheim used the term "traumatic neurosis," but linked it to organic factors occurring at the molecular level. In contrast, Charcot believed that traumatic neuroses were psychogenic in origin, pointing to the effectiveness of hypnosis in inducing similar symptoms. During the American Civil War, Da Costa described a syndrome that became known as "soldier's heart," owing to the presence of autonomic cardiac symptoms (e.g., palpitations, chest tightness, etc.). In World War I, the notion of "shell shock" came into vogue and was thought to result from the traumatic effects of exploding bombshells. Posttraumatic syndromes were seen in World War II following the atomic bombings of Japan and the liberation of the Nazi concentration camps. Around the same time, survivors of the Coconut Grove fire (1941) showed many symptoms of what we now call PTSD. In DSM-I, the designation "gross stress reaction" appeared, but was dropped from DSM-II. PTSD emerged in DSM-III (American Psychiatric Association 1980) largely as a result of the Vietnam veterans' experience.

The Biopsychosocial Perspective

Biological Factors

A role for heredity in PTSD is suggested by some animal data; for example, stress response to inescapable shock varies among different strains of mice raised in identical environments (Wieland et al. 1986). In an important recent study involving 4,042 Vietnam veteran twin pairs, True et al. (1993) demonstrated a significant genetic influence on PTSD symptom liability. Even after controlling for combat exposure, genetic factors accounted for 13% to 34% of the variance in PTSD symptom clusters in this population. On the other hand, there was no evidence that shared environment contributed to the development of PTSD symptoms (True et al. 1993).

You have probably noticed that many PTSD symptoms resemble those we have already seen in panic disorder. Thus, it may not surprise you that SNS hyperarousal and locus coeruleus dysfunction have been implicated in PTSD. PTSD patients often have higher urinary norepinephrine levels than do control subjects, as well as higher baseline heart rate and blood pressure (M. J. Friedman 1988). Van der Kolk et al. (1985) proposed that massive trauma alters locus coeruleus activity. Potentiation of locus coeruleus pathways to the hippocampus and amygdala then results in hyperarousal, traumatic nightmares, and flashbacks. Kolb (1987) advanced a complex neuropsychological theory of PTSD in which the locus coeruleus is but one element. Kolb proposed that in PTSD, lower brain stem structures such as the medial hypothalamic nuclei and locus ceruleus "escape from inhibitory cortical control." These lower brain centers in turn "repeatedly reactivate the perceptual, cognitive, affective, and somatic clinical expressions related to the original traumata" (p. 994). Fluctuations in endogenous opioid levels may also play a role in PTSD (Van der Kolk et al. 1985).

More recently, Ross et al. (1989) hypothesized that dysfunctional REM sleep mechanisms may be involved in PTSD-related flashbacks and nightmares. Indeed, these workers speculated that PTSD is essentially a disorder of REM sleep. Decreased REM latency in some PTSD patients suggests a physiological link with affective disorders, but not all studies have confirmed this (Ross et al. 1989).

Psychological Factors

Freud postulated two broad responses to trauma: 1) attempts to remember or repeat the trauma and 2) attempts to avoid or fend off such memories and repetitions (Brett et al. 1988). Both mechanisms may be involved in the development of PTSD. In essence, the psycho-analytic view holds that a particular trauma in the here and now may reactivate an unresolved childhood conflict. The ego is overwhelmed, and the aggressive drives of the id gain the upper hand. (Note the analogy between this view and Kolb's hypothesis that lower brain centers "escape" cortical inhibition.) Through the use of regression and such primitive defenses as repression, denial, and undoing, the ego attempts to "fend off" the emergent id anxiety (Andreasen 1980; Kaplan and Sadock 1988). At the same time, the ego struggles to "master" the anxiety by repeatedly confronting it. Note that the emphasis here is on anxiety. A different and rather controversial view stresses "dissociation" as the dynamic nucleus of PTSD—a plausible argument if one focuses on phenomena like flashbacks and emotional "numbing." Thus, whether to classify PTSD as an anxiety disorder or a dissociative disorder remains unsettled (Brett et al. 1988).

Our psychological understanding of PTSD must also incorporate the notion of "conditioned fear" (Kolb 1987). Anderson and Parmenter (1941) long ago showed that "experimental neuroses" could be induced in both sheep and dogs. These researchers used electric shocks as the unconditioned stimulus and the sound of a metronome as the conditioned stimulus, producing long-term behavioral and physiological hyperactivity in the animals (e.g., hyperalertness to touch, restlessness, and persistent tachycardia). As Kolb (1987) points out, this response "was remarkably similar to that noted in the chronic posttraumatic stress disorder of combat veterans with conditioned emotional response" (p. 991). In some combat veterans, the mere sight of an army-green jacket is capable of serving as the conditioned stimulus for panic-type symptoms.

Nadelson (1992) has outlined the complex biopsychosocial factors that lead some traumatized combat veterans to become emotionally "attached" to their violent combat experiences.

Preexisting psychopathology may also play a role in the later development of PTSD. The Epidemiologic Catchment Area survey (Helzer et al. 1987) showed that childhood behavioral problems predict a greater risk of PTSD after exposure to a traumatic event. Early work by Andreasen et al. (1972) showed that persons with difficulty handling dependency needs may be prone to develop PTSD after industrial and auto accidents—perhaps because they more easily assume the "sick role." McFarlane (1989) looked at predisposing factors for PTSD in firefighters exposed to a bushfire disaster in southeastern Australia. "Neuroticism" and a history of treatment for psychological disorder were better predictors of posttraumatic morbidity than was the degree of exposure to the disaster. Thus, although everyone may have a psychological "breaking point," there is good evidence suggesting that PTSD is more common in the emotionally vulnerable.

Horowitz (1985) has summarized the premorbid characteristics that may interfere with an adaptive response after a disaster. The person may have had 1) a belief in magical causation, leading to the idea that "past bad thoughts brought present harm"; 2) an active conflict with a theme similar to those of the present disaster; 3) a tendency to use pathological defenses such as projection, leading to distorted memories of the disaster; and 4) a habit of using fantasy to repair personal "ego blows," thus hindering realistic coping skills after the disaster.

Sociocultural Factors

The availability of social supports may influence the development, severity, and duration of PTSD (Andreasen 1980; Lifton 1973). The disorder is more likely to occur in the single, divorced, widowed, and socioeconomically deprived (A. Adler 1945). Furthermore, Horowitz (1989) has noted that

> cultures that provide support only after a threshold of illness is crossed will increase the likelihood that such illness will occur. The most important social ingredient after a disaster is extended care-giving as modulated by shared values. Failures in social coherence will increase the rate of non-resolution of stress responses. Something of this sort occurred after the war in Vietnam. Returning American servicemen were sometimes socially ignored or treated as if they were responsible for the war. (p. 2072)

The interpersonal aspects of PTSD may be understood through the concept of the "trauma membrane" (Lindy 1985). Like the newly developing surface of an injured cell, the trauma membrane protects the victim's inner reparative processes from noxious stimuli. It also permits the entry of agents perceived as curative. As Lindy (1985) notes, "For individual survivors, the surface of the membrane is guarded by the spouse, parent, or close friend. When populations of traumatized survivors have the opportunity to form an informal survivor network, a common trauma membrane forms" (p. 155). Such group "membranes" may promote a sense of safety among the survivors—for example, in a group of Vietnam veterans who get together to play cards—but they may prove quite impermeable to well-meaning mental health workers. Thus, the psychiatrist who "never even set foot in ''Nam'" will sometimes be greeted with considerable (and understandable) mistrust by a group of Vietnam veterans.

Pitfalls in the Differential Diagnosis

The differential diagnosis of PTSD includes 1) other anxiety disorders, 2) affective (mood) disorders, 3) various psychotic disorders, 4) dissociative disorders, 5) organic amnestic disorders, and 6) adjustment disorders with anxious or depressive features. Let's see how this differential is applied (or misapplied) in the following vignette.

Vignette

A 38-year-old Vietnam veteran presented in the ER with marked anxiety, agitation, and irritability. He gave a 15-year history of moderate anxiety and depression, sometimes accompanied by insomnia and feelings of estrangement from others. These symptoms followed a tour of duty in which the patient had seen "six of my buddies blown away." A week before admission, the patient had been eating in Chinatown, where he witnessed an altercation between a group of Chinese youths and a Caucasian taxi driver. Although, as the patient related it, "the cabbie started the fight," the Chinese youths had retaliated by "beating the crap out of the guy." The patient had witnessed this from within the restaurant and "felt paralyzed . . . like I was frozen in my chair. I wanted to go out and help the cabbie, but I couldn't." Although the patient considered himself "a fair guy" with no prejudice toward Chinese individuals, he admitted, "All I saw out that window was a bunch of gooks." Shortly after this incident, the patient felt "panicky . . . like somebody was following me." He began to hear "voices like . . . yelling in my head . . . I'm not sure what they were saying . . . maybe they were saying, 'Watch out!' Anyway, it feels like there's some kind of damn radio in my head." The resident in the ER, noting the patient's disorganized thought processes and disheveled appearance, made a diagnosis of paranoid schizophrenia. However, treatment with antipsychotic medication had no effect on the patient's core symptoms and led to marked parkinsonian side effects.

You can easily see how the resident might have reached this erroneous conclusion—after all, didn't the patient present with paranoia, auditory hallucinations, and a somatic delusion? The answers, of course, are "No," "No," and "No." Note the patient's use of the word "like": he felt "like" somebody was following him and "like" a radio was in his head. The resident didn't explore the patient's ability to reality-test these feelings. Most likely, the patient would have retained at least a marginal grasp on reality. The "auditory hallucinations" were most probably pseudo-hallucinations or intensely experienced auditory recollections of actual combat experiences (in which "Watch out!" would have been heard frequently).

The differential diagnosis of PTSD and other psychiatric syndromes is summarized in Table 6–9. But, be warned: DSM-III-R noted that "symptoms of depression and anxiety are common [in PTSD], and in some instances may be sufficiently severe to be diagnosed as an anxiety or depressive disorder" (American Psychiatric Association 1987, p. 249). Thus, although we include panic disorder in the differential diagnosis, it is possible that someone could meet the criteria for both PTSD and panic disorder. The same is true of PTSD and major depressive disorder.

Adjunctive Testing

Psychophysiological Testing

Kolb (1987) has reviewed the data suggesting that combat veterans with PTSD show a variety of psychophysiological abnormalities in

Table 6–9. Differential diagnosis of PTSD and other psychiatric disorders

Disorder	Features differentiating it from PTSD
Panic disorder	Attacks more often "out of the blue" in PD vs. set off by trauma-specific stimuli in PTSD.
	PD is more often associated with general agoraphobia vs. avoidance of trauma-specific stimuli/places in PTSD.
Major depressive episode	MDE may or may not be related to a clear precipitant; there are more neurovegetative features in MDE (early A.M. awakening, weight loss, diurnal variation, etc.).
Paranoid or other psychotic disorder	Greater loss of reality testing is evident in paranoid (delusional) disorder and schizophrenia. Affect and thought process are more inappropriate/disorganized in schizophrenia (but affect may be constricted in PTSD).
Dissociative disorders	Basic integrity of personality in PTSD is evident compared with multiple personality disorder (MPD). (But many MPD patients do have a history of childhood trauma/abuse.)
	Sudden travel and assumption of new identity are unlikely in PTSD compared with fugue.
	Psychogenic amnesia patient is less likely to have flashbacks, hypervigilance, etc., though some may meet criteria for PTSD.
	Depersonalization disorder patient is less likely to have hyperarousal and flashbacks, though stressor may predispose to depersonalization.
Organic amnestic disorder	In OAD, there is usually a history of head trauma, alcohol abuse/thiamine deficiency, cerebral hypoxia, etc. OAD is more often associated with confabulation, inability to learn new information.
Adjustment disorder	In adjustment disorder, the stressor is usually less severe and the flashbacks, hypervigilance, etc., are less common.

comparison to non-PTSD combat veterans. When exposed to "combat sounds," the PTSD group shows abnormal increases in heart rate, systolic blood pressure, and diastolic pressure (Blanchard et al. 1986). Other studies have shown increases in respiratory rate and skin resistance and decreases in alpha rhythm when combat veterans are exposed to various audiovisual stimuli (Dobbs and Wilson 1960; Malloy et al. 1983). Kolb concluded that such testing "offers strong potential not only for diagnostic identification . . . but also for assessment of the severity of [PTSD]" (p. 991). Although not routinely used, such tests may prove useful in diagnostically confusing cases. However, it remains to be seen how applicable these findings are to patients with non-combat-induced PTSD and to patients whose traumata occurred early in childhood.

Neuroendocrine Testing

M. J. Friedman (1988) has reviewed the neuroendocrine data in relation to PTSD, noting that PTSD patients may have a significantly higher urinary norepinephrine/cortisol ratio than do patients with other psychiatric disorders (e.g., bipolar and paranoid schizophrenic patients) (Mason et al. 1985, 1986). The higher norepinephrine levels are consistent with increased SNS activity, and lower urinary cortisol levels suggest "that denial and psychological defenses can exert a strong suppressive effect on urinary corticosteroid levels" (M. J. Friedman 1988, p. 282). Charney et al. (1993) have recently provided an excellent review of psychobiological mechanisms in PTSD. They cite an abundance of preclinical data pointing to stress-induced aberrations in the noradrenergic, dopaminergic, and endogenous opiate systems. The noradrenergic system is implicated by studies showing exaggerated responsiveness to yohimbine in combat veterans with PTSD. For example, the yohimbine-induced increase in plasma MHPG (3-methoxy-4-hydroxyphenylglycol), the main metabolite of central norepinephrine, is more than twice as great in PTSD patients than in normal control subjects (Charney et al. 1993). The evidence for involvement of the endogenous opiate system in PTSD is less direct—for example, the clinical observation that opiates are preferred substances of abuse in many traumatized individuals—but one study, by Pitman et al. (1990), supports this hypothesis. These workers found that the opiate antagonist naloxone reversed the analgesia ("numbing") induced by stressful combat films in Vietnam veterans with PTSD. It remains to be seen how effective such opiate antagonists will prove in clinical practice.

Sleep Studies

We have already alluded to abnormalities in the sleep patterns of some PTSD patients. A number of sleep studies of veterans with combat-related PTSD show increased REM latency, decreased REM sleep, decreased stage 4 sleep, and reduced sleep efficiency (Kramer and Kinney 1985; Lavie et al. 1979; Schlossberg and Benjamin 1978). (Recall that in major depression there is often decreased REM latency and excessive REM sleep.) In addition to abnormal sleep patterns, chronic PTSD patients may also show disturbed dreaming. Thus, M. J. Friedman (1981) noted that traumatic nightmares associated with PTSD do not fit into the category of REM-related dream anxiety attacks, nor into the stage 4 "night terror" syndrome. Van der Kolk et al. (1984) showed that traumatic nightmares may arise out of various stages of sleep and are not confined to REM sleep. Finally, Ross et al. (1989) have argued that sleep disturbance is a "hallmark" of PTSD. Specifically, "dysfunctional REM sleep mechanisms may be involved in the pathogenesis of the posttraumatic anxiety dream" (p. 697) Ross et al. also hypothesize that dysfunctional REM mechanisms may result in the exaggerated startle response seen in many PTSD patients. We shall say more about REM mechanisms in our discussion of treatment approaches.

Imaging Studies

There appears to be very little to report in the area of PET, brain electrical activity mapping (BEAM), or other imaging studies of PTSD.

Psychological Testing

On the MMPI, patients with PTSD resemble patients with panic disorder but have fewer signs of disruption in overall personality functioning (Meyer 1983). Recent psychometric evaluation of PTSD has involved the use of specific scales to measure combat exposure. For example, the Combat Exposure Scale (CES; Keane et al. 1989) consists of 47 items designed to measure the subjective report of wartime stressors and appears to be useful in the diagnosis of PTSD. Another scale, the Structured Interview for PTSD (SI-PTSD), developed by Davidson et al. (1989), utilizes DSM-III criteria for PTSD in a structured interview. The SI-PTSD measures symptom severity on a scale from 0 to 52, and its measure appears to correlate well with ratings of subjective stress.

Treatment Directions and Goals

Somatic Approaches

M. J. Friedman (1988), in reviewing the pharmacotherapy of PTSD, concluded that "pharmacotherapy alone is rarely sufficient to provide complete remission of PTSD." Rather, "symptom relief provided by medication facilitates the patient's participation in individual, behavioral, or group psychotherapy" (p. 283). Nonetheless, medication can provide substantial symptomatic relief in many cases. Friedman argues that "antipsychotic agents have no place in the routine treatment of PTSD" (p. 283), which rarely presents with frank psychosis. Occasionally, however, the paranoid and hallucinatory symptoms of the PTSD patient may require brief treatment with an antipsychotic agent. Benzodiazepines may be helpful, particularly if panic-type symptoms predominate. However, the presence of comorbid substance abuse commonly seen in PTSD patients is a relative contraindication.

Perhaps the most useful agents for PTSD are the heterocyclic antidepressants and the MAOIs (M. J. Friedman 1988; Silver et al. 1990). Although there are few controlled studies, several reports attest to the usefulness of tricyclics in dampening hyperarousal, reducing intrusive recollections, suppressing flashbacks, and reducing traumatic nightmares. (Recalling our earlier discussion, it seems surprising that tricyclics, which decrease REM sleep, should be useful in patients whose putative sleep abnormality is diminished REM sleep. Ross et al. [1989] have discussed this seeming paradox.) Obviously, tricyclics would also be of value in PTSD patients who in addition fit the criteria for major depression. In a recent placebo-controlled study of 46 veterans with chronic PTSD, Davidson et al. (1990) found that amitriptyline yielded better results than placebo on two measures: the Hamilton Depression Rating Scale and the Clinical Global Impression (CGI) scale. There was no evidence for amitriptyline's superiority on the SI-PTSD (a structured interview for PTSD, discussed in the previous subsection). Response to medication was reduced in patients with comorbid alcohol abuse. Even these modest benefits of amitriptyline took about 8 weeks to emerge. Several reports (e.g., Hogben and Cornfield 1981) suggested that MAOIs may be useful in PTSD— perhaps reflecting, in part, the powerful antipanic properties of these drugs. Of course, MAOIs pose substantial risk if the PTSD patient is prone to alcohol abuse. Lithium and the anticonvulsants carbamazepine and valproate have also been found effective in treating chronic PTSD (Kitchner and Greenstein 1985; Silver et al. 1990; Van der Kolk 1983). Finally, there are theoretical reasons for supposing that fluoxetine may prove useful in PTSD; for example, it appears to have both antipanic and antiobsessional properties (Jenike et al. 1989). In a recent open, prospective trial of fluoxetine for PTSD, Nagy et al. (1993) found the drug effective on a number of PTSD symptom scales. It appears that higher doses of fluoxetine (up to 80 mg/day) may be needed for PTSD than are commonly used to treat depression.

Psychosocial Approaches

Horowitz (1986, 1989) advocates a multimodal, phased treatment approach to PTSD that emphasizes interpersonal and social support as well as the "healthy working through" of the traumatic events. This approach is summarized in Table 6–10.

It is difficult to describe a single "correct" form of psychotherapy for PTSD, because patients present with a wide variety of traumata at various stages of evolution or resolution. As a general principle, Horowitz notes that psychotherapy of PTSD begins with the establishment of a "safe relationship" and with the patient's "telling the story" of the traumatic events. Because patients usually seek treatment during the "intrusive" phase of PTSD, therapeutic efforts are aimed at helping the patient modulate the often overwhelming flood of memories, feelings, and ideas surrounding the trauma. This may involve the use of behavioral approaches, such as relaxation techniques or systematic desensitization. The following vignette illustrates this approach.

Vignette

A 23-year-old female graduate student was held at knife point and sexually molested while walking back to her dorm. She presented 1 week later with complaints of insomnia, "flashbacks" of the assailant's touching her, tearfulness, and inability to attend classes. She stated that she "can't set foot anywhere near" the scene of the crime. Moreover, she complained that "I can't get near men now without thinking of them all as rapists or perverts." A course of brief, time-limited psychotherapy was initiated at the student health center. The therapist first listened carefully to the student's tearful recollection of the event and then offered some directive suggestions (e.g., spending time with a close female friend). The therapist taught the patient some breathing techniques to help control her "panicky" feelings. In the third of 10 sessions, the patient was

Table 6–10.   Multimodal treatment approach to PTSD

Patient's current state	Treatment goal
Is under continuing impact of traumatic events.	Provide safety, support, help with making decisions.
Has intolerable mood swings, intrusive recollections, denial, numbness.	Help patient "dose" recollection by putting out of mind, remembering, putting out of mind, etc.
Is able to tolerate waves of emotion and recollection.	Help patient work through implications of trauma to self-image, relations to others, prior traumata.
Is able to work through ideas emotions on one's own.	Work through loss of therapeutic relationship; end treatment.

Source. Extensively modified from Horowitz 1989.

instructed to imagine herself walking past the scene of the trauma while feeling confident and relaxed. This "imaging" technique was extended to her attending class, and even to spending time with men. Eventually, the patient was encouraged to walk by the scene of the attack in the company of her friend. This was repeated several times until the patient was able to resume classes.

Sometimes, a more psychodynamic approach is necessary. For example, let's say that our patient in the vignette above had complained of feeling "dirty . . . like a whore who deserved what she got." After the initial intrusive symptoms were under control, it may have been useful to explore how the current trauma related to the patient's previous life experiences and self-concept. For example, could she have been molested as a child by a family member? Had the current sexual assault reawakened the feelings of unworthiness and guilt? If so, the therapist would have tried to relate past and present and then "work through" the attendant feelings.

Conclusion

Our understanding of anxiety disorders and their treatment has expanded enormously in the past decade. While the biological underpinnings of panic disorder have been investigated more extensively than those of the other anxiety disorders, we are beginning to understand the neurophysiology of PTSD, GAD, and OCD as well. The use of benzodiazepines, tricyclics, MAOIs, and SSRIs in these disorders has become increasingly refined. At the same time, the alternative or adjunctive use of cognitive-behavioral techniques is finding more and more support. The most successful approach to the anxious patient will almost certainly entail the careful integration of biological and psychosocial treatments.

References

Adler A: Understanding Human Nature. New York, Greenberg Press, 1927
Adler A: Mental symptoms following head injury: a statistical analysis of 200

cases. Archives of Neurology and Psychiatry 53:34, 1945

Adler G: Borderline Psychopathology and Its Treatment. New York, Jason Aronson, 1985

Akiskal HS, Lemmi H: Sleep EEG findings bearing on the relationship of anxiety and depressive disorders, in Anxious Depression: Assessment and Treatment. Edited by Racagni B, Esmeraldi E. New York, Raven, 1987, pp 153–159

American Psychiatric Association: Diagnostic and Statistical Manual of Mental Disorders, 3rd Edition. Washington, DC, American Psychiatric Press, 1980

American Psychiatric Association: Diagnostic and Statistical Manual of Mental Disorders, 3rd Edition, Revised. Washington, DC, American Psychiatric Association, 1987

American Psychiatric Association: Benzodiazepine Dependence and Withdrawal. Washington, DC, American Psychiatric Association, 1989

American Psychiatric Association: Diagnostic and Statistical Manual of Mental Disorders, 4th Edition. Washington, DC, American Psychiatric Association, 1994

Anderson OD, Parmenter R: Long term study of the experimental neurosis in the sheep and dog: with nine case histories. Psychosom Med Monogr 2(3,4a), 1941

Andreasen NC: Posttraumatic stress disorder, in Comprehensive Textbook of Psychiatry/III, 3rd Edition, Vol 2. Edited by Kaplan HI, Freedman AM, Sadock BJ. Baltimore, MD, Williams & Wilkins, 1980, pp 1517–1525

Andreasen NC, Noyes R, Hartford CE: Factors influencing adjustment of burn patients during hospitalization. Psychosom Med 34:517, 1972

Avery DH, Osgood TB, Ishiki DM, et al: The DST in psychiatric outpatients with generalized anxiety disorder, panic disorder, or primary affective disorder. Am J Psychiatry 142:844–848, 1985

Barlow DH: Current models of panic disorder and a view from emotion theory, in American Psychiatric Press Review of Psychiatry, Vol 7. Edited by Frances AJ, Hales RE. Washington DC: American Psychiatric Press, 1988, pp 10–28

Baxter LR Jr, Phelps ME, Mazziotta JC, et al: Local cerebral glucose metabolic rates in obsessive-compulsive disorder: a comparison with rates in unipolar depression and normal controls. Arch Gen Psychiatry 44:211–218, 1987

Baxter LR Jr, Schwartz JM, Mazziota JC, et al: Cerebral glucose metabolic rates in nondepressed patients with obsessive-compulsive disorder. Am J Psychiatry 145:1560–1563, 1988

Baxter LR Jr, Schwartz JM, Bergman MP, et al: Caudate glucose metabolic rate changes with both drug and behavior therapy for OCD. Arch Gen Psychiatry 49:681–689, 1992

Beck AT: Cognitive Therapy and the Emotional Disorders. New York, International Universities Press, 1976

Beck AT, Emery G: Anxiety Disorders and Phobias: A Cognitive Perspective. New York, Basic Books, 1985

Blanchard EB, Kolb LC, Gerardi RJ, et al: Cardiac response to relevant stimuli as an adjunctive tool for diagnosing posttraumatic stress disorder in Vietnam veterans. Behavior Therapy 17:592–606, 1986

Blazer D, Hughes D, George LK: Stressful life events and the onset of generalized anxiety syndrome. Am J Psychiatry 144:1178–1183, 1987

Breier A, Charney D, Heninger: The diagnostic validity of anxiety disorders and their relationship to depressive illness. Am J Psychiatry 142:787–798, 1985

Brett EA, Spitzer RL, Williams JW: DSM-III-R criteria for posttraumatic stress disorder. Am J Psychiatry 145:1232–1236, 1988

Buchsbaum MS, Wu J, Haier R, et al: Positron emission tomography assessment of effects of benzodiazepines on regional glucose metabolic rate in patients with anxiety disorder. Life Sci 40:2393–2400, 1987

Burnam MA, Hough RL, Escobar JI, et al: Six-month prevalence of specific psychiatric disorders among Mexican-Americans and non-Hispanic whites in Los Angeles. Arch Gen Psychiatry 44:687–694, 1987

Cameron OG, Lee MA, Curtis GC, et al: Endocrine and physiological changes during "spontaneous" panic attacks. Psychoneuroendocrinology 12:321–331, 1987

Canino GJ, Bird HR, Shrout PE, et al: The prevalence of specific psychiatric disorders in Puerto Rico. Arch Gen Psychiatry 44:727–735, 1987

Carr DB, Sheehan DV: Panic anxiety: a new biologic model. J Clin Psychiatry 45:323–330, 1984

Casas M, Alvarez E, Duro P, et al: Antiandrogenic treatment of obsessive compulsive disorder. Acta Psychiatr Scand 73:221–222, 1986

Chambless DL, Caputo GC, Bright P, et al: The assessment of fear in agoraphobics: the Body Sensations Questionnaire and the Agoraphobics Cognitions Questionnaire. J Consult Clin Psychol 52:1090–1097, 1984

Charney DS, Deutch AY, Krystal JH, et al: Psychobiologic mechanisms of posttraumatic stress disorder. Arch Gen Psychiatry 50:294–305, 1993

Christie KA, Burke JD, Reiger DA: Epidemiologic evidence for early onset of mental disorders and higher risk of drug abuse in young adults. Am J Psychiatry 145:971–975, 1988

Clary C, Schweizer E: Treatment of MAOI hypertensive crisis with sublingual nifedipine. J Clin Psychiatry 48:249–250, 1987

Cohen ME, White PD: Life situations, emotions and neurocirculatory asthenia. Psychosom Med 13:335–357 1951

Cowley DS, Dager SR, McClellan J, et al: Response to lactate infusion in generalized anxiety disorder. Biol Psychiatry 40:9–14, 1988

Craske MG: Cognitive-behavioral treatment of panic, in American Psychiatric Press Review of Psychiatry, Vol 7. Edited by Frances AJ, Hales RE. Washington, DC, American Psychiatric Press, 1988, pp 121–137

Cummings JL. Clinical Neuropsychiatry. Orlando, FL, Grune & Stratton, 1985

Davidson JRT, Smith RD, Kudler HS: Validity and reliability of the DSM-III criteria for post-traumatic stress disorder: experience with a structured interview. J Nerv Ment Dis 177:336–341, 1989

Davidson JRT, Kudler H, Smith R, et al: Treatment of posttraumatic stress disorder with amitriptyline and placebo. Arch Gen Psychiatry 47:259–269, 1990

DeVeaugh-Geiss J, Katz RJ, Landau P, et al: Preliminary results from a multicenter trial of clomipramine in obsessive-compulsive disorder. Psychopharmacol Bull 25:36–40, 1989

DiNardo PA, O'Brien GT, Barlow DH, et al: Reliability of DSM-III anxiety disorder categories using a new structured interview. Arch Gen Psychiatry 40:1070–1074, 1983

Dobbs D, Wilson WP: Observations on persistence of war neurosis. Diseases of the Nervous System 21:686–691, 1960

Dubovsky SL: Generalized anxiety disorder: new concepts and psychopharmacologic therapies. J Clin Psychiatry 51(No 1, Suppl):3–10, 1990

Ellis A: Reason and Emotion in Psychotherapy. New York, Lyle Stuart, 1962

Ellis A, Harper RA: A New Guide to Rational Living. North Hollywood, CA, Wilshire Book Co, 1975

Fenichel O: The Psychoanalytic Theory of Neurosis. New York, WW Norton, 1945

Fisher S, Greenberg RP: The Scientific Credibility of Freud's Theories and Therapy. New York, Basic Books, 1977

Fishman GG: Psychoanalytic psychotherapy (of anxiety disorders), in Treatments of Psychiatric Disorders, Vol 3. Washington, DC, American Psychiatric Association, 1989, pp 2010–2024

Foa EB, Steketee GS, Ozarrow BJ: Behavior therapy with obsessive-compulsives: from theory to treatment, in Obsessive Compulsive Disorder: Psychological and Pharmacological Treatment. Edited by Mavissakalian M, Turner SM, Michelson L. New York, Plenum, 1985, pp 49–129

Frankel FH, Orne MT: Strategies of relaxation, self-control, and fear-mastery, in Treatments of Psychiatric Disorders, Vol 3. Washington, DC, American Psychiatric Association, 1989, pp 2052–2092

Freud S: On the grounds for detaching a particular syndrome from neurasthenia under the description "anxiety neurosis" (1895[1894]), in The Standard Edition of the Complete Psychological Works of Sigmund Freud, Vol 3. Translated and edited by Strachey J. London, Hogarth Press, 1962, pp 85–115

Friedman MJ: Post-Vietnam syndrome: recognition and management. Psychosomatics 22:931–943, 1981

Friedman MJ: Toward rational pharmacotherapy for posttraumatic stress disorder: an interim report. Am J Psychiatry 145:281–285, 1988

Friedman P, Goldstein J: Phobic reactions, in American Handbook of Psychiatry, 2nd Edition, Vol 3. New York, Basic Books, 1974, pp 110–140

Fyer AJ, Sandberg D: Pharmacologic treatment of panic disorder, in American Psychiatric Press Review of Psychiatry, Vol 7. Edited by Frances AJ, Hales RE. Washington, DC, American Psychiatric Press, 1988, pp 88–120

Fyer AJ, Mannuzza S, Gallops MS, et al: Familial transmission of simple phobias and fears: a preliminary report. Arch Gen Psychiatry 47:252–256, 1990

Fyer AJ, Mannuzza S, Chapman TF, et al: A direct interview family study of social phobia. Arch Gen Psychiatry 50:286–293, 1993

Gaffney FA, Feneon BJ, Lane LD, et al: Hemodynamic ventilatory and biochemical responses of panic patients and normal controls with sodium lactate infusion and spontaneous panic attacks. Arch Gen Psychiatry 45:53–60, 1988

Ganesan S, Fine S, Lin TY: Psychiatric symptoms in refugees families from Southeast Asia: therapeutic challenges. Am J Psychother 23:218–228, 1989

Gittelman R, Klein DR: School phobia: diagnostic considerations in the light of imipramine effects. J Nerv Ment Dis 156:199–215, 1973

Goodman WK, Price LH, Rasmussen SA, et al: The Yale-Brown Obsessive-Compulsive Scale (Y-BOCS), Part I: development, use, and reliability. Arch Gen Psychiatry 46:1006–1011, 1989

Gorman JM, Fyer AJ, Glicklich J, et al: Effect of imipramine on prolapsed mitral valves of patients with panic disorder. Am J Psychiatry 138:997–998, 1981

Gorman JM, Liebowitz MT, Fyer AJ: Lactate infusions in obsessive-compulsive disorder. Am J Psychiatry 142:864–866, 1985

Gorman JM, Liebowitz MT, Fyer AJ, et al: Possible respiratory abnormalities in panic disorders. Psychopharmacol Bull 2:797–801, 1986

Gorman JM, Liebowitz MT, Fyer AJ, et al: An open trial of fluoxetine in the treatment of panic attacks. J Clin Psychopharmacol 7:329–332, 1987

Greist J: Treating the anxiety: therapeutic options in obsessive-compulsive disorder. J Clin Psychiatry 51 (No 11, Suppl):29–34, 1990a

Greist JH: Treatment of obsessive-compulsive disorder: psychotherapies, drugs, and other somatic treatments. J Clin Psychiatry 51 (No 8, Suppl):44–50, 1990b

Greist JH, Jefferson JW: Anxiety disorders, in Review of General Psychiatry, 2nd Edition. Edited by Goldman HH. Norwalk, CT, Appleton & Lange, 1988, pp 349–364

Griez E, van den Hout MA: CO$_2$ inhalation in the treatment of panic attacks. Behav Res Ther 24:145–150, 1986

Grunhaus L, Gloger S, Birmacher B: Clomipramine treatment for panic attacks in patients with mitral valve prolapse. J Clin Psychiatry 45:25–27, 1984

Helzer JE, Robins LN, McEvoy L: Post-traumatic stress disorder in the general population: findings of the Epidemiologic Catchment Area survey. N Engl J Med 317:1630–1634, 1987

Hogben GL, Cornfield RB: Treatment of traumatic war neurosis with phenelzine. Arch Gen Psychiatry 38:440–445, 1981

Horowitz M: Disasters and psychological responses to stress. Psychiatric Annals 15:135–142, 1985

Horowitz MJ: Stress Response Syndromes, 2nd Edition. New York, Jason Aronson, 1986

Horowitz MJ: Posttraumatic stress disorder, in Treatments of Psychiatric Disorders, Vol 3. Washington, DC, American Psychiatric Association, 1989, pp 2065–2082

Insel TR: Phenomenology of obsessive compulsive disorder. J Clin Psychiatry 51 (No , Suppl):4–8, 1990

Insel TR, Kalin NH, Guttmacher LB, et al: The dexamethasone suppression test in patients with primary obsessive-compulsive disorder. Psychiatry Res 6:153–160, 1982

Jackson SW: Melancholia and Depression: From Hippocratic Times to Modern Times. New Haven, CT, Yale University Press, 1986

Jacob RG, Turner SM: Panic disorder: diagnosis and assessment, in American Psychiatric Press Review of Psychiatry, Vol 7. Edited by Frances AJ, Hales RE. Washington, DC, American Psychiatric Press, 1988, pp 67–87

Jagger J, Prusoff BA, Cohen DJ, et al: The epidemiology of Tourette's syndrome: a pilot study. Schizophr Bull 8:267–278, 1982

Janet P, Raymond R: Les Neuroses et Ideés Fixes. Paris, Alcan, 1898

Jenike MA: Obsessive-compulsive and related disorders: a hidden epidemic (editorial/comment). N Engl J Med 321:539–541, 1989

Jenike MA, Buttol PHL, Baer L, et al: Fluoxetine in obsessive-compulsive disorder: a positive open trial. Am J Psychiatry 46:909–911, 1989

Kaplan HI, Sadock BJ: Synopsis of Psychiatry, 5th Edition. Baltimore, MD, Williams & Wilkins, 1988

Keane TM, Fairbank JA, Caddell JM, et al: Clinical evaluation of a measure to assess combat exposure. J Consult Clin Psychol 57:53–55, 1989

Kernberg O: Borderline Conditions and Pathological Narcissism. New York, Jason Aronson, 1975

Kierkegaard S: The Concept of Dread. Translated by Lowrie W. Princeton, NJ, Princeton University Press, 1944

Kitchner I, Greenstein R: Low dose lithium carbonate in the treatment of post traumatic stress disorder: brief communication. Milit Med 150:378–381, 1985

Klein D: The pathophysiology of panic anxiety (abstract). J Clin Psychiatry 52 (No 2, Suppl):10–11, 1991

Klein D: False suffocation alarms, spontaneous panics, and related conditions: an integrative hypothesis. Arch Gen Psychiatry 50:306–317, 1993

Koegel P, Burnam A, Farr RK: The prevalence of psychiatric disorders among homeless individuals in the inner city of Los Angeles. Arch Gen Psychiatry 45:1085–1093, 1988

Kolb LC: A neuropsychological hypothesis explaining posttraumatic stress disorders. Am J Psychiatry 144:989–995, 1987

Kramer M, Kinney L: Is sleep a marker of vulnerability to delayed posttraumatic stress disorder? Sleep Research 14:181, 1985

Kupfer DJ, Frank E, Grochocinski VJ, et al: Electroencephalographic sleep profiles in recurrent depression: a longitudinal investigation. Arch Gen Psychiatry 45:678–681, 1988

Lasch C: The Culture of Narcissism. New York, Warner Books, 1979

Lavie P, Hefez A, Halperin G, et al: Long-term effects of traumatic war-related events on sleep. Am J Psychiatry 136:175–178, 1979

Lieberman JA, Kane JM, Sarantakos MD, et al: Dexamethasone suppression test in patients with obsessive-compulsive disorder. Am J Psychiatry 142:747–751, 1985

Liebowitz MR, Fyer AJ, Gorman JM, et al: Specificity of lactate infusions in social phobia versus panic disorders. Am J Psychiatry 142:947–949, 1985

Liebowitz MR, Gorman JM, Fyer AJ, et al: Pharmacotherapy of social phobia: an interim report of a placebo-controlled comparison of phenelzine and atenolol. J Clin Psychiatry 49:252–257, 1988

Liebowitz MR, Schneier F, Campeas R: Phenelzine and atenolol in social phobia. Psychopharmacol Bull 26:123–125, 1990

Liebowitz MR, Schneier F, Campeas R, et al: Phenelzine vs atenolol in social phobia. Arch Gen Psychiatry 49:290–300, 1992

Lifton RJ: Home From the War. New York, Simon & Schuster, 1973

Lindy J: The trauma membrane and other clinical concepts derived from psychotherapeutic work with survivors of natural disasters. Psychiatric Annals 15:153–160, 1985

Lishman WA: Organic Psychiatry, 2nd Edition. Oxford, UK, Blackwell Scientific, 1987

Lucey JV, Butcher G, Clare , et al: Elevated growth hormone responses to pyridostigmine in obsessive-compulsive disorder: evidence of cholinergic supersensitivity. Am J Psychiatry 150:961–962, 1993

Luxenberg JS, Swedo SE, Flament MF, et al: Neuroanatomical abnormalities in obsessive-compulsive disorder detected with quantitative X-ray computed tomography. Am J Psychiatry 145:1089–1093, 1988

MacDonald M: Mystical Bedlam: Madness, Anxiety and Healing in Seventeenth-Century England. Cambridge, UK, Cambridge University Press, 1981

MacKinnon RA, Michels R: The Psychiatric Interview in Clinical Practice. Philadephia, PA, WB Saunders, 1971

Mahler MS, Pine F, Bergman A: The Psychological Birth of the Human Infant: Symbiosis and Individuation. New York, Basic Books, 1975

Malloy PF, Fairbank JA, Keane TM: Validation of a multi-method assessment of posttraumatic stress disorders in Vietnam veterans. J Consult Clin Psychol 51:488–494, 1983

Margalit M, Heiman T: Family climate and anxiety in families with learning disabled boys. Journal of the American Academy of Child Psychiatry 25:841–846, 1986

Markowitz JS, Weissman MM, Ouellette R, et al: Quality of life in panic disorder. Arch Gen Psychiatry 46:984–992, 1989

Marks IM, Gelder MG: The common ground between behavior therapy and psychodynamic methods. Br J Med Psychol 39:11, 1966

Mason J, Giller EL, Kosten TR, et al: Elevated norepinephrine/cortisol ratio in PTSD, in New Research Program and Abstracts, 138th Annual Meeting of the American Psychiatric Association, Dallas, TX, May 1985, NR172, p 94

Mason JW, Giller EL, Kosten TR, et al: Urinary free cortisol in postraumatic stress disorder. J Nerv Ment Dis 174:145–149, 1986

Mavissakalian M, Perel JM: Protective effects of imipramine maintenance treatment in panic disorder with agoraphobia. Am J Psychiatry 149:1053–1057, 1992

May R: The Meaning of Anxiety. New York, WW Norton, 1977

McDermott JF, Werry J, Petti T, et al: Anxiety disorders of childhood or adolescence, in Treatments of Psychiatric Disorders, Vol 1. Washington, DC, American Psychiatric Association, 1989, pp 401–442

McDougle CJ, Goodman WK, Price LH, et al: Neuroleptic addition in fluvoxamine-refractory obsessive-compulsive disorder. Am J Psychiatry 147:283–294, 1990

McFarlane AC: The aetiology of post-traumatic morbidity: predisposing, precipitating, and perpetuating factors. Br J Psychiatry 154:221–228, 1989

McNeil GN: Anxiety, in Handbook of Psychiatric Differential Diagnosis. Edited by Soreff SM, McNeil GM. Littleton, MA, PSG Publishing, 1987, pp 127–163

Mellman TA, Uhde TW: Electroencephalographic sleep in panic disorder: a focus on sleep-related panic attacks. Arch Gen Psychiatry 46:178–184, 1989

Meltzer HY: Editorial and commentary, in Yearbook of Psychiatry and Applied Mental Health. Chicago, IL, Year Book Medical, 1989, p 35

Meth JM: Exotic psychiatric syndromes, in American Handbook of Psychiatry, Vol 3. Edited by Arieti S. New York, Basic Books, 1974, pp 723–739

Meyer RG: The Clinician's Handbook: Psychopathology of Adulthood and Late Adolescence. Boston, MA, Allyn & Bacon, 1983

Mountz JM, Modell JG, Wilson MW, et al: Positron emission tomographic evaluation of cerebral blood flow during state anxiety in simple phobia. Arch Gen Psychiatry 46:501–504, 1989

Nadelson T: Attachment to killing. J Am Acad Psychoanal 20:130–141, 1992

Nagy LM, Morgan CA, Southwick SM, et al: Open prospective trial of fluoxetine for posttraumatic stress disorder. J Clin Psychopharmacol 13:107–113, 1993

Nemiah JC: Anxiety state, in Comprehensive Textbook of Psychiatry/III, 3rd Edition, Vol 2. Edited by Kaplan HI, Freedman A, Sadock BJ. Baltimore, MD, Williams & Wilkins, 1980a, pp 1483–1492

Nemiah JC: Obsessive-compulsive disorder, in Comprehensive Textbook of Psychiatry/III, 3rd Edition, Vol 2. Edited by Kaplan HI, Freedman A, Sadock BJ. Baltimore, MD, Williams & Wilkins, 1980b, pp 1504–1516

Nemiah JC: Phobic disorder, in Comprehensive Textbook of Psychiatry/III, 3rd Edition, Vol 2. Edited by Kaplan HI, Freedman A, Sadock BJ. Baltimore, MD, Williams & Wilkins, 1980c, pp 1493–1503

Nemiah JC: Anxiety states (anxiety neuroses), in Comprehensive Textbook of Psychiatry/IV, 4th Edition, Vol 1. Edited by Kaplan HI, Sadock BJ. Baltimore, MD, William & Wilkins, 1985a, pp 883–894

Nemiah JC: Obsessive-compulsive disorder (obsessive-compulsive neurosis), in Comprehensive Textbook of Psychiatry/IV, 4th Edition, Vol 1. Edited by Kaplan HI, Sadock BJ. Baltimore, MD, William & Wilkins, 1985b, pp 904–917

Nemiah JC: Phobic disorders (phobic neuroses), in Comprehensive Textbook of Psychiatry/IV, 4th Edition, Vol 1. Edited by Kaplan HI, Sadock BJ. Baltimore, MD, William & Wilkins, 1985c, pp 894–904

Newmark CS: Major Psychological Assessment Instruments. Boston, MA, Allyn & Bacon, 1985

Ontiveros A, Fontaine R: Social phobia and clonazepam. Can J Psychiatry 35:439–441, 1990

Ortiz A, Rainey JM, Frohman R, et al: Effects of imipramine on lactate-induced panic anxiety. Abstract of presentation at World Congress of Biological Psychiatry, Philadelphia, PA, September 1985

Ost L: One-session treatment for specific phobias. Behav Res Ther 27:1–7, 1989

Paul SM: Anxiety and depression: a common neurological substrate? J Clin Psychiatry 49 (No 10, Suppl):13–16, 1988

Pies R: Distinguishing obsessional from psychotic phenomena. J Clin Psychopharmacol 4:345–347, 1984

Pitman RK, van der Kolk BA, Orr SP, et al: Naloxone-reversible analgesic response to combat-related stimuli in posttraumatic stress disorder. Arch Gen Psychiatry 47:541–544, 1990

Pitts FN, McClure JN: Lactate metabolism in anxiety neurosis. N Engl J Med 277:1328–1336, 1967

Raj AR, Sheehan DV: Medical evaluation of panic attacks, J Clin Psychiatry 48:309–313, 1987

Rapoport JL: Obsessive-compulsive disorder and basal ganglia dysfunction. Psychol Med 20:465–469, 1990

Rapoport JL, Elkins R, Langer DH, et al: Childhood obsessive-compulsive disorder. Am J Psychiatry 138:1545–1554, 1981

Rasmussen SA: Lithium and tryptophan augmentation in clomipramine-resistant obsessive-compulsive disorder. Am J Psychiatry 141:1283–1285, 1984

Rasmussen SA, Eisen JL: Epidemiology of obsessive-compulsive disorder. J Clin Psychiatry 51 (No 8, Suppl):20–23, 1990

Rasmussen SA, Eisen JL: Epidemiology and differential diagnosis of obsessive-compulsive disorder. J Clin Psychiatry 53 (No 4, Suppl):4–10, 1992

Reich J, Noyes R, Yates W: Anxiety symptoms distinguishing social phobia from panic and generalized anxiety disorders. J Nerv Ment Dis 176:510–513, 1988

Reiman EM, Raichle ME, Robins E, et al: The application of positron emission tomography to the study of panic disorder. Am J Psychiatry 143:469–477, 1986

Reiman EM, Raichie ME, Robins E, et al: Neuroanatomical correlates of a lactate-induced anxiety attack. Arch Gen Psychiatry 46:493–500, 1989

Reiser M: Theoretical concepts in psychosomatic medicine, in American Handbook of Psychiatry, Vol 4. Edited by Arieti S, Reiser M. New York, Basic Books, 1975, pp 477–500

Riblet LA, Eison AS, Eison MS: Neuropharmacology of buspirone. Psychopathology 17 (suppl 3):69–78, 1984

Ross RJ, Ball WA, Sullivan DA, et al: Sleep disturbance as the hallmark of posttraumatic stress disorder. Am J Psychiatry 146:697–707, 1989

Roth M: The phobic anxiety-depersonalization syndrome. Proc Royal Soc Med 52:587–595, 1959

Roth M, Burney C, Garside RF, et al: The relationship between anxiety states and depressive illnesses. Br J Psychiatry 121:147–161, 1972

Roy-Byrne P, Geraci M, Uhde TW: Life events preceding the onset of panic disorder. J Affect Disord 9:103–105, 1986

Schlesinger EG, Devore W: Ethnically sensitive social work practice in health care. Paper presented at the annual meeting of the American Public Health Association, Detroit, MI, October 1980

Schlossberg A, Benjamin M: Sleep patterns in three acute combat fatigue cases. J Clin Psychiatry 39:546–549, 1978

Shader RI: Stress, fear, and anxiety, in Handbook of Clinical Psychopharmacology, 2nd Edition. Edited by Tupin JP, Shader RI, Harnett DS. Northvale, NJ, Jason Aronson, 1988, pp 73–96

Shear MK, Fyer MF: Biological and psychopathologic findings in panic disorder, in American Psychiatric Press Review of Psychiatry, Vol 7. Edited by Frances AJ, Hales RE. Washington, DC, American Psychiatric Press, 1988, pp 29–53

Shear MK, Cooper AM, Klerman GL, et al: A psychodynamic model of panic disorder. Am J Psychiatry 150:859–866, 1993

Sheehan DV, Raj AB, Sheehan KH, et al: Is buspirone effective for panic disorder? J Clin Psychopharmacol 10:3–11, 1990

Siever LJ, Insel TR, Jimerson DC, et al: Growth hormone response to clonidine in obsessive-compulsive patients. Br J Psychiatry 142:184–187, 1983

Silver JM, Sandberg DP, Hales RE: New approaches in the pharmacotherapy of posttraumatic stress disorder. J Clin Psychiatry 51 (No 10, Suppl):33–38, 1990

Sitaram N, Dube S, Jones D: Acetylcholine and alpha adrenergic sensitivity in the separation of depression and anxiety. Psychopathology 17:24–39, 1984

Snell B: The Discovery of the Mind. New York, Dover, 1982

Spitz R: The First Year of Life: A Psychoanalytic Study of Normal and Deviant Development of Object Relations. New York, International Universities Press, 1965

Stark P, Hardison CD: A review of multicenter controlled studies of fluoxetine vs imipramine and placebo in outpatients with major depressive disorder. J Clin Psychiatry 46:53–58, 1985

Starkman MN, Zelnick TC, Nesse RM, et al: A study of anxiety in patients with pheochromocytoma. Arch Intern Med 145:248–252, 1985

Stein MB, Uhde TW: Thyroid indices in panic disorder. Am J Psychiatry 145:745–747, 1988

Stewart RS, Devous MD, Rush AJ, et al: Cerebral blood flow changes during sodium-lactate-induced panic attacks. Am J Psychiatry 145:442–450, 1988

Swedo SE, Rapoport JL, Leonard HL, et al: Obsessive-compulsive disorder in children and adolescents. Arch Gen Psychiatry 46:335–341, 1989

Swedo SE, Pietrini P, Leonard HL, et al: Cerebral glucose metabolism in childhood-onset obsessive-compulsive disorder: revisualization during pharmacotherapy. Arch Gen Psychiatry 49:690–694, 1992

Taylor CB, Sheikh J, Agras WS, et al: Ambulatory heart rate changes in patients with panic attacks. Am J Psychiatry 143:478–482, 1986

True WR, Rice J, Eisen SA: A twin study of genetic and environmental contributions to liability for posttraumatic stress symptoms. Arch Gen Psychiatry 50:257–265, 1993

Uhde AT, Roy-Byrne P, Gillin JC, et al: The sleep of patients with panic disorder: a preliminary report. Psychiatry Res 12:251–259, 1984

Van der Kolk BA: Psychopharmacologic issues in posttraumatic stress disorder. Hosp Community Psychiatry 34:683–691, 1983

Van der Kolk B, Blit R, Burr W, et al: Nightmares and trauma: a comparison of nightmares after combat with lifelong nightmares in veterans. Am J Psychiatry 141:187–190, l984

Van der Kolk B, Greenberg M, Boyd H, et al: Inescapable shock neuro-transmitters, and addiction to trauma: toward a psychobiology of post-traumatic stress. Biol Psychiatry 20:314–325, 1985

Van Valkenburg C, Akiskal HS, Puzantian V, et al: Anxious depression: clinical family history and naturalistic outcome-comparisons with panic and major depressive disorder. J Affect Disord 6:67–82, 1984

Vaughan DA: Interaction of fluoxetine with tricyclic antidepressants (letter). Am J Psychiatry 145:1478, 1988

Volkow ND, Harper A, Swann AC: Temporal lobe abnormalities and panic attacks. Am J Psychiatry 143:1484–1485, 1986

Von Korff MR, Eaton WW, Keyl PM: The epidemiology of panic attacks and panic disorder: results of three community surveys. Am J Epidemiol 122:970–981, 1985

Walder CP, McCracken JS, Herbert M, et al: Psychological intervention in civilian flying phobia: evaluation and a three year follow up. Br J Psychiatry 151:494–498, 1987

Watson CG, Kucala T, Manifold V, et al: Differences between posttraumatic stress disorder patients with delayed and undelayed onsets. J Nerv Ment Disease 176:568–572, 1988

Watson JB, Rayner R: Conditioned emotional reactions. Journal of Experimental Psychology 3:1–14, 1920

Weissman MM. The epidemiology of anxiety disorders: rates, risks, and familial patterns. J Psychiatr Res 22 (No 1, Suppl):99–114, 1988

Whytt R: Observations on the nature, causes, and cure of those disorders which are commonly called nervous, hypochondriac, or hysteric (1764), in The Works of Robert Whytt, M.D. Edinburgh, Becket, DeHondt, & Balfour, 1768

Wieland S, Boren JL, Consroe PF, et al: Stock differences in the susceptibility of rats in learned helplessness training. Life Sci 39:939–944, 1986

Wilson T: Behavior therapy, in Treatments of Psychiatric Disorders, Vol 3. Washington, DC, American Psychiatric Association, 1989, pp 2025–2035

Winnicott DW: Collected Papers: Through Paediatrics to Psychoanalysis. New York, Basic Books, 1958

Woodward R, Jones RB: Cognitive restructuring treatment: a controlled trial with anxious patients. Behav Res Ther 18:401–407, 1989

Zohar J, Mueller EA, Insel TR, et al: Serotonergic responsivity in obsessive-compulsive disorder: comparisons of patients and healthy controls. Arch Gen Psychiatry 44:946–951, 1987

7

Somatoform Disorders

> I have headaches from time to time . . . sometimes
> I seem to have a sort of mist before my eyes . . . at
> other times I've a pain at my heart . . . at other
> times I'm weary in every limb . . . then I have pains
> in my stomach—as if I had colic!
>
> > Argan to Toinette, in Molière's
> > *Le Malade Imaginaire*

Molière had a good deal of fun at the expense of "hypo-chondriacs"—and even more at the expense of doctors and their "cures." We still find hypochondriasis funny—as Woody Allen's character proves in the movie *Hannah and Her Sisters*. Yet the somatoform disorders—which include hypochondriasis, somatization disorder, conversion disorder, body dysmorphic disorder, and pain disorder—exact a very serious toll on those who suffer from them. Smith et al. (1986) note that somatization disorder is "chronic and disabling," with a recovery rate of only 31% at 15-year follow-up assessment. The per capita expenditure for health care of "somatizing" patients is up to nine times the average per capita amount. On the other hand, great harm may come from assuming a psychogenic origin of somatic complaints; as an old clinical maxim notes, "Hysteria is the last diagnosis the patient will ever receive." Koranyi (1979), in his classic studies, discovered that 43% of patients in psychiatric clinics suffered from one or more physical disorders and that almost half of these disorders had not been diagnosed by the referring physician. Among the cases cited by Koranyi are patients with undiagnosed digitalis poisoning, hypoglycemia, thyrotoxicosis, and medulloblastoma. Thus, we should have a very high "threshold" for diagnosing the disorders discussed in this chapter. Once recognized, the somatoform disorders require a patient, supportive, and yet vigilant approach, keeping in mind the other maxim we have espoused, "The body can have as many diseases as it pleases!"

All of the somatoform disorders involve the presentation of some physical complaint, sign, or symptom that cannot be explained by any known physiological mechanism or "organic" disease process. All, in other words, are related to some presumed psychological factor, but none arises from an act of voluntary control or feigning of symptoms. Thus, the somatoform disorders are not to be confused with malingering or factitious disorders.

Somatization Disorder

The Central Concept

Vignette

A 23-year-old female college student presented to the emergency room with the chief complaint of "burning in my urethra." She reported that this problem had begun quite suddenly after she returned from a "wild party" the previous night, and the patient theorized in a very animated fashion, "It must have been that weird punch—God, I'm probably gonna get AIDS or something!" She denied any use of illicit drugs. In addition to the chief complaint, the patient voiced numerous ancillary problems, including nonmenstrual abdominal pain of several years' duration, frequent lower back pain, shortness of breath on exertion, episodic dizziness, chronic difficulty swallowing, episodic vomiting, weakness and pain in her arms and legs for many years, frequent blurry vision (she wore no corrective lenses), and "incredibly painful periods—like my insides are being eaten alive." All previous medical and laboratory tests to determine an organic etiology for these complaints had been negative. On physical examination, the patient showed no abnormalities, and a gynecological consultant could find no physical cause for the patient's "burning."

As you can see, somatization disorder often presents as a kind of "organ recital," usually involving the reproductive, digestive, or cardiopulmonary organs. DSM-III-R (American Psychiatric Association 1987) required 13 symptoms from a list of 35 (in females). DSM-IV (American Psychiatric Association 1994) has condensed things considerably, requiring a total of 8 symptoms from four categories: pain, gastrointestinal, sexual, and pseudoneurological. Two symptoms that in DSM-III-R were considered "cardiopulmonary"—chest pain and nonexertional dyspnea—have in DSM-IV been subsumed, respectively, under "pain symptoms" and "pseudoneurological symptoms." The 7 symptoms most strongly correlated with somatization disorder are shown in Table 7–1. In DSM-III-R these symptoms were considered "screening" criteria for the disorder.

Associated features in somatization disorder commonly include anxiety, depression, and pseudopsychotic features such as hearing one's name being called, without delusional elaboration. The patient often presents the complaints in a dramatic or vague fashion, usually in the context of a long and complicated medical history. (To "count" a symptom as diagnostic of somatization disorder, it must not be fully explained by a known medical condition.)

Somatization disorder often begins in the teen years and shows a chronic, fluctuating course with considerable incapacity. Often, somatization disorder patients have been "doctor-shoppers" for many years and have undergone extensive medical testing. Many have developed a concomitant substance use disorder, related either to pre-

Table 7–1.   "Screening" items for somatization disorder

Vomiting (other than during pregnancy)

Pain in extremities

Nonexertional dyspnea

Amnesia

Difficulty swallowing

Burning sensation in sexual organs or rectum, other than during intercourse

Painful menstruation

scribed or to over-the-counter sedative drugs. This disorder is rarely diagnosed in males (see subsection on the biopsychosocial perspective later in this section).

Historical Development of the Disorder

Somatization disorder has its origins in the hoary and much-abused term "hysteria" (from the Greek *hystera*, or "womb"). Hippocrates had theorized that a "wandering uterus" caused the symptoms of hysteria, and he recommended marriage as the best remedy! However, our modern concept of somatization disorder arose from the work of Paul Briquet, based on his examination of over 400 patients, nearly all of whom were women (Nemiah 1985). *Briquet's syndrome* is still used as a synonym for somatization disorder, and Briquet's description of the disorder in 1859 has been elegantly represented by Mai and Merskey (1980).

Briquet noted nine predisposing factors to what he (rather reluctantly) referred to as "hysteria" (*l'hysterie*): female gender, youth (onset before age 20), family history of the disorder, low social class, sexual intercourse (contrary to the prevailing view that abstinence promoted hysteria), emotional/impressionable temperament, harsh upbringing, strong negative emotions, and poor health prior to onset of the syndrome (see Mai and Merskey 1980). For Briquet, the "core" features of hysteria included epigastric pain, left-sided chest or vertebral pain, hyperesthesias (e.g., headache, neuralgia), anesthesias, hallucinatory experiences, muscular or behavioral "spasms" (e.g., hyperventilation, vocal tics), and seizures.

Similar descriptions of hysteria were given by Savill in 1909 and Purtell et al. in 1951; the latter group emphasized the often dramatic and vague presentation of complaints in this disorder (Nemiah 1985). In the 1960s, Samuel Guze and his colleagues further refined our concept of somatization disorder (though Guze still termed it "hysteria"). Guze made the important distinction between "conversion reaction" and "hysteria" (essentially, somatization disorder), noting that "conversion symptoms are individual symptoms while hysteria is a polysymptomatic disorder" (Guze 1967, p. 493). In the most recent editions of DSM, the term "hysteria" has been abandoned, owing to its womb-centered (some would say "sexist") implications. Interestingly, Briquet himself, while anxious to disprove the "uterine" theory of hysteria, clearly established that hysteria was at least 20 times more likely in females than in males (Mai and Merskey 1980).

The Biopsychosocial Perspective

Biological Factors

Somatization disorder is seen in about 15% of female first-degree relatives of females with this disorder; interestingly, the male relatives of females with somatization disorder show an increased risk of antisocial personality disorder and psychoactive substance use disorders (American Psychiatric Association 1987). These data suggest that a genetic factor plays a role in somatization disorder and perhaps that somatization disorder and antisocial personality disorder are phenotypic variants of the same genotypic (biochemical?) disorder. Whether the different "outcome" in men and women relates to differing hormonal or psychosocial factors is not known (see discussion of sociocultural factors later in this section).

Flor-Henry (1983) has pointed out that "there has been virtually no systematic study . . . of possible alterations of cerebral functions in hysteria" (p. 272). Flor-Henry, using the criteria developed by Perley and Guze (1962) for hysteria, studied neuropsychological function in 10 patients (9 female, 1 male) with what we would now call somatization disorder. Compared with normal and schizophrenic control subjects, the somatization disorder subjects demonstrated more bilateral frontal lobe and nondominant frontotemporal dysfunction. Anterior brain regions were affected more than posterior regions. However, the Flor-Henry findings are more complicated than these data would suggest. Specifically, he notes that "dominant hemisphere dysfunction is fundamentally related to the syndrome of hysteria [somatization disorder] and . . . dysfunction of the nondominant hemisphere is brought about by associated features: the female excess, the emotional instability and dysphoric mood, the presence of asymmetrical pain, and conversion symptomatology" (p. 293).

In essence, when you clear the wheat from the chaff, somatization disorder per se is related to dominant hemisphere dysfunction. Based on some of his other studies, Flor-Henry argues further that "hysteria in the female is a syndrome equivalent to psychopathy in the male (who also exhibits dominant hemisphere dysfunction)" (p. 293).

A broader neuropsychological hypothesis holds that somatization disorder patients have "characteristic attentional and cognitive impairments that result in the faulty perception and assessment of somatosensory input . . . [e.g.,] excessive distractibility, inability to habituate to repetitive stimuli, the grouping of cognitive constructs on an impressionistic basis, and partial and circumstantial associations" (Kaplan and Sadock 1988, p. 335). Translated into everyday terms: If your brain habitually focuses on every itch and twitch in your body, and can't "think through" what these ordinary sensations really mean, you may end up experiencing a host of bodily complaints in the absence of any bodily pathology.

There are no known neuroendocrine abnormalities in somatization disorder, but Orenstein et al. (1986), noting the overlap between Briquet's syndrome and polycystic ovary (PCO) disease, has advanced a bold hypothesis: that "Briquet's syndrome also may be associated with CNS dysfunction . . . [and] may be as much a physical as a psychological illness" (p. 771). Orenstein and colleagues note possible hypothalamic dysfunction in PCO that resulted in decreased dopaminergic function, as well as the association of PCO and temporal lobe epilepsy. Because Briquet's was associated with PCO in 5 of 39 patients studied by Orenstein et al., they infer (perhaps across a rather wide information gap) a possible biological connection between the syndromes. Although speculative, the notion of Briquet's syndrome or somatization disorder as a neurophysiological disorder is supported by at least one single-photon emission computed tomography (SPECT) study (Lazarus and Cotterell 1989), in which the scan of a 44-year-old man with somatization disorder showed reduced tracer uptake in the right posterior parietal region. Another study, by James et al. (1987), showed increased blood flow in the right posterior region of somatization disorder patients, suggesting a disorder of attentional processing. It is too early to conclude much from these (seemingly contradictory) studies, but, taken together, they may suggest a disorder of the nondominant hemisphere in somatization disorder.

Psychological Factors

Once again, it is hard to sort out "psychological" from "social" influences (see below), but here we will focus on intrapsychic factors thought to be related to somatization disorder. Kellner (1990) has admirably summarized the chief psychosocial theories of "somatization" in general.

The psychoanalytic understanding of somatization disorder begins with the observation that "somatization" is one of the so-called immature defense mechanisms (see Meissner 1985). In this context, "somatization" is "the defensive conversion of psychic derivatives into bodily symptoms." From a psychodevelopmental perspective, "[i]nfantile somatic responses are replaced by thought and affect during development (desomatization): regression to earlier somatic forms of response (resomatization) may result from unresolved conflicts and may play an important role in psychological reactions" (Kaplan and Sadock 1988, p. 143). Thus, Maxmen (1986) notes that "somatization is often considered a defense mechanism, in which the patient unconsciously avoids painful affects by experiencing physical discomfort. Supposedly, in somatization disorder, the central defense mechanism is somatization, and the painful affect, depressive" (p. 241).

But other kinds of (repressed) affects have been posited. Fenichel (1945), in describing "conversion symptoms" (discussed later in this chapter), actually described the psychoanalytic understanding of what we would call somatization disorder. Fenichel stated that "in all these [somatic] symptoms, the entire cathexis of the objectionable impulses seems to be condensed into a definite physical function" (p. 227). The "choice of the afflicted region" depends on four factors: 1) the unconscious sexual fantasies and the corresponding erogeneity of the afflicted part (e.g., a person with oral fixations will develop oral symptoms, a person with anal fixations, anal ones, etc.); 2) premorbid disposition (e.g., "an individual of strong vasomotor lability will be more subject to vasomotor symptoms; an organically myopic individual is more likely to produce eye symptoms"); 3) the "situation in which the decisive repression occurred" (e.g., if the individual was breathing heavily at the time an unacceptable [e.g., sexual] impulse occurred, he or she might develop psychogenic dyspnea); and 4) the "ability of the . . . organ to express symbolically the unconscious drive in question" (e.g., "concave organs like mouth, anus, nostrils . . . may symbolize the vagina and represent feminine wishes") (p. 228).

How much evidence is there that somatization disorder arises from the repression of depressed affect? Despite the frequent co-morbidity of somatization and depression, Kellner (1990) notes that "there is no conclusive evidence that somatization is a true depressive equivalent, meaning that it has the same etiology, course, and re-sponse to treatment as depression" (p. 152). Indeed, a linguistic analysis of patients with somatization disorder (Oxman et al. 1985) revealed that "rather than repressing or defending against unbearable depression, our primary-care patients with somatization disorder ex-hibited the capacity to express their unhappiness quite overtly" (p. 1154). Oxman et al. found that the somatization disorder patients showed in their language usage evidence of excessive self-absorption and mild narcissistic traits, including a "basic preoccupation with self-identity." These authors concluded that somatization disorder "is not reducible" to a masked form of depression. Nevertheless, the co-occurrence of somatization and depression is undeniable. Lipowski (1988) notes that most patients who seek medical care for depressive symptoms complain of somatic rather than psychological symptoms. While this may reflect an alternate psychic mechanism of some sort, Lipowski points out that some depressed patients present with somatic complaints "because they do not wish to be given psychiatric diagno-ses and hence be stigmatized" (p. 1363).

What about a more general mechanism in somatization disorder, involving "the denial and repression of distressing emotions"? Sum-marizing the literature, Kellner (1990) notes that there is "an associa-tion of repression, denial, the inhibition of emotion, and the lack of confiding . . . [with] somatic symptoms, and the incidence of disease" (p. 156).

Like depression, anxiety is commonly associated with somatiza-tion disorder, and some have held the view that "somatic sensations are mainly the bodily manifestations of anxiety states" (Kellner 1990, p. 152). Indeed, somatic symptoms are much more common in patients with anxiety disorders than in normal control subjects; these symptoms tend to decrease when the anxiety remits. Lipowski (1988) notes that patients with panic disorder (see subsecton on differential diagnosis) often present with many somatic complaints (e.g., chest pain, palpitations, dyspepsia, headache, dizziness, fainting, and dyspnea). It is possible that such patients exhibit excessive or selective attention to bodily sensations and a "negative bias" in appraising their health (see Chapter 6).

Sociocultural Factors

Kellner (1990) has summarized the literature suggesting that somatization is a form of "learned behavior" in a social context. For example, children's somatic symptoms are often "copies" of those symptoms occurring in other members of the family; moreover, somatization in later years may be correlated with parental attention to the individual's somatic symptoms in childhood. Viewed somewhat differently, these observations suggest that somatization disorder is essentially a conditioned response, whereby "somatizing behavior" is made more likely by the "positive reinforcer" of parental attention or perhaps the attention of well-meaning physicians (Kellner 1990; Lipowski 1988).

Morrison (1983) discovered that "birth order" (i.e., order of birth within a sibship) in 90 female patients with Briquet's syndrome was significantly earlier than the theoretical mean for a normally distributed population. At that time, Morrison speculated that some early environmental influence might play a role in the etiology of somatization disorder; for example, perhaps "older children in a sibship grow up with younger, possibly more volatile parents" (p. 1597). Subsequent work by Morrison (1989) showed something more alarming. In a study of 60 female patients with somatization disorder and 31 females with primary affective disorder, significantly more of the subjects with somatization disorder gave histories of having been sexually molested as children. This finding is of great theoretical, as well as clinical, interest, because of how sexual abuse predisposes to dissociative disorders (see Chapter 8). Indeed, Bliss (1980) noted that most patients with multiple personality disorder could be diagnosed as having somatization disorder; however, as Morrison (1989) points out, "there is no convincing evidence that patients with somatization disorder dissociate more than average" (p. 241). Thus, in the study by Morrison (1989), only 3 of 60 patients with somatization disorder had multiple personality disorder.

Aside from the matter of sexual abuse per se, the early environment of patients with somatization and related disorders is often chaotic:

> The home was frequently marked by marital strife. Physical abuse and violence were not uncommon . . . one or the other of the parents may have been involved with an addictive drug, particularly alcohol . . . patients frequently made premature excursions into sexual behavior, often had pregnancies at an early age . . . as a consequence, the developmental tasks of later adolescence were frequently uncompleted at the expense of premature responsibility for children." (Ford 1987, pp. 225–226)

We have already noted that somatization disorder is much more common in women than in men. It is also more common among the less educated, the poor, and those of lower occupational status (Kaplan and Sadock 1988). With respect to the gender difference, Briquet himself offered what at first glance might sound like a woefully "sexist" hypothesis: that "women are more sensitive, impressionistic, and more easily distressed" than men (Briquet 1859, p. 301, translated by and quoted in Mai and Merskey 1980, p. 1402). But Briquet made a more perceptive point when he added, "A man with these faculties could also become hysterical. An hysterical man represented a reversal of the basic rules of society" (Briquet 1859, p. 301, translated by and quoted in Mai and Merskey 1980, p. 1402). This raises the question—suggested in our earlier discussion of somatization disorder and sociopathy—of whether differential societal expectations and "roles" shape the outcome of some common, underlying tendency. This view is compatible with the hypothesis of Lilienfeld et al. (1986) that "histrionic" individuals develop antisocial traits if they are males and somatization disorder if they are females. And after all, aren't men in most Western cultures expected, even encouraged, to express strong emotion through self-assertion or aggression? Conversely, aren't women encouraged to "hold in" anger—to "be sweet" and docile? And couldn't such "bottling up" of negative emotions lead to "discharge" through various bodily organs? At this point, all these rhetorical questions remain unanswered by well-designed empirical studies. Moreover, another possibility suggests itself: perhaps the differential hormonal influences on men and women account for the different "presentations" of histrionic traits. Androgen levels have been linked with aggression in male adolescents (Susman et al. 1987), and we need to consider this in our understanding of male sociopathy versus female somatization.

Do cultural or ethnic factors play a role in somatization disorder? There is a widespread view among clinicians (in my experience) that Hispanic patients are much more likely to express feelings "somatically" and that somatization disorder is commonly seen in Hispanic females of low socioeconomic status. In an epidemiological study of Puerto Rican households, Canino et al. (1987) found a somewhat higher lifetime prevalence of somatization disorder than that seen in American populations: roughly 0.7% in Puerto Rico (males and females showed no difference) versus about 0.1% in the United States (American Psychiatric Association 1987; Kellner 1990). Interestingly, the prevalence of somatization disorder in Puerto Rico declined with increasing years of education. We have very few data on the prevalence of specific somatization disorders (by DSM-III-R or DSM-IV criteria) in other cultures. However, Barsky (1979) notes that somatization is more common in Jewish populations and also "among ethnic groups that discourage and disparage the undisguised expression of emotional distress." Barsky adds that "the tendency to generalize and dramatize a given symptom is determined culturally" (p. 66).

Pitfalls in the Differential Diagnosis

Medical Conditions

We have already discussed the trap of assuming that a pattern of multiple somatic complaints represents "hysteria." There are, unfortunately, several "medical" illnesses that may present with a confusing polysymptomatic picture suggesting somatization disorder. Let's consider the following vignette.

Vignette

A 27-year-old female graduate student presented to her family practitioner with a long, complicated medical history. She complained of pain in her arms, legs, and back; acute incapacitating abdominal pain; episodic nausea and vomiting; "horrible" headaches; "fits of falling"; depression; and numbness in her extremities. A previous physician had suspected multiple sclerosis (MS), but a complete neurological evaluation 2 years ago had been negative. Of note in the patient's history was a brother with remarkably similar symptoms. The physician's initial diagnosis was "hysterical hypochondriasis." However, when the patient became seriously ill after having "a couple of beers" at a party, the physician became suspicious of an organic process. A test of the patient's urine revealed high levels of porphobilinogen, and a provisional diagnosis of acute intermittent porphyria (AIP) was made.

Several "organic" conditions besides AIP and MS may be confused with somatization disorder; systemic lupus erythematosus, hyperparathyroidism, and systemic mastocytosis are often cited (Ford 1987). Ford (1987) makes the important point that somatization disorder patients are often using or abusing a variety of non-psychotropic, psychotropic, and "street" drugs (e.g., analgesics, sedative-hypnotics, and alcohol). Intoxication or withdrawal from these drugs may produce physical symptoms that complicate diagnosis of somatization disorder (e.g., alcoholic gastritis may be dismissed as "hysterical abdominal pain"). Conversely, a "million-dollar workup" of every symptom presented by a somatization disorder patient is both cost-ineffective and potentially hazardous (see discussion on treatment later in this section).

Finally, we should note that so-called chronic fatigue syndrome (CFS)—an illness of unknown etiology but probably related in some cases to several different types of viral infection—may also present with a picture resembling somatization disorder (see Komaroff and Buchwald 1991). Patients with CFS may present with myalgias, depression, headache, sore throat, blurry vision, nocturia, dizziness, paresthesias, diarrhea, and a multitude of other somatic complaints. The relationship of CFS to depression remains very controversial.

Psychiatric Disorders

Various psychiatric disorders may be confused with somatization disorder (Table 7–2). Let's consider the following vignette in light of this differential diagnosis.

Vignette

A 19-year-old male college student presented to his family physician with a large number of physical complaints—for example, "frighteningly loose bowel movements," chest pain, tingling in the extremities, "grand mal seizures," sudden loss of voice, and difficulty urinating. Complete physical and laboratory examinations were negative. A psychiatric consultant noted that the patient showed no thought process disorder or peculiarities of affect. However, on more specific questioning, the consultant elicited the following beliefs from the patient: "The whole thing . . . I mean these physical problems I have . . . they all stem from this high-tension power line that runs right outside my dorm. The electromagnetic resonances are causing . . . like a vibration, a resonance, in my organs." The patient had shown a pattern of increasing social withdrawal and poor self-care over the preceding 6 months. Family history was positive for a sister diagnosed with schizophrenia. The consultant's provisional diagnosis was "psychotic disorder NOS [not otherwise specified], r/o paranoid schizophrenia."

Major depression or dysthymia may precede, follow, or coexist with symptoms of somatization disorder; the notion of a "masked" or

Table 7–2. Psychiatric disorders that may be confused with somatization disorder

---
Other somatoform disorder (e.g., hypochondriasis, conversion)

Major depression or dysthymia

Panic disorder or another anxiety disorder

Schizophrenia with somatic delusions

Factitious disorder with physical symptoms

"atypical" depression has already been discussed (see Chapter 4). How can you differentiate between somatization disorder and depression? In some cases, the exercise is largely academic, since you will end up treating the total symptom picture. But as a general rule, major depressive episodes tend to be more episodic than somatization disorder, with periods of complete or near-complete remission; in contrast, somatization disorder patients are rarely entirely asymptomatic, and it is unusual for them to go more than a year without seeking medical attention (Kaplan and Sadock 1988). In major depression, the depressed mood is usually more "autonomous" (unvarying) than in somatization disorder, in which "it is remarkable how often these dysphoric feelings remit when circumstances in the patient's environment change for the better" (Ford 1987, p. 229).

While patients with panic disorder often voice somatic concerns and amplify somatic sensations, these traits usually follow the onset of frank panic attacks, in my experience. Moreover, panic disorder patients generally experience their somatic symptoms (e.g., dizziness, paresthesias, nausea, etc.) only during the actual panic attack and thus for more circumscribed periods than do patients with somatization disorder. When somatic symptoms "spill over" into time periods outside the actual panic attacks, both diagnoses—somatization disorder and panic disorder—may be made.

The differential between somatization disorder and the other somatoform disorders is discussed in the relevant subsections in the remainder of this chapter.

"Malingering" and factitious disorders, such as Munchausen's syndrome, are also in the differential diagnosis of somatization disorder. The differences between patients with somatization disorder and malingerers are summarized in Table 7–3.

Adjunctive Testing

There are, as yet, no clinically useful neuroendocrine, electrophysiological, or neuroimaging studies diagnostic of somatization disorder. We noted earlier one instance of an abnormal SPECT scan in a patient with somatization disorder (Lazarus and Cotterell 1989); it remains to be seen whether such findings will be confirmed in large-scale studies and whether such right-hemisphere abnormalities are specific to somatization disorder.

The Amytal interview has been used in the diagnosis of "hysterical" symptoms and, in theory, could be useful in the diagnosis of somatization disorder. However, the available literature does not make mention of this.

Neuropsychological Testing

Meyer (1983) has summarized the Minnesota Multiphasic Personality Inventory (MMPI) findings in patients with somatization disorder and related disorders. Typically, these patients show elevation of scales 1, 2, 3, and 7. Elevation of scale 2 reflects the depression that frequently accompanies somatization disorder. Elevation of scale 7 (psychasthenia) is an indication of the "passivity and complaining" often seen in these patients. The 1-4/4-1 pattern reflects not only many physical complaints but excessive narcissism and egocentricity as well, which is consistent with the findings of Oxman et al. (1985). On the Rorschach, somatization disorder patients typically do not provide a high number of responses, and the percentage of W or complex M responses is usually low (Meyer 1983).

We have already discussed Flor-Henry's (1983) extensive neuropsychiatric examination of patients with Briquet's syndrome. Among

Table 7–3. Differential diagnosis of malingering and somatization disorder

Malingering	Somatization disorder
Conscious simulation of illness	Unconscious solution to intrapsychic conflict (?)
Obvious secondary gain (e.g., disability payments)	No evident secondary gain except attention, care
Past history of antisocial behavior/drug abuse	No past history of antisocial behavior
Threatening or abusive behavior when confronted with deception	Indignation, anxiety, or tearfulness when psychological cause is suggested

Source. Adapted from Dubovsky 1988.

the tests that were used to discriminate Briquet's patients from control subjects were trail making A and B; finger-tapping test; tactual performance test; seashore rhythm test; porteus maze test, and the Wechsler Adult Intelligence Scale (WAIS) (Flor-Henry 1983). Though Flor-Henry's results are intriguing, it is not clear that such a battery of tests will reliably distinguish patients with somatization disorder from other psychiatric patients or that such extensive testing is practical in a clinical setting.

Treatment Directions and Goals

The overall approach to the patient with somatization disorder is "conservative" and comprehensive. As Barsky (1992) summarizes, "Psychosocial treatment must be closely integrated with medical management. It entails providing practical psychosocial support while acknowledging the patient's suffering rather than trying to eliminate it. The focus of medical management should be shifted from definitive diagnosis and outright cure to symptom palliation and assistance in coping."

Somatic Approaches

Shader (1994) states that "psychopharmacological treatment [of somatization disorder] is not indicated unless the patient has concomitant anxiety of depression; medication use is then directed at these conditions" (p. 19). There is, in other words, no specific pharmacological treatment for the overall somatization disorder syndrome and the various dynamics that generate it. Nevertheless, as Kellner (1990) notes, "Antidepressant as well as antianxiety drugs relieve somatic symptoms in depressed as well as anxious patients" (p. 157). On a more cautious note, Lipowski (1988) points out that sedatives and hypnotics should be used cautiously in this population, "as persistent somatizers readily become addicted to them" (p. 1366). Murphy (1982) makes the important additional point that "one has to have treated several hysterics before coming to the realization that an effort to 'control' or abolish a complaint will usually lead to prescribing greater and greater amounts of medication to no avail" (p. 2562).

Psychosocial Approaches

There is a supervening issue that confronts the psychiatrist faced for the first time with a "somatizing" patient: who should be the patient's primary caregiver? Smith et al. (1986) provide convincing arguments for treatment by primary physicians, after a thorough psychiatric consultation. Regularly scheduled appointments with the primary physician—roughly every 4 to 6 weeks—may reduce the patient's tendency to develop new and more complicated symptoms in order to see the physician. Physicians are encouraged not to tell patients "it's all in your head," and to be conservative in ordering diagnostic procedures.

Although we may agree with Smith et al. that the primary physician should see the somatization disorder patient routinely, psychiatrists should still be familiar with the general psychotherapeutic approach to somatization disorder. Murphy (1982) emphasizes the following principles:

1. Listen attentively to the patient but do not dwell on the minute details of each somatic complaint.
2. Avoid conveying the sense that the patient's symptoms are the most interesting thing about him or her.
3. Acknowledge that you are "uncertain" about how to treat a particular complaint, especially when the patient requests medication; ask for time to "think about it."
4. Understand that "seductiveness" by the patient is not an invitation to sexual intimacy, but an attempt to retain the physician's interest.
5. Provide the patient with a definitive time for a follow-up appointment; do not "wait" for the patient to develop new problems.

Murphy emphasizes that the chief goal with somatizing patients is to avoid "errors of commission" (e.g., unnecessary procedures, operations, or medications).

Barsky (1979) emphasizes the assessment of three psychological factors in the somatizing patient: traumatic childhood experiences, the personal significance of symptoms, and the psychological stressors that may precipitate or amplify somatic complaints. It is useful to inquire, for example, about early experiences of suffering or pain in both the patient and family members; specifically, was the patient (or sibling) given "extra attention" when he or she complained of physical symptoms? Because such symptoms often have very deep personal meanings to somatization disorder (and other) patients, it's useful to ask, "What worries you most about your symptom?" In my own experience, the patient frequently has a relative or friend who either died or became severely incapacitated after developing "exactly the same thing I have." Finally, Barsky notes that losses, separations, or "defeats" may exacerbate the somatizing patient's physical complaints, and these issues need to be explored in therapy.

There are few well-controlled studies looking at group and family therapy in the treatment of somatization disorder (Kellner 1989). Although there is some pessimism about the effectiveness of group therapy, one (uncontrolled) study by Valko (1976) showed that patients with Briquet's syndrome benefited from a supportive form of group therapy. Family therapy—though largely untested—should be of help to some somatization disorder patients, at least in theory. (For example, it could help family members understand the nature of the disorder while avoiding undue "reinforcement" of the patient's complaints.)

We conclude this section with the principles outlined by Kellner (1989), summarized in Table 7–4.

Pain Disorder

The Central Concept

Vignette

Ms. Meg Algos was a 45-year-old accountant with a 5-year history of severe craniofacial pain of unknown etiology. An extensive neurological and rheumatological evaluation 3 years ago had failed to uncover any "organic" cause for the pain, which Ms. Algos described as "a constant drilling, grinding misery." Despite the "negative" medical workup, the patient had sought further advice, diagnostic tests, and medications from at least 12 physicians in the past 2 years, all "without getting any help at all." The patient added, "You're my last hope for a cure, Doctor. Otherwise, I just don't know if it pays to go on . . . I've had it." Discussion with the patient's daughter revealed that Ms. Algos had alienated most of her family with her constant demands for attention and care, which, very ambivalently, they continued to attempt to provide. "When she calls, we come, even though we think this whole thing is all in her head," the daughter stated.

As the vignette suggests, patients with DSM-IV pain disorder (in DSM-III-R, somatoform pain disorder) are typically women in their 30s or 40s with a long history of "doctor shopping," diagnostic evaluations, and largely unsuccessful treatments (Blackwell et al. 1989; Kaplan and Sadock 1988). Their pain usually begins suddenly and increases in severity over weeks or months and persists for several years. The person with pain disorder has usually been unable to work and has assumed the role of "invalid." Pain disorder is often accompanied by localized paresthesias or muscle spasm, and dependence on analgesics or tranquilizers is common. Symptoms of depression often accompany pain disorder, and a history of conversion symptoms (see

Table 7–4. Psychotherapy of somatization disorder

1. The therapist must be prepared to accept empathically the patient's ongoing descriptions of pain and suffering.
2. The therapist should explain that his or her role is to help the patient deal with the emotional consequences of bodily symptoms, not necessarily to provide immediate relief.
3. Coexisting anxiety and depressive disorders need to be treated, often with appropriate medication.
4. The therapist should try to persuade the patient to limit his or her visits to one physician.
5. The therapist should communicate as needed with the primary physician, especially around issues such as "weaning" the patient off a medication.

Source. Extensively modified from Kellner 1989.

below) is often elicited. Typically, the pain disorder patient resists a psychological understanding of his or her pain.

Whereas DSM-III-R emphasized the absence of adequate physical findings or a known disease entity in (then) somatoform pain disorder, DSM-IV takes a less "Cartesian" approach to pain disorder. It requires only that "psychological factors are judged to have an important role in the onset, severity, exacerbation, or maintenance of the pain" (American Psychiatric Asociation 1994, p. 461). Depending on the *predominance* of psychological factors or a concomitant medical condition, you may "code" pain disorder as either "associated with psychological factors" or "associated with both psychological factors and a general medical condition." Pain disorder may be either "acute" or "chronic," depending on whether it has been present for less than or more than 6 months.

Historical Development of the Disorder

The notion of "imaginary" or "psychogenic" pain goes back well before Molière's "imaginary invalid," whose bodily pain (probably part of his hypochondriasis) was noted in the epigraph to this chapter. In DSM-III, the category of "psychogenic pain disorder" implied that some (often unspecified) psychological conflict or dynamic played a causal role in the patient's pain; the designation of somatoform pain disorder in DSM-III-R acknowledged that this disorder "frequently appears in the absence of clear evidence of the etiologic role of psychological factors" (American Psychiatric Association 1987, p. 424). Meanwhile, in the early 1980s, Blumer and Heilbronn (1982) began to develop the notion of "dysthymic pain disorder" (see next section), which has many features in common with the profile of the pain disorder patient.

The Biopsychosocial Perspective

Biological Factors

There are few biological studies of pain disorder based on DSM-III-R or DSM-IV criteria; however, Blumer (1987) has summarized several lines of investigation suggesting biological factors in what he calls "dysthymic pain disorder." Essentially, patients qualify for this diagnosis when "no somatic origin for their pain [can] be determined by well-accepted clinical standards." These patients share several of the biological markers seen in major depression, though to a lesser extent; for example, urinary cortisol levels are abnormal in about 17% of dysthymic pain patients versus about 80% of patients with major depression (Blumer 1987). Similarly, nonsuppression on the dexamethasone suppression test (DST) is 24% among the pain patients versus 57% in the group with major depression. Ten percent of the chronic pain patients show abnormally shortened REM latency, versus 44% among the depressed patients. These markers tend to be more strongly positive in the more severely depressed chronic pain patients.

Blumer also notes that high levels of endorphins have been seen in both depressed patients and chronic pain patients. In a small-scale study of chronic pain patients with various psychiatric diagnoses, depressed psychiatric patients, and normal control subjects, Atkinson et al. (1983) found a possible gradient of plasma beta-endorphin immunoreactivity: it was highest in the pain patients, intermediate in the depressed patients, and lowest in the control subjects. Whether this finding represents a cause or an effect of chronic pain is difficult to determine, and its applicability to pain disorder per se is not clear. However, the findings of Almay et al. (1978) add weight to the role of endorphins in chronic ("psychogenic") pain. These workers compared cerebrospinal fluid (CSF) endorphin levels in patients with predominantly "organic" pain with levels in patients with "psychogenic" pain. The mean level of CSF endorphin was significantly lower in the patients with organic pain.

The relationship of pain disorder to a syndrome known as "rheumatic pain modulation disorder" (RPMD), and the relationship of both conditions to depression, remain an intriguing puzzle (Gupta and Moldofsky 1986; Moldofsky et al. 1984). RPMD is characterized by dysphoria, fatigue, and chronic musculoskeletal pain with no evident organic basis for the pain. While RPMD has been conceptualized by some as an atypical or "masked" form of depression, Gupta and Moldofsky have shown (in a study of 12 patients) that RPMD and dysthymia have differing sleep physiology. Dysthymic patients, for example, had much longer latency to stage 2 sleep and more awakenings per hour than did the RPMD patients. Moreover, Moldofsky has noted a specific abnormality in the sleep physiology of RPMD patients—the so-called alpha-delta pattern, in which alpha activity intrudes into "deep" (i.e., delta) sleep. (Low-dose tricyclics may ameliorate this problem.)

In discussing biological factors in pain disorder, we need to consider the interaction of premorbid "organic" processes with the patient's current somatic complaints. Blackwell et al. (1989) state that in pain disorder "some medical or surgical event has invariably contributed to the initiation of chronic pain, and these disturbances may continue to interact and account for behavioral changes" (p. 2123). It is even possible that earlier "bona fide" peripheral nerve damage led to abiding changes in the reactivity of the CNS in as many as a third of chronic pain states (Bouckoms and Hackett 1991). Thus, it is important to elicit a history of, e.g., back injury, trauma, myocardial infarction, angina, rheumatoid arthritis, and so forth, in patients with pain disorder.

Finally, we must take note of the role of serotonin (5-hydroxytryptamine) in chronic pain. We will say more about this neurotransmitter in discussing somatic approaches to the treatment of pain disorder, but for now we should note that serotonin has been strongly implicated in at least one chronic pain syndrome—namely, migraine headache. Indeed, serotonergic projections from the dorsal raphe to the forebrain may be overactive in migraine and may possibly be "turned off" by certain antimigraine drugs (N. H. Raskin, undated monograph). Although patients with migraine should not be diagnosed with pain disorder, it is likely that serotonergic dysfunction is involved in both conditions.

Psychological Factors

The traditional psychoanalytic understanding of psychogenic pain involved the concepts of repression and "feared instinctual excitement" (Fenichel 1945). Here is a representative vignette of Fenichel's:

> A patient suffered from pain in the lower abdomen. The pain repeated sensations she had felt as a child during an attack of appendicitis. At that time, she had been treated with unusual ten-

derness by her father. The abdominal pain expressed simultaneously a longing for the father's tenderness and a fear that an even more painful operation might follow a fulfillment of this longing. (Fenichel 1945, p. 220)

In essence, psychogenic pain was understood as a conversion reaction (see discussion of conversion disorder later in this chapter). There is little empirical evidence to support such a formulation in pain disorder, though Blumer (1987) implicates "the conflict of guilt with concealed rage and aggression" in the genesis of dysthymic pain disorder. Specifically, Blumer cites psychological test data showing that dysthymic pain patients usually manifest the following profile:

Underneath a detached attitude, a different set of core issues lies at the base of the patient's dilemma: the patient has strong needs to be accepted, to depend on others, to receive affection, and to be cared for. Nonetheless, the patient has never acknowledged these basic childlike needs. Guilt is easily provoked by anything socially un-acceptable . . . any hostile-aggressive trends are also denied. Anger and aggression, being overcontrolled, are turned inward . . . a phys-ical pain is viewed as honorable victimization, while a pain of mental origin is felt to be . . . proof of a weak mind. (pp. 4–5)

In addition, the patient with dysthymic pain disorder is thought to show "alexithymia" (i.e., the inability to appreciate and verbalize feelings) (Blumer 1987). Thus, Nemiah (1985) suggests that "symp-tom production in psychogenic pain is related to major defects in ego functions underlying the experience and expression of feelings, rather than to the psychological conflicts found in the common neurotic disorders" (p. 937).

Sociocultural Factors

Pain disorder is diagnosed almost twice as frequently in females as in males, although "dysthymic pain disorder" seems to be equally com-mon in men and women (Blumer 1987).

Nemiah (1985) states that the pain associated with pain disorder is "clearly related to environmental stress—often, a significant change in human relationships" (p. 937). In a similar vein, Blumer has found that dysthymic pain patients

> tend to come from families troubled by divorce, unfaithful parents, alcoholism, depression, or chronic pain. They assumed precociously adult roles in support of the family . . . their work for the family is well-motivated, but it is excessive, as is their inherent self-sacrifice . . . [e.g.,] in having submitted to an unfaithful, alcoholic, or physically abusive spouse for a prolonged period of time." (p. 2)

In analyzing "psychogenic pain" and the "pain-prone patient," Engel (1959) discerned seven predisposing psychosocial factors:

1. One or both of the patient's parents were physically or verbally abusive, either to each other or to the patient.
2. One parent was "brutal" and the other "submissive," the former often an alcoholic father.
3. A parent typically punished the patient often and then "compensated" with excessive affection, thus inculcating the idea that "pain and suffering gain love."
4. A "cold and distant" parent typically became more affectionate when the child was ill or suffering pain.
5. A parent suffered illness or pain for which the child (patient) felt somehow responsible.
6. The patient, as a child, was habitually aggressive or hurtful, until some event forced an end to such behavior, usually with much guilt.
7. The patient, as a child, habitually deflected the anger of one parent away from the other, redirecting it toward himself or herself.

Pitfalls in the Differential Diagnosis

Medical Disorders

Obviously, the most serious error in the treatment of pain is to overlook a treatable, "organic" cause, such as a covert malignancy, spinal cord compression, rheumatoid arthritis, and so on. The classical description of "psychogenic" pain emphasizes its "dramatic" nature (Ford 1987); for example, "It feels like someone stuck a hot knife into my back, then turned it around a couple of dozen times." However, in my experience, such descriptions may represent the patient's habitual histrionic style and may not necessarily betoken a "psychogenic" problem. In discussing the differential diagnosis between "psychogenic" and "organic" pain, Weddington (1982) notes that the former is "temporally related to psychological stress, usually an unresolved grief reaction" (p. 46). Weddington also points out that "patients with [psychogenic] pain steadfastly resist the exploration of a possible connection between psychological stress and the pain symptom, whereas patients with organically induced pain are usually open to the idea that psychological factors affect their symptoms. Indeed, patients with organic symptoms may even suggest a psychological explanation" (p. 46).

Weddington makes the important point that "psychogenic pain" is not a diagnosis of exclusion made on the basis of "negative" physical and laboratory findings. For such patients, the proper conclusion is "diagnosis not determined."

Blumer (1987) compared patients with dysthymic pain disorder and those with documented rheumatoid arthritis. The results are summarized in Table 7–5. How applicable these differences are to pain disorder is not clear, but we might expect many similarities.

Table 7–5. Rheumatoid arthritis and dysthymic pain disorder: a comparison

Rheumatoid arthritis	Dysthymic pain disorder
Onset of pain mostly gradual	Onset usually sudden
Pain variable in intensity	Pain usually continuous
Depressive traits not common	Depressive traits common
Rare history of past physical abuse	Physical abuse history more common
Normal work history	Excessive work history

Source. Extensively modified from Blumer 1987.

As noted earlier, DSM-IV permits separate coding for "pain disorder associated with psychological factors" and "pain disorder associated with both psychological factors and a general medical condition," depending on the predominant etiological factor.

Psychiatric Disorders

The psychiatric disorders often confused with pain disorder are listed in Table 7–6. Let's consider the following vignette.

Vignette

A 66-year-old Hispanic male presented to his family physician with the complaint of "dolor de cabeza" (headache) of 5 months' duration. He described bilateral occipital "pressure" and bitemporal pain that sometimes radiated down the neck. There was no history of unilateral head pain, teichopsia, or nausea associated with the headache. A complete physical and laboratory workup was "negative," as were cervical films and a computed tomography (CT) scan of the brain. The patient had recently been forced to retire from his job as a meat cutter, which he had always enjoyed. He lived alone, complaining that "I have no life anymore." He reported poor concentration, loss of appetite, and difficulty staying asleep. He had lost about 15 pounds in the past 6 months and frequently had the feeling that "there's not much point in going on." Yet when asked by his Spanish-speaking physician, "Esta deprimido?" ("Are you depressed?"), the patient shrugged and replied, "No, it's just

Table 7–6. Differential diagnosis of pain disorder

Somatization disorder

Hypochondriasis

Conversion disorder

Dysthymia or major depression

Schizophrenia (with somatic delusions)

Narcotic addiction and/or malingering

Factitious disorder (e.g., Munchausen's syndrome)

this miserable headache." The physician began the patient on doxepin up to 150 mg/day; in 5 weeks the patient no longer complained of headache, insomnia, or anorexia and had gained back 7 pounds.

You have probably had little difficulty in making the diagnosis of major depressive episode, despite the patient's red-herring denial of depression. It would not be uncommon for an elderly male of Hispanic background to present his depression in overtly somatic terms. The diagnosis of major depression, in this case, supersedes the diagnosis of pain disorder in so far as treatment is concerned; however, both diagnoses may be coded on Axis I.

Incidentally, although we often associate headaches with "tension and anxiety," Weatherhead (1980) states that "probably depression in all its forms contributes to as many headaches as does anxiety" (p. 52).

Chronic pain may be part of schizophrenic and related psychotic disorders (Ford 1987). In such cases, the pain complaint has a bizarre and/or delusional quality, and is embedded in the other common features of schizophrenia (i.e., thought process disorder, blunted affect, etc.).

Differentiation of pain disorder from the other somatoform disorders is discussed elsewhere in this chapter. Remember that pain is among the symptoms of somatization disorder and that both diagnoses may be given if the patient meets criteria for both. However, in pain disorder, pain dominates the emotional picture. Furthermore, whereas somatization disorder is almost always seen in females and has an onset before age 30, pain disorder may occur in males or females (though females predominate) and usually begins in the third through fifth decades.

Ford (1987) points out that "complaints of persistent pain may be associated with narcotic addiction and/or malingering" (p. 221). Suspicion should arise when a patient demands a specific agent for pain, claims to be "allergic" to any other agent, and rejects alternative treatment approaches to the pain. These patients often have vague medical histories and make it difficult to obtain previous records.

Finally, factitious disorders may present with pain as the chief complaint. (Remember that in factitious disorders, unlike malingering, there is no evident "secondary gain," but rather a need to assume the "sick" role.) The Munchausen's patient, for example, classically presents with severe right lower quadrant pain, a history of nausea and vomiting, a dramatically detailed history, and an extensive "medical vocabulary." Of course, you should resist applying this diagnosis unless you have made a diligent effort to rule out "genuine" physical illness. Patients with factitious disorders commonly evoke strong negative feelings in would-be caregivers, as do many patients with chronic pain disorders.

Adjunctive Testing

Neuroendocrine and Neuroimaging Tests

As with somatization disorder, we have no "sensitive and specific" neuroendocrine or neuroimaging test for pain disorder. We have already noted the incidence of abnormal cortisol function and sleep abnormalities in this disorder. In patients with "unexplained" musculoskeletal pain—particularly when accompanied by poor quality sleep, daytime somnolence, morning stiffness, and headaches—it pays to get a polysomnogram: you may pick up the "rheumatic pain modulation disorder" described by Moldofsky, and its associated "alpha-delta" electroencephalogram (EEG) abnormality. There are a few preliminary studies suggesting that cortical evoked potentials and EEG patterns may help differentiate "organic" from "psychogenic" pain (Meyer 1983), but these techniques have not evolved to the point of clinical utility.

Neuropsychiatric Testing

The literature on dysthymic pain disorder (Blumer 1987) suggests that the MMPI may be a useful adjunctive test. Typically, dysthymic pain patients show abnormally high scores on the "left" side of the scale (hysteria, depression, and hypochondriasis). Elevations in scales 1, 2, and 3 (in order of degree) are common. (Insomnia due to pain will cause an elevation in the depression scale [Blackwell et al. 1989].)

Interestingly, patients with a single pain complaint often score higher on these scales than do patients with multiple pain complaints (Meyer 1983; Strassberg et al. 1981). Meyer distinguishes two groups of "somatoform pain" patients: those who show high scores on scales 1, 3, 7, and 8, and those who show high scores on scale K and scale 1, with a low score on scale 6. The first group is characterized by somatic preoccupation, obsessive thinking, isolation, and denial of psychological problems. The second group shows interpersonal insensitivity, naïveté, and strong denial of psychological difficulties. Interestingly, in a sample of 104 consecutive pain patients, Aronoff and Evans (1982) found that the initial MMPI score did not correlate with the pain total or pain sensory scores of the McGill-Melzack Pain Questionnaire (MPQ), but did correlate with the affective score. Moreover, the amount of pain change in treatment correlated with the amount of improvement in mood—once again suggesting the link between chronic pain and depression. (Not all of these patients would have fit the DSM-IV criteria for pain disorder, however.)

Several scales are useful in measuring the effects of chronic pain (e.g., the Sickness Impact Profile and the West Haven–Yale Multidimensional Pain Inventory (Blackwell et al. 1989). Blackwell et al. also recommend the use of a daily behavioral diary so that the relationship of pain to environmental events may be assessed.

Treatment Directions and Goals

Somatic Approaches

The traditional management of chronic pain has utilized bedrest, physical therapy, potent analgesic medications, nerve blocks, surgery, and—in some cases—ablative surgery in parts of the CNS. While bedrest and physical therapy may have a limited role in patients with pain disorder, the other treatments mentioned are clearly contraindicated. As Blumer (1987) advises vis-à-vis dysthymic pain disorder, "Curb somatic investigations and avoid unnecessary procedures" (p. 9). Analgesics, sedatives, and antianxiety agents are usually not helpful for pain disorder patients and may even make matters worse; for example, benzodiazepines may worsen depression and/or become addictive in pain disorder. As you might expect, the most useful agents in pain disorder seem to be the antidepressants, though their mechanism of action is not precisely known; they may work as antidepressants per se or by stimulating efferent inhibitory pain pathways (Kaplan and Sadock 1988). Tricyclics—alone or in combination with neuroleptics—are increasingly being used to manage chronic pain (Weddington 1982). (Neuroleptics, of course, carry the long-term risk of tardive dyskinesia.) While some clinicians favor more serotonergic agents, Blumer (1987) considers the noradrenergic agent desipramine the drug of choice for chronic (dysthymic) pain; he finds that amitriptyline and doxepin may be too sedating and are prone to induce weight gain. On the other hand, Weatherhead (1980) favors amitriptyline for psychogenic headache associated with depression. Blackwell et al. (1989) note that, despite the theoretical utility of serotonergic agents, two of the most serotonergic drugs—clomipramine and zimelidine—have not been particularly useful in the management of chronic pain. On the other hand, in one case of premenstrual pain and another of atypical facial pain, I found the serotonergic drug fluoxetine helpful. (Large-scale controlled studies on the selective serotonin reuptake inhibitors [SSRIs] [e.g., sertraline, fluvoxamine] will be necessary before the utility of these compounds is known.) Bouckoms and Hackett (1991) note that monoamine oxidase inhibitors (MAOIs) may be especially helpful for the atypical pain associated with atypical depression. In general, these authors favor the use of standard "antidepressant" doses of tricyclics for chronic pain patients (e.g., up to 300 mg/day of imipramine or the equivalent).

Other studies (see Blackwell et al. 1989) suggest that tricyclics at lower doses (e.g., 100 mg of imipramine per day) may be effective for most chronic pain patients, and have an earlier onset of action than the 3 to 5 weeks seen with their use in depression.

Nonpharmacological somatic strategies for pain disorder include electromyographic feedback ("biofeedback"), relaxation training, transcutaneous nerve stimulation, and acupuncture (Kaplan and Sadock 1988; Weddington 1982). Blackwell et al. (1989) have reviewed the mixed results achieved with these various modalities.

Finally, part of the somatic treatment of many chronic pain patients entails detoxification from, and reduction of dependence on, analgesic or sedative medications.

Psychosocial Approaches

The pain disorder patient typically resists psychological explanations for his or her pain, making a psychotherapeutic approach difficult and frustrating. The empirical basis for choosing a dynamically versus a cognitively oriented approach to pain disorder is quite shaky (Blackwell et al. 1989). There is some evidence that traditional psychodynamic techniques, such as free association, dream analysis, and evocation of fantasies, are unhelpful in this type of patient. The cornerstone of any psychotherapeutic approach to pain disorder embodies two basic tenets: developing a strong empathic bond with the patient and accepting the "reality" of the patient's pain.

Blackwell et al. (1989) emphasize the "shift to a rehabilitative approach" in pain disorder. The key features of this approach are summarized in Table 7–7.

Blumer (1987) has detailed some of the behavioral approaches useful in the chronic pain patient's treatment:

> Activity needs to be prescribed in initially modest, well-tolerated quotas that are then gradually increased, with rest allowed after a set period of work rather than upon the occurrence of pain. The family must be instructed not to be solicitous of the pain but supportive of all attempts of the patient to become more active . . . the patients must be steadily advised to ignore the pain as much as possible and to distract themselves by renewing their old interests or seeking new endeavors. (p. 10)

Table 7–7. Rehabilitative approach to pain disorder

1. *Alter pain behavior:* avoid excessive caregiving or other reinforcement of the patient's "sick role" and encourage patient's autonomy.

2. *Enhance healthy behavior:* employ skills training, assertiveness training, and/or individual psychotherapy.

3. *Redeploy environmental rewards:* modify behavior of spouse, family, and primary physician to minimize "reinforcement" of pain behavior.

Source. Extensively modified from Blackwell et al. 1989.

Finally, although not a form of "psychotherapy," hypnosis may be a useful approach with a few highly receptive chronic pain patients (Blackwell et al. 1989). Hypnosis is probably effective, however, only when it is part of a comprehensive treatment program incorporating the other modalities discussed in this section.

Integrated Case History

Ms. Sohtap is a 32-year-old married mother of two who presented with a complaint of "severe lower back pain" for the past year. A thorough orthopedic and neurological workup (including myelogram and magnetic resonance imaging [MRI] of the lumbosacral region) had revealed no significant active pathology; however, there was evidence of past lumbosacral injury and subsequent surgery to fuse two lumbar vertebrae, performed 12 years earlier. Since her present illness began, the patient had self-medicated with a variety of nonsteroidal anti-inflammatory agents, and she had recently been using a narcotic analgesic "from a friend" on a daily basis. The present illness began in the context of significant marital strain, precipitated by "infidelity" on the part of the patient's husband 15 months prior to evaluation. It also emerged that the patient subsequently "had an affair . . . maybe out of revenge" but had not acknowledged this to her husband. She commented in the course of psychiatric evaluation, "I suppose I've become too used to my husband to think about leaving him," but found it very difficult to express her feelings about him. An interview with the patient's husband produced the following description of the patient: "She hardly ever says how she feels about me . . . I mean, she won't really use the word 'love.' But boy, if she gets sick or a little depressed, I can't even leave the house. I mean, she's all over me, asking me if I still love her, and on and on." The husband acknowledged that "I do kind of pamper her when she gets the back pain . . . I don't know . . . I guess I feel like I need to make up for some of the lousy things I've done in the marriage."

The patient had come from what she described as "a pretty rough family." Her father was "a white-collar alcoholic" who used to hit the patient "if I ever stepped out of line." Her mother was a relatively passive woman who had lavished attention on the patient whenever she (the patient) had been hit by her father. When the patient's father required lengthy hospitalization for cirrhosis, the patient "pretty much took over the household," including the care of her three younger siblings.

On psychological testing, the patient's MMPI showed a general elevation on the "left" (hysteria, depression, and hypochondriasis). There was also evidence of denial of psychological problems.

A provisional diagnosis of pain disorder (associated with psychological factors) was made. The patient was gradually weaned off the narcotic analgesic and then was begun on desipramine 50 mg/day. She also began psychotherapy with a psychologist in order to explore her feelings about her marriage and to undergo "assertiveness training." The therapist also met with the patient's husband, both to explore his need to "pamper" his wife when she complains of pain, and to teach him how to avoid excessive reinforcement of her "sick role." Over the ensuing 2 months, the patient's pain improved significantly.

Hypochondriasis

The Central Concept

Vignette

Mr. Edalam, a 40-year-old business executive, presented to a family practitioner with the complaint that "I've got some kind of stomach cancer . . . I'm sure of it." The patient went on to describe how he came to this conclusion. "For the past year, I've been hearing this sort of whistling sound every time I move my bowels . . . and at the same time, I feel a sort of pang in my stomach." The patient had no formal psychiatric history but did "get some counseling" in college for "some anxiety I was having after my father died." The patient's father had died of a myocardial infarction, but, as the patient recalled, his father "had complained of nausea just before we took him to the hospital. We all thought it was his stomach." When pressed vigorously by a psychiatric consultant, the patient acknowledged that "I could be wrong, I suppose, but the odds are about one in a million . . . why doesn't anyone take me seriously?" Indeed, the patient had consulted three physicians over the past year and had undergone an extensive GI workup, with entirely negative results. This outcome had not reassured the patient, who stated, "You know as well as I do, Doctor, that they never level with you. They tell you it's all in your head."

Cassem and Barsky (1991) summarize this condition as follows:

> Hypochondriasis is fundamentally an overconcern about illness, a fearful attitude toward one's health, and a way of thinking about one's body. . . . [These patients'] physical health becomes a salient aspect of their self-identity, a nonverbal language they use for communicating with other people, and a way of reacting to life's stresses and demands. (p. 150)

Hypochondriasis is diagnosed about equally in males and females, with the peak onset usually after age 25. DSM-IV requires that the duration of the disturbance is at least 6 months. The course of the disorder may be phasic, fluctuating, or constant, with most patients showing a progressive decline (Cassem and Barsky 1991). On the other hand, recovery can occur. The condition is often accompanied by anxiety, depression, obsessive-compulsive traits, and a detailed medical history with much "doctor shopping." Social and occupational functioning is often impaired, and complications may occur as a result of multiple medical procedures.

Note that Mr. Edalam—unlike, for example, the patient with a somatic delusion—retains at least a modicum of reality testing regarding his condition. Also note that the hypochondriacal patient's belief system is based, to a large degree, on actual interoceptive stimuli—bowel sounds, for example—and not on imaginary or hallucinatory experiences. In effect, it is the cognitive interpretation of reality that is flawed. Finally, note that the hypochondriacal patient is not reassured by reassurance; reams of "medical evidence" do not alter the patient's conviction that a serious illness is being ignored. DSM-IV specifies that a patient has "poor insight" if for most of the time during the current episode he or she fails to recognize that the fear of having a serious illness is excessive or unreasonable. Clearly, this lack of insight can shade into a bona fide somatic delusion (see discussion of differential diagnosis later in this section).

Historical Development of the Disorder

From the time of Galen on, scholars have described the syndrome that Robert Burton (1577–1640) called "hypochondriacal or flatulous melancholy" (Nemiah 1985). Falret (1794–1870) noted that hypochondriacal persons—unlike classical "hysterics"—often present their complaints with stubborn and anxious insistence, rather than la belle indifférence. Freud heightened this distinction by considering hypochondriasis an "actual neurosis," as opposed to the psychogenic type typified by hysteria; that is, he saw hypchondriasis as "a condition in which somatic factors played a predominant causal role" (Nemiah 1985, p. 938). In DSM-II (American Psychiatric Association 1968), "hypochondriacal neurosis" was seen as distinct from hysterical neurosis (conversion and dissociative types). In DSM-III (American Psychiatric Association 1980), hypochondriasis was shunted into the somatoform disorders.

Historically, hypochondriasis has been seen through two divergent lenses: as a disorder in its own right and as a manifestation of some other (usually affective) syndrome. We will say more of this in our section on differential diagnosis.

The Biopsychosocial Perspective

Biological Factors

Cassem and Barsky (1991) note that hypochondriacal patients tend to amplify somatic and visceral sensation more than nonhypochondriacal patients. Is there a pathophysiological basis for this trait, or is it purely a matter of cognitive style? We know that a medical disorder can predispose a patient to hypochondriasis; for example, persons with primary hypochondriasis often have had more childhood medical illnesses than have control subjects (Kaplan and Sadock 1988). Is it possible that the repeated occurrence of "actual" illness in childhood—during which the nervous system is still developing—"biases" the adult nervous system so as to "amplify and augment visceral sensation"? At this point, such questions are largely rhetorical and heuristic. However, the "kindling" model of seizures and bipolar disorder may serve as an instructive analogy. It may be, for example, that the repeated firing of neuronal clusters associated with interoceptive stimuli—in response, say, to repeated GI illness in childhood—sensitizes surrounding brain regions and that, eventually, weaker and weaker interoceptive stimuli are required to set off the neurons. This "kindling hypothesis" has some indirect support. Thus, Ging et al. (1964) found a significant correlation between paroxysmal EEG abnormalities and multiple physical complaints as scored on the MMPI. Ervin et al. (1955) had earlier suggested that the frequency of hypochondriasis found in temporal lobe epilepsy might be due to ictal visceral sensations. Shimoda (1961) studied 2,500 patients with episodic somatic disturbances and found a high incidence of paroxysmal EEG abnormalities (see Monroe 1974). All of these data, of course, are merely suggestive; thus far, we can't point to any neurophysiological mechanism underlying hypochondriasis.

Of some theoretical interest is the observation of Flor-Henry (1983), based on earlier work by Kenyon (1964), that hypochondriacal symptoms are often unilateral (16% of cases) and that, of this percentage, 74% are left-sided. Moreover, this left-sided distribution seems to be correlated with increasing depression or anxiety. We will discuss the possible meaning of this "lateralization" when we discuss conversion disorder.

Psychological Factors

The traditional psychodynamic formulation of hypochondriasis implicated the following mechanisms: 1) repression of anger toward others, 2) displacement of anger onto the body, 3) the use of pain and suffering as punishment for guilt-provoking impulses, and 4) somatic complaints as a form of "undoing"—presumably, of some perceived transgression (Kaplan and Sadock 1988). Essentially, aggressive and hostile wishes toward others are transformed (via repression and displacement) into somatic complaints. (As we will see below, this model merges imperceptibly into a more "social" or interpersonal theory of hypochondriasis.) In a somewhat more "ego-centered" approach, Sullivan viewed hypochondriacal symptoms as a kind of protective distraction "that prevents persons from experiencing the pain of directly facing a dangerously low self-esteem" (Nemiah 1985, p. 939). In a similar vein, Nemiah (1985) notes the importance of narcissistic personality traits in hypochondriasis—as Molière seems presciently to have grasped in his portrayal of Argan in *Le Malade Imaginaire*.

Barsky and Klerman (1983) have reviewed the putative "cognitive" abnormalities in hypochondriacal patients. Thus, these individuals are thought to "incorrectly assess and misinterpret the somatic symptoms of emotional arousal and of normal bodily function" (p. 276), much as we have seen in panic disorder patients. For example, a minor inconsistency in breast tissue is misinterpreted as cancer. The role of "cognitive set" in hypochondriasis is typified by the well-known tendency of second-year medical students to misattribute normal bodily sensations to serious illness (Barsky and Klerman 1983).

Sociocultural Factors

Hollingshead and Redlich (1958) suggested that hypochondriacal or somatic concerns tend to cluster in the lower middle class or in the upper portion of the lower class. There is also evidence that hypochondriasis is more likely in cultures that discourage direct expression of emotion or psychological understanding of distress (Barsky 1979; Ford 1987). Familial factors also seem important; for example, many hypochondriacal patients come from families in which "there was a model for the hypochondriacal complaints" (Ford 1987, p. 201). Perhaps such patients have learned that illness "pays," in the form of extra attention, nurturance, and so forth. Stressful life events also appear to precipitate or worsen hypochondriacal complaints.

On a more interpersonal level, Brown and Vaillant (1981) suggest that hypochondriasis entails the "transformation of reproach toward others, arising from bereavement, loneliness, or unacceptable aggressive impulses, into . . . self-reproach and then complaints to others of pain" (p. 723). Specifically, "In lieu of openly complaining that others have ignored or hurt him, the hypochondriac settles on belaboring those present with his genuinely felt, but misplaced, bodily pains or discomforts" (p. 724).

A related hypothesis has been put forth by Adler (1981):

> Hypochondriacal patients all share two important characteristics: their sense of self-worth is shaky and easily disrupted; and they are vulnerable to feelings of incompleteness in that a solid sense of their identity depends on the presence of another person. . . . To feel complete, some may desperately need a supporting relationship with an idealized person. . . . losses are especially threatening to these vulnerable people. (pp. 1394–1395)

Pitfalls in the Differential Diagnosis

Medical Disorders

Any of the medical disorders we have discussed thus far (covert malignancy, rheumatoid arthritis, acute intermittent porphyria, etc.) must be considered in the differential diagnosis of hypochondriasis. DSM-III-R noted that early stages of neurological disorders (e.g., MS), endocrine disorders (e.g., thyroid or parathyroid disease), and illnesses that affect multiple body systems (e.g., systemic lupus erythematosus) may easily be confused with hypochondriasis. It is wise to remember Ford's (1987) dictum that "hypochondriasis does not confer immunity from [physical] disease" (p. 203). In addition to frank diseases, Ford (1987) has also noted that a variety of physical or organic factors may contribute to hypochondriacal concerns or to apparent hypochondriasis (Table 7–8).

Consider the following vignette.

Vignette

A 34-year-old chemical plant worker suffered severe burns over 60% of his body in an industrial accident. He required extensive skin grafts and experienced intense pain for several months. Shortly after being released from the hospital, he phoned his general practitioner complaining of tingling in his extremities. He wondered if "nerve damage" had occurred as a result of his burns or the skin grafts. Despite reassurance from the doctor, the patient became extremely anxious. He was referred for psychiatric consultation with the diagnosis of "hypochondriasis."

In fact, as Ford (1987) notes, a "post-traumatic syndrome" commonly follows physical trauma and/or surgical procedures. Such patients commonly experience anxiety, grief, and preoccupation with bodily vulnerability; this should be considered a normal response to trauma and not a pathological condition per se. Of course, in severe cases, a diagnosis of posttraumatic stress disorder might be warranted if the criteria for that condition are met.

The patient in our vignette, however, should not be given a diagnosis of hypochondriasis at the early stage described; he would have to voice the complaint for at least 6 months, and not have an organic (e.g., postsurgical) cause for his "tingling." (Some genuinely hypochondriacal patients who undergo unnecessary surgical procedures may wind up with "real" somatic problems, such as nerve damage or intra-abdominal adhesions.)

Psychiatric Conditions

Psychiatric conditions that may be confused with hypochondriasis are listed in Table 7–9.

Let's look at the following vignette.

Table 7–8. Somatic-organic factors contributing to hypochondriasis

Nonpsychotropic medications (adverse reactions)

Psychotropic medications

Covert alcohol/substance abuse

Surgical complications (e.g., intra-abdominal adhesions)

Physical trauma (psychological aftereffects)

Source. Extensively modified from Ford 1987.

Vignette

Mr. Kwetch, a 72-year-old German-born immigrant, complained to an internist that he suffered from "a bad liver . . . God only knows, it could be cancer." A thorough physical and laboratory examination failed to uncover any organic basis for these complaints. This information was only somewhat reassuring to the patient, who said, "I'm sorry for causing you all this trouble, Doctor. But I don't know . . . maybe all the tests missed the cancer." The patient gave a history of poor appetite and weight loss for the past 6 months, which he interpreted as evidence of a malignancy. He worried excessively at night and experienced both initial and midcycle insomnia. The internist told the patient, "You're fine. You're just worrying too much," and prescribed diazepam 2 mg at hs. This helped the patient fall asleep but seemed to worsen his mood. The internist diagnosed "hypochondriasis" and asked for a psychiatric consultation. The consultation revealed that Mr. Kwetch had felt "fine" up to about 8 months prior to consultation, at which time his 34-year-old nephew in Germany had died of liver cancer. Mr. Kwetch did not find out about the death until 2 weeks after his nephew's funeral and felt "very, very bad" that he had been unable to attend. His medical history prior to the current episode had been unremarkable, and there was no history of "doctor shopping" or many instances of "nonorganic" somatic complaints. A diagnosis of

Table 7–9. Psychiatric disorders that may be confused with hypochondriasis

Major depression/dysthymia

Anxiety disorders
  Generalized anxiety disorder
  Panic disorder
  Obsessive-compulsive disorder

Schizophrenia (with somatic delusions)

Other somatoform disorders (e.g., conversion disorder)

"Psychosomatic" syndromes

Factitious disorder with physical symptoms

"masked" major depression with atypical features was made, and the patient was referred for psychiatric treatment. This treatment focused on the patient's unresolved feelings about his nephew's death. The patient was also begun on trazodone 50 mg at hs, with subsequent increases up to 150 mg at hs. Over the ensuing 6 weeks, the patient's sleep, mood, and "hypochondriacal" complaints improved significantly.

Depression is both a common underlying disorder in patients with hypochondriacal complaints and a frequent "mimic," in its atypical forms, of hypochondriasis. As Ford (1987) notes, however, "The diagnosis of primary hypochondriasis is based on the features of a pervasive long-standing life-style that has emphasized preoccupation with health and illness. With a somatizing depression, there should be a time of onset, even if it extends back 2 or 3 years" (p. 204).

Adler (1981) has provided another clue to the differential diagnosis; namely, "hypochondriacal patients tend to blame others rather than themselves" (p. 1394). Our Mr. Kwetch, in contrast, was all too contrite. Moreover, a careful history revealed the presence of a "depressogenic" precipitant (the patient's guilt over his nephew) and a fairly discrete onset of symptoms—all more consistent with major depression than primary hypochondriasis. In practice, of course, these conditions are often much more difficult to "tease out."

Patients with anxiety disorders—particularly panic disorder—may infer serious bodily illness via misinterpretation of autonomic stimuli; for example, the patient may reason, "I must be having a heart attack," on the basis of simple palpitations.

The hypochondriacal patient, in contrast, demonstrates obsessive thinking about the body but rarely has physiological changes such as dyspnea or palpitations. It is sometimes difficult to distinguish primary obsessive-compulsive disorder from hypochondriasis when the former involves obsessions about bodily illness. However, the patient with true obsessive-compulsive disorder usually views the intrusive thoughts as ego-alien or senseless; the hypochondriacal patient, on the other hand, experiences his or her bodily concerns as ego-syntonic and ragards them as eminently sensible. As Meyer (1983) puts it, "In one sense, hypochondriacs do not fear being sick; they are certain they already are" (p. 139). (Hence the old joke about the hypochondriac's epitaph: "See! I told you I was sick!")

The psychotic patient with somatic delusions may sound like the hypochondriacal patient at first, but usually is distinguished from the latter by the bizarre and "unshakable" quality of the somatic preoccupation (e.g., "My liver is being eaten up by worms! You know it's true, Doctor!") (Adler 1981). But again, the hypochondriacal patient may transiently show poor reality testing—especially when under increased stress—or become more fixed in his or her belief over time.

Adjunctive Testing

We have no neuroendocrine, imaging, or electrophysiological "test" for hypochondriasis; indeed, a late 1992 computerized search of the literature looking for neuroimaging and neuroendocrine studies of hypochondriasis turned up virtually nothing. However, EEG abnormalities and peculiarities of left-sided lateralization associated with hypochondriasis have been reported (Flor-Henry 1983; Monroe 1974). It remains to be seen whether any adjunctive tests that take advantage of these findings will be devised.

Neuropsychiatric Testing

Meyer (1983) notes that, compared with somatization disorder patients, hypochondriacal patients tend to be "more focused and intellectualized" (p. 141). Thus, scores on scales 1, 7, and 8 of the MMPI tend to be lower, but with scale 1 remaining at least moderately elevated. The 3-1/1-3 profile is common, as is the 2-7/7-2 pattern (Meyer 1983). The latter is common in individuals who are "guilt-ridden, intropunitive, generally fearful, and obsessively preoccupied with their personal deficiencies" (Newmark 1985, p. 42). On the revised WAIS (WAIS-R), hypochondriacal patients (who, as Meyer notes, are "people who cope with words") often show a higher score on the verbal than on the performance scale. Blatt et al. (1970) found that a low score on object assembly was predictive of high bodily concern, including hypochondriacal patterns. On the Rorschach, it is no surprise that anatomical responses are common.

Treatment Directions and Goals

The general approach to the hypochondriacal patient is guided by the principle enunciated by Adler (1981): "The hypochondriacal patient does not seek a cure, but palliation through a long-term relation with the physician. If cure is the goal of physicians, they will almost certainly be disappointed" (p. 1395). Like patients with other somatoform disorders, hypochondriacal patients are usually best managed in a "medical" rather than "psychiatric" setting (Brown and Vaillant 1981). Exceptions to this caveat include the presence of serious depression or suicidality, or in the relatively unlikely event that the patient requests adjunctive psychiatric care. However, the psychiatrist may play an important collaborative/consultative role with the primary physician. There are very few controlled studies of the treatment of hypochondriasis (Kellner 1989); what follows is a synopsis of mostly clinical experience and uncontrolled reports.

Somatic Approaches

Kellner (1989) has pointed out that "there is no evidence that drug treatment is effective in primary hypochondriasis, yet drug treatment is often indicated when the patient is severely distressed and not benefitting adequately from psychotherapy" (p. 2144). In such cases, medication is usually aimed at symptoms of major depression, pronounced anxiety, or both. There is now compelling evidence that MAOIs are specifically useful in cases of "atypical depression," which is often characterized by anxiety and somatic preoccupations (Pies 1988); because there is considerable overlap of atypical depression and hypochondriasis, an MAOI may be worth trying in cases of the latter. To the extent that obsessive features characterize the hypochondriacal patient, it may be worth considering one of the SSRIs (e.g., fluoxetine, sertraline) or clomipramine. Because hypochondriacal patients may tolerate anticholinergic side effects poorly (Shader 1994), the tertiary tricyclics should be used conservatively. We will discuss the pharmacological treatment of so-called monosymptomatic hypochondriasis in the section on body dysmorphic disorder.

Psychosocial Approaches

As Lipsitt (1970) has noted, patients with hypochondriacal features can present a true psychotherapeutic challenge. The core elements of the psychosocial treatment of hypochondriasis are summarized in Table 7–10.

As with other "somatizing" patients, it is best to schedule regular appointments with hypochondriacal individuals; this reduces the need for the (unconscious) "production" of symptoms in order to secure the therapist's time and interest. As Brown and Vaillant (1981) note, "After the physician is reasonably assured that the patient is not suffering from a new organic pathologic condition, everything turns on understanding why the patient is using his or her somatic ticket of entry into the medical system at this particular moment" (p. 725). The clinician also needs to monitor countertransference feelings, because hypochondriacal patients often evoke feelings of anger or helplessness (Adler 1981). Quasi-paradoxical interventions may sometimes be appropriate. For example, rather than saying, "I hope your stomach feels a little better today," it may be more useful to "turn up the volume" a bit, for example, by saying, "I don't know how you can stand such pain" (Brown and Vaillant 1981). In my experience, it is also useful to explore how patients typically cope with their problem in a "positive" way, for example, by asking, "What do you do to get through the day

Table 7–10.   Psychosocial approaches to hypochondriasis

Keep in mind that after rapport is established, reassurance may be helpful.

Explore fears and beliefs about bodily complaints.

Provide education regarding relationship between emotion and somatic problems.

Use cognitive restructuring and "distraction."

Explore feelings of grief, loss, anger, and helplessness without dismissing patient's somatic explanations.

Empathically set limits on patient's demands for therapist's time, attention, etc.

Source. Adler 1981; Brown and Vaillant 1981; Kellner 1989.

with all these physical problems?" The patient's response (e.g., "Well, I go for a walk or watch TV") can then be positively reinforced. Family interventions and group therapy also have a place in treatment of the hypochondriacal patient, for example, through exploring how the family unwittingly reinforces the patient's somatizing tendencies. Shader (1994) recommends the use of "charts that identify the timing and character of [hypochondriacal] symptoms"; these may provide information regarding temporally related stressors. Finally, you should realize that in treating the hypochondriacal patient, you are in for "the long haul." Cassem and Barsky (1991) note that many hypochondriacal patients, aside from their general "neediness," have significant Axis II disorders—including hostile, obsessive-compulsive, masochistic, and paranoid traits—that do not lend themselves to short-term approaches.

Conversion Disorder

The Central Concept

Vignette

A 22-year-old mother of a 4-year-old boy was brought to the ER with the complaint "I got no feeling or movement in my right leg." The patient reported that the problem began when she awakened that morning and found, to her surprise (but not horror), that she could not move her right leg; she also lacked sensation from the knee down. A neurological examination revealed completely normal reflexes, as well as normal muscle strength (downward pressure on examiner's hand when placed beneath the patient's heel) in the affected leg when asked to lift the contralateral ("good") leg from a prone position. Decreased sensation on the affected leg conformed to a "stocking" distribution beneath a clearly demarcated line 1 inch below the kneecap. The patient had a psychiatric history consistent with one major depressive bout at age 19, which had resolved without treatment. She could not remember any precipitating stressors to her current problem, when first asked. Under hypnosis, however, it emerged that the patient had recently been "ditched" by her common-law husband and had become very angry with her young son. She lost control after the boy spilled paint all over the living room carpet, and had kicked the boy "in the butt" using her right foot. She subsequently felt quite guilty about this, took "a couple of sleeping pills," and went to bed. The next morning, she awoke with her presenting problem. Her affect seemed curiously blasé, and she opined that "it's something that you just get, I guess."

Conversion disorder was one of the only categories in DSM-III-R that posited a "psychodynamic" etiology (i.e., when a psychosocial stressor related to a psychological "conflict" or "need" is temporally related to the conversion symptom). DSM-III-R posited that psychological factors are "etiologically related" to the conversion symptom. DSM-IV has backed off from this slightly, stating simply that psychological factors are thought to be "associated" with the symptom.

Typically, conversion disorder presents with one of several sensory or motor impairments not explicable in terms of genuine neurological dysfunction; examples include anesthesia/paresthesia, deafness or blindness, gait disturbance (classically, the wildly ataxic "astasia-abasia"), paresis or paralysis, and "hysterical seizures." As the foregoing vignette demonstrates, the symptom often has symbolic value: in effect, our patient's paralyzed leg "embodied" her conflict over kicking her son (the relief thereby obtained being termed "primary gain"). Often, there is also evident "secondary gain" (e.g., being excused from the responsibilities of motherhood, career, etc.). Typically, an acute psychosocial stressor antedates the conversion symptom (Ford 1987). In its classic presentation, conversion disorder is accompanied by la belle indifférence—the seeming unconcern we witnessed in our vignette ("It's something that you just get, I guess"). However, this finding is neither very sensitive nor very specific; for example, it is often absent in conversion disorder patients and present in various organic brain syndromes. Most presentations of conversion disorder are monosymptomatic (i.e., only one specific dysfunction is present). The condition usually remits spontaneously after a short period but may recur in around 25% of cases over the ensuing 5 years, with either the same or a different symptom (Kaplan and Sadock 1988). Actually, the most common form of conversion disorder seen in American clinical practice may be the hysterical exacerbation of physical illness (Merskey 1989); as we will see, this means that the clinician must avoid the temptation to write off a physical complaint as "just hysterical."

Historical Development of the Disorder

Conversion disorder has a cherished place in the annals of psychoanalytic theory; it was in connection with this disorder that many of Freud's seminal ideas developed (see subsecton on psychological factors in discussion of the biopsychosocial perspective). Charcot, Bernheim, and Janet all made important contributions to our current concept of conversion disorder (Freedman et al. 1972). Both Charcot and Janet posited a hereditary degenerative process in conversion disorder, but Janet also proposed the concept of "dissociation" in this disorder—that "specific networks of ideas are lost to conscious attention and volition but continue to produce the sensory and motor affects" of conversion disorder (Freedman et al. 1972, p. 336). We will say more of Freud's views in the next section.

Guze (1967) has pointed out that "disorders diagnosed as hysteria have been encountered for about 2500 years" (p. 491), though the implications of this diagnosis have been much debated. In the first place, many clinicians use the term "conversion symptom" in a generic way, without reference to either a specific disease entity or a specific etiology (Guze 1967). Indeed, conversion symptoms occur in a variety of psychiatric disorders (see discussion of differential diagnosis).

In DSM-II, "hysterical neurosis, dissociative type" was distinguished from "hysterical neurosis, conversion type." DSM-III and DSM-III-R, as we have seen, distinguished dissociative from somatoform disorders and shunted the two hysterical "neuroses," respectively, into these new categories—arguably a mistake from the psychodynamic viewpoint, as will be discussed in the next section.

The Biopsychosocial Perspective

Biological Factors

The overrepresentation of conversion disorder in women and in certain families suggests—but by no means demonstrates—a biological component in this disorder. (It could be argued that both findings arise from various sociocultural factors, as discussed later in this section.) There are a number of lines of evidence aside from these that point to biological factors in conversion disorder. Flor-Henry (1983), drawing on the work of Stern, Galin, and others, suggests that conversion symptoms show a left-sided predominance and that this lateral distribution is determined by the presence of females in the samples studied. Flor-Henry hypothesizes a "special vulnerability" of the nondominant hemisphere in the female and cited a variety of neuroanatomical and neuropsychological data to bolster this claim. Cummings (1985) notes that between 50% and 70% of patients with conversion symptoms presenting in medical or neurological settings will go on to develop bona fide neurological conditions within the next several years. Thus, Cummings regards the conversion reaction as "an important harbinger of an underlying condition that must be identified and treated" (see discussion of the differential diagnosis). In some conversion disorder patients, neuropsychological testing reveals "subtle cerebral impairments in verbal communication and memory, affective incongruity, suggestibility, vigilance, and attention" (Kaplan and Sadock 1988, p. 337); these findings may reflect abnormal interaction between the cortex and the reticular formation in the brain stem (Kaplan and Sadock 1988).

Finally—though an "indirect" biological factor—premorbid medical illness can influence or determine the specific presentation of conversion disorder (Cassem and Barsky 1991). Thus, hysterical vertigo or seizures may be "modeled" on a preexisting organic process. Interestingly, Merskey (1989) notes that "patients with epilepsy appear to be more prone to conversion seizures than patients without brain damage and are also liable to produce additional seizures if they think their existing condition is being inadequately treated" (p. 2155).

Psychological Factors

In its most simplistic form, the psychoanalytic model of conversion disorder characterizes it as a compromise formation "between a strong instinctual drive (e.g., anger) and the superego prohibition of the expression of such a drive" (Ford 1987, p. 208). Thus, our patient's paralyzed leg would represent the wish to strike out in anger—directed, perhaps, at her absent husband but displaced onto her son—and the countervailing superego prohibition against such violence. Ford (1987) also points to the role of "identification" in conversion disorder; for example, a young woman develops hysterical blindness soon after her mother—who had had severe retinal disease—dies of smoke inhalation in the daughter's house. Unconscious dependency needs may also play a role in conversion disorder, as when a conversion symptom results in the alleviation of ordinary responsibilities and the provision of nurturing care. Freud, of course, posited a more complex psychosexual etiology of hysterical conversion phenomena, involving a fixation at the oedipal level and a failure to relinquish incestuous ties to the loved parent (Freedman et al. 1972). This would lead to conflicts over sexual drives in adult life and, in a particularly stressful or frustrating situation, would result in the conversion symptom (e.g., inability to relax the muscles of the legs and thighs). This particular symptom would both protect the patient from conscious awareness of the sexual drive and symbolize that same forbidden impulse.

Finally, Cassem and Barsky (1991) note that preexisting psychopathology increases the risk of conversion symptoms (if not conversion disorder proper). The most commonly associated Axis I disorders are depression, anxiety disorders, and schizophrenia. On Axis II, histrionic, passive-dependent, and passive-aggressive traits are common predisposing factors.

Sociocultural Factors

We have already noted the female predominance in conversion disorder and speculated about a biological factor to account for this. But perhaps the predominance—if it is not due to a simple diagnostic bias on the part of (mostly male) clinicians—arises from sociocultural forces that impinge mainly on females. Ford (1987) suggests as much when he notes that "if there are cultural prohibitions of certain types of behavior, e.g., the expression of anger by a woman, then conversion symptoms may serve as a means for her to communicate in a more socially acceptable manner the feelings which she is experiencing" (p. 209).

Interestingly, Cassem and Barsky (1991) note that the sex ratio of conversion disorder in children is equal, becoming disproportionately a "female" problem (by a ratio of about 3:1) only in adult populations. Whether this evolution reflects a sociocultural adaptation or a biological divergence of some sort is not clear. Ford (1987) also noted that conversion disorders seem to be more common among "rural, unsophisticated persons"—individuals, perhaps, who have not learned more adaptive ways of communicating their distress. Indeed, Chodoff (1974) has conceptualized hysteria as a form of nonverbal communication between patient and physician by which the former covertly transmits personal distress and needs.

Pitfalls in the Differential Diagnosis

Medical Conditions

Let's consider the following vignette, freely adapted from an actual case investigated by the "medical detective" Burton Roueche (1982):

> A 22-year-old woman presented to her family practitioner with the insidious progression of several symptoms: "shakiness," fainting, anxiety, depression, slurred speech, imbalance, "muscle tightening" on her right side, and drooling. A basic neurological examination showed normal reflexes and gait. Laboratory tests, with the exception of a mildly elevated serum glutamic-oxaloacetic transaminase (SGOT), were normal. Because the patient had expressed some difficulties adjusting to her marriage, the family practitioner referred her to a psychiatrist. He, in turn, diagnosed "hysterical neurosis with secondary depression." However, the patient had a poor response to psychotherapy and tricyclic antidepressants. A follow-up liver profile 1 year later showed further elevation of liver functions. A ceruloplasmin level came back markedly low, and urinary copper levels were elevated. A slit-lamp examination of the patient's cornea showed the characteristic Kayser-Fleischer ring of Wilson's disease.

This cautionary tale reminds us that "hysteria" as a diagnosis should be viewed with extreme skepticism. Other conditions that must be ruled out when a patient presents with apparent conversion disorder are MS (in which transient optic neuritis is often misdiagnosed as "hysterical blindness"), CNS malignancy, myasthenia gravis, polymyositis, temporal lobe epilepsy, and a variety of drug or heavy metal intoxications. Some specific adjunctive tests that may aid in the differential diagnosis are discussed later in this section.

Psychiatric Disorders

The psychiatric disorders sometimes confused with conversion disorder are listed in Table 7–11.

Let's consider the following vignette.

Vignette

Mr. Niag, a 22-year-old Cambodian immigrant who had recently moved to the United States, presented to the local hospital ER with the complaint "I can't move my right arm." The patient gave a somewhat contradictory history (despite adequate translation by a Cambodian-speaking clinician) and became irritable when probed for more details. It seemed that the paralysis had begun 1 day prior to admission, when the patient was struck by a baseball bat wielded by "a kid in one of the neighborhood gangs." Orthopedic and neurological exams were essentially normal, although there was a large ecchymotic area on the patient's right arm, consistent with blunt trauma. When unobserved, the patient demonstrated full

Table 7–11. Differential diagnosis of conversion disorder

Other somatoform disorders (e.g., Briquet's syndrome)
"Catatonia" secondary to affective or schizophrenic disorder
Major depression
Panic disorder
Schizophrenia
Malingering

range of motion of the affected arm. Confronted with this fact, the patient began to cry, acknowledging that he was "afraid the police will pick me up" for having been involved in a fight with the aforementioned gang member. A diagnosis of malingering was made, but the patient's evident fear prompted social work intervention, leading to resolution of the presenting problem.

Patients with panic disorder may sometimes complain of tingling, numbness, or even transient weakness of the arms or legs, suggesting the diagnosis of "hysteria" or conversion disorder. However, the panic disorder patient's symptoms occur on a shorter timescale than do those of the conversion disorder patient, and are accompanied by marked autonomic dysfunction and extreme psychic anxiety (not la belle indifférence).

Conversion symptoms sometimes occur as a prodrome of schizophrenia, or as part of the actual schizophrenic syndrome. However, more severe disruption of ego function and thought processes would be expected in schizophrenia.

Ford (1987) notes that conversion symptoms may serve as a defense against a major depressive episode. Thus, an elderly widow who develops hysterical loss of function in her left arm shortly after her husband dies of a heart attack (with pain radiating into his left arm) may well be fending off the onset of major depression.

Adjunctive Testing

As we have seen with the other somatoform disorders, we have no specific neuroimaging or other laboratory test that helps us make a "positive" diagnosis of conversion disorder. Interestingly, in a study of 84 children with conversion disorder, Spierings et al. (1990) found slight to moderate EEG abnormalities in roughly half the sample; however, the abnormalities did not appear to be related to the main conversion symptom. On the other hand, Drake et al. (1988), in a study of EEG frequency in conversion disorder and what these workers termed "somatoform disorder," concluded that "patients with conversion disorder and somatoform disorder may differ from each other in several quantitative EEG parameters, and are different in several respects from normal controls" (p. 124). Specifically, comparison of left-right power deviation in frontal and posterior regions showed quite different patterns in the three groups; however, it is not clear what patients were included in the "somatoform disorder" group, because this is not a specific diagnostic category. (This report is also useful for its review of other electrophysiological studies of "hysterical" disorders.)

Drake (1985) investigated the use of saline infusion in patients suspected of (hysterical) pseudoseizures. Three groups were distinguished: patients who had their typical attacks with saline infusion, patients who failed to respond to infusion, and patients who upon infusion had attacks different from their characteristic spells. The first group showed female predominance and a high frequency of somatoform disorders. The other groups more often consisted of males with various personality disorders. The author concluded that saline infusion may have at least a limited role in confirming the nonepileptic origin of some seizures, but noted various pragmatic and ethical limitations. Pritchard et al. (1985) presented what may be a more practical means of detecting pseudoepileptic attacks. They found that in six patients with bona fide epilepsy, a twofold increase in serum prolactin levels followed true epileptic seizures, whereas no significant change in serum prolactin followed pseudoepileptic attacks in six other patients.

There are a number of helpful neurological findings that point toward a diagnosis of conversion disorder (Table 7–12). As a general rule, remember that "hysterical" symptoms often correspond to "popular" or "intuitive" notions of neurological function, show marked inconsistency over time, tend to occur only or mainly when others are present, and are highly susceptible to suggestion.

Neuropsychological Testing

Meyer (1983) notes two characteristic MMPI profiles in conversion disorder: the classic "conversion V," in which scales 3 and 1 are both high and scale 2 is relatively low; and the 2-1-7 pattern, with a high score on scale 3. Another profile occasionally seen in acute conversion reactions accompanied by moderately high anxiety levels is the

3-9/9-3 pattern. On the WAIS-R, conversion disorder patients (especially those with la belle indifférence) tend to do poorly on tests of subtle intellectual discrimination, such as comprehension, similarities, and picture arrangement. On the Rorschach, conversion disorder patients often react with "emotional distancing," for example, with comments like "That's weird" or "They are ugly" (Meyer 1983).

We have already mentioned Flor-Henry's hypothesis regarding nondominant hemisphere dysfunction in females with hysteria. However, Flor-Henry takes note of Bendefeldt et al.'s (1976) study of cognitive performance in conversion hysteria (7 men, 10 women). On the whole, these tests revealed more dominant hemisphere dysfunction in conversion hysteria patients than in control subjects (Flor-Henry 1983).

Table 7–12.　A comparison of hysterical and neurological conditions

	Conversion disorder	Neurological disorder
Sensory symptoms	"Stocking-and-glove" anesthesia and hemi-anesthesia are evident beginning precisely at midline; all sensory modalities are affected at same level.	Normal dermatomes are involved; borders of anesthesia are imprecise, with differing levels for touch and pinprick.
Motor symptoms	"Paralyzed" leg is dragged and used for leverage when "good" leg is raised from supine position. Gait is wildly ataxic with flailing arms; falls occur only rarely. Reflexes are normal.	Leg is circumducted with upper motor neuron lesion; paralyzed leg is not used for leverage; falls may occur if gait impaired. Reflexes are abnormal.
Seizures	Irregular, thrashing "coital" movements are present; incontinence and postictal somnolence/confusion are rare.	Tonic-clonic movement is evident; incontinence and postictal somnolence/confusion may be evident.

Source.　Cummings 1985; Freedman et al. 1972.

Finally, we should note that the Amytal interview (described in Chapter 8) is sometimes useful in obtaining a history of trauma in conversion disorder patients (Kaplan and Sadock 1988), and it may also aid in treatment (see below).

Treatment Directions and Goals

Somatic Approaches

The Amytal interview may help the conversion disorder patient to reexperience the precipitating trauma, and permits the therapist to "suggest" that the conversion symptom will soon go away (Kaplan and Sadock 1988). Merskey (1989) notes that in acute cases of conversion, amobarbital injection followed by methylamphetamine may occasionally be of help; however, with "established chronic conversion symptoms," such measures are of little help. A case report by Stevens (1990) found that intravenous lorazepam, in combination with hypnotic suggestion, was helpful in restoring function in a case of conversion paralysis.

Although pharmacological intervention is rarely recommended for conversion disorder per se, the presence of a concomitant or possibly "underlying" illness may warrant a trial of anxiolytics, antidepressants, or mood stabilizers (Kaplan and Sadock 1988; Merskey 1989). Merskey (1989) also notes the use of a single session of electroconvulsive therapy (ECT) in extreme or refractory cases of conversion disorder; presumably, the acute confusional state of the procedure helps break down the patient's defensive system long enough to mobilize her or him, or otherwise helps restore normal function. (This is not, however, a generally recognized use of ECT and should certainly be preceded by consultation and informed consent.)

Psychosocial Approaches

The traditional approach to conversion disorder has emphasized an insight-oriented or psychoanalytic approach. Abse (1974) has suggested that psychoanalysis is probably most successful in those patients with adequate ego strength, "oedipal" rather than preoedipal level fixations, and good self-esteem. Abse has also noted, however, that "in instances of conversion . . . which follow a severely stressful precipitating situation, the simpler supportive methods of psychotherapy may suffice for recovery to the status quo ante" (pp. 189–190). Indeed, this is the approach advocated by Cassem and Barsky (1991):

> Suggesting that the conversion symptom will improve is the commonest form of treatment. This ordinarily begins with the reassuring news that tests of the involved body system show no damage and therefore recovery is certain. Predicting that recovery will be gradual, with specific suggestions [e.g., "You'll first notice a little strength returning to your hand"] . . . will usually succeed. (pp. 143–144)

It may also be important to explore recent life stresses and the type of nonverbal interpersonal communication the patient uses to convey distress. Marital or family counseling may be helpful when the precipitant resides in one of these systems.

Direct confrontation (e.g., "Your arm is paralyzed because you're unable to convey your needs to others") is seldom helpful (Cassem and Barsky 1991). Merskey (1989), citing the work of Lazarus and others, notes that behavioral approaches may be helpful (e.g., identifying and eliminating any reinforcing factors) (Shader 1994). Shader (1994) points out further that "an effort should be made to redirect the patient's attention and focus away from the impairment and to shift it toward the events and issues that provoked it." Kaplan and Sadock (1988) note that "the longer that [conversion disorder] patients have been in the sick role and the more that they have regressed, the more difficult the treatment will be" (p. 37).

Let's examine a brief vignette to see how some of these various approaches can be integrated.

Vignette

Harold was a 22-year-old unemployed male with "borderline low" intelligence and a history of poor tolerance of stress. While packing boxes in a sheltered workshop, Harold suddenly lost strength in his right arm and then "felt my legs give out." He was rushed to the ER in order to rule out a suspected seizure; however, the patient showed no postictal fatigue or weakness other than total paralysis of his right arm. An EEG was normal. Harold was seen by a psychiatric consultant, who was able to elicit a history of recent sexual advances by Harold's supervisor at the workshop. Harold revealed that "I was real pissed at him . . . I wanted to smash his face in . . . but I need that job . . . it's the only money I get." The psychiatric consultant commented, "When we get too stressed out or angry, our bodies sometimes blow the time-out whistle. I think you're going to get your strength back quite soon. In the meantime, I'll look into getting you set up at another workshop." The consultant also gave Harold some "special exercises" to do with his "good arm" in order to "build your strength back up." The patient was kept overnight for observation and was seen the next day by the consultant; by that time, the patient had recovered nearly all motor function in his right arm.

Body Dysmorphic Disorder

We will depart from our usual format in discussing body dysmorphic disorder because comparatively little has been determined about this diagnosis; indeed, it is a category that was not present in DSM-III and has more recently been described as "little-known" (Phillips 1991). Phillips (1991) summarizes body dysmorphic disorder nicely in the title of her article "The Distress of Imagined Ugliness."

In essence, body dysmorphic disorder entails the "preoccupation with some imagined defect in appearance in a normal-appearing person" (DSM-III-R; American Psychiatric Association 1987, p. 256). The belief is not "of delusional intensity," though the distinction between body dysmorphic disorder and somatic delusions is not always straightforward. Indeed, as Phillips notes, the European literature uses the term "monosymptomatic hypochondriacal psychosis" to describe a syndrome quite like body dysmorphic disorder. The essentials of body dysmorphic disorder (as modified from Phillips 1991 and the DSM-IV) are summarized in Table 7–13.

Probably the most convincing evidence thus far links body dysmorphic disorder with diseases along the "obsessive-compulsive spectrum" (which includes obsessive-compulsive disorder, trichotillomania, onychophagia, and various types of self-injurious behavior) (Hollander et al. 1989; Phillips 1991). It remains to be seen whether

Table 7–13. Body dysmorphic disorder

Demographics	Prevalence possibly as high as 20% in nonclinical populations; age at onset usually 18 to 25; roughly equal male:female ratio.
Family history	Possible association with family history of mood disorder, OCD, schizophrenia.
Biological markers	Unknown.
Associated features	Depressive, obsessive-compulsive, avoidant traits; repeated visits to plastic surgeons.
Complications	Difficulties in social, marital, occupational functioning common; suicidal ideation and suicide attempts reported; unnecessary surgery common.
Etiology	Unitary explanation unlikely. Theories include 1) unconscious displacement of guilt, low self-esteem onto body part; 2) disturbed family system that overemphasized appearance; 3) distressing life event or interpersonal "slight"; and 4) serotonergic abnormality, as in "OCD spectrum" disorders.[a]
Differential diagnosis	Includes delusional disorder, somatic subtype; "normal" adolescent concern with appearance; OCD; hypochondriasis; major depression with somatizing features; social phobia; avoidant personality disorder.
Treatment	Uncertain. Approaches used include dynamically oriented, behavioral, and "supportive" psychotherapies; plastic surgery[b]; serotonin reuptake inhibitors (e.g., clomipramine, fluoxetine, possibly pimozide).

Note. OCD = obsessive-compulsive disorder.
[a]See Hollander et al. 1989.
[b]Caution: careful selection of patient is critical.
Source. Extensively modified from Phillips 1991.

common biological, familial, and pharmacological factors will ultimately unify body dysmorphic disorder and these other disorders. In the meantime, you will probably do little harm and possibly considerable good by treating a body dysmorphic disorder patient with a serotonergic antidepressant and involving the patient in some form of supportive psychotherapy.

Conclusion

The somatoform disorders present the clinician with challenging, and sometimes frustrating, diagnostic and therapeutic issues. Of paramount importance is the diligent search for physical factors in the patient's presenting complaint—remembering that "functional" and "organic" conditions may (and often do) coexist. Equally important is the nature of the therapeutic relationship: it must be based on the premise that adaptation and relief—not "cure"—are the goals of treatment. To this end, the psychiatrist will need to work closely with the patient's primary care physician.

References

Abse WD: Hysterical conversion and dissociative syndromes and the hysterical character, in American Handbook of Psychiatry, 2nd Edition, Vol 3. Edited by Arieti S. New York, Basic Books, 1974, pp 155–194

Adler G: The physician and the hypochondriacal patient. N Engl J Med 304:1394–1396, 1981

Almay BG, Johansson R, Von Knorring, et al: Endorphins in chronic pain, I: differences in CSF endorphin levels between organic and psychogenic pain syndromes. Pain 5:153–162, 1978

American Psychiatric Association: Diagnostic and Statistical Manual, 2nd Edition, Revised. Washington, DC, American Psychiatric Association, 1968

American Psychiatric Association: Diagnostic and Statistical Manual, 3rd Edition. Washington, DC, American Psychiatric Association, 1980

American Psychiatric Association: Diagnostic and Statistical Manual, 3rd Edition, Revised. Washington, DC, American Psychiatric Association, 1987

American Psychiatric Association: Diagnostic and Statistical Manual, 4th Edition. Washington, DC, American Psychiatric Association, 1994

Aronoff GM, Evans WO: The prediction of treatment outcome at a multidisciplinary pain center. Pain 14:67–73, 1982

Atkinson JH, Kremer EF, Risch SC, et al: Neuroendocrine function and endogenous opioid peptide synthesis in chronic pain. Psychosomatics 24:899–913, 1983

Barsky AJ: Patients who amplify bodily sensations. Ann Intern Med 91:63–70, 1979

Barsky A: The somatoform disorders (abstract). Practical Reviews in Psychiatry (audiotape). Birmingham, AL, Educational Reviews, Inc, February 1992

Barsky AJ, Klerman GL: Overview: hypochondriasis, body complaints, and somatic styles. Am J Psychiatry 140:273–283, 1983

Bendefeldt F, Miller L, Ludwig A: Cognitive performance in conversion hysteria. Arch Gen Psychiatry 33:1250–1254, 1976

Blackwell B, Merskey H, Kellner R: , in Treatments of Psychiatric Disorders, Vol 3. Washington, DC, American Psychiatric Association, 1989, pp 2120–2137

Blatt S, Baker, B, Weiss J: Wechsler Object Assembly Subtest and bodily concern. J Consult Clin Psychol 34:269–274, 1970

Bliss EL: Multiple personalities: a report of 14 cases with implications for schizophrenia and hysteria. Arch Gen Psychiatry 37:114–123, 1980

Blumer D: The Dysthymic Pain Disorder: Chronic Pain as Masked Depression. Biomedical Information Corporation, 1987

Blumer D, Heilbronn M: Chronic pain as a variant of depressive disease: the pain prone disorder. J Nerv Ment Dis 170:381–406, 1982

Bouckoms A, Hackett TP: The pain patient: evaluation and treatment, in Handbook of General Hospital Psychiatry. Edited by Cassem NH. Boston, MA, Mosby Year Book, 1991, pp 39–68

Briquet P: Traité de l'Hysterie. Paris, JB Bailliere, 1859

Brown HN, Vaillant GE: Hypochondriasis. Arch Intern Med 141:723–726, 1981

Canino GJ, Bird HR, Shrout PE, et al: The prevalence of specific psychiatric disorders in Puerto Rico. Arch Gen Psychiatry 44:727–735, 1987

Cassem NH, Barsky AJ: Functional somatic symptoms and somatoform disorders, in Massachusetts General Handbook of General Hospital Psychiatry. Edited by Cassem NH. Boston, MA, Mosby Year Book, 1991, pp 131–158

Chodoff P: Diagnosis of hysteria: an overview. Am J Psychiatry 131:1073–1078, 1974

Cummings JL: Clinical Neuropsychiatry. Orlando, FL, Grune & Stratton, 1985

Drake ME: Saline activation of pseudoepileptic seizures: clinical EEG and neuropsychiatric observations. Clin Electroencephalogr 16:171–176, 1985

Drake ME, Padamadan H, Pakalnis A: EEG frequency analysis in conversion and somatoform disorder. Clin Electroencephalogr 19:123–128, 1988

Dubovsky SL: Concise Guide to Clinical Psychiatry. Washington, DC, American Psychiatric Press, 1988

Engel G: Psychogenic pain and the pain-prone patient. Am J Med 26:899–918, 1959

Ervin R, Epstein AW, King HE: Behavior of epileptic and nonepileptic patients with temporal spikes. Archives of Neurology and Psychiatry 74:488, 1955

Fenichel O: The Psychoanalytic Theory of Neurosis. New York, WW Norton, 1945

Flor-Henry P: Cerebral Basis of Psychopathology. Boston, MA, John Wright, 1983

Ford CV: Somatization, in Handbook of Psychiatric Diagnosis. Edited by Soreff SM, McNeil GN. Littleton, MA, PSG Publishing, 1987, pp 195–235

Freedman AM, Kaplan HI, Sadock BJ: Modern Synopsis of the Comprehensive Textbook of Psychiatry. Baltimore, MD, Williams & Wilkins, 1972

Ging RJ, Jones E, Manis M: Correlation of electroencephalograms and multiple physical symptoms. JAMA 187:579–582, 1964

Gupta MA, Moldofsky H: Dsythymic disorder and rheumatic pain modulation disorder (fibrositis syndrome): a comparison of symptoms and sleep physiology. Can J Psychiatry 31:608–616, 1986

Guze SB: The diagnosis of hysteria: what are we trying to do. Am J Psychiatry 124:77–84, 1967

Hollander E, Liebowitz MR, Winchel R, et al: Treatment of body-dysmorphic disorder and serotonin reuptake blockers. Am J Psychiatry 146:768–770, 1989

Hollingshead AB, Redlich FC: Social Class and Mental Illness. New York, Wiley, 1958

James L, Singer A, Zurynski Y, et al: Evoked response potentials and regional cerebral blood flow in somatization disorder. Psychother Psychosom 47:190–196, 1987

Kaplan HI, Sadock BJ: Synopsis of Psychiatry, 5th Edition. Baltimore, MD, Williams & Wilkins, 1988

Kellner R: Somatoform and factitious disorders, in Treatments of Psychiatric Disorders, Vol 3. Washington, DC, American Psychiatric Association, 1989, pp 2119–2146

Kellner R: Somatization: theories and research. J Nerv Ment Dis 178:150–160, 1990

Kenyon FE: Hypochondriasis: a clinical study. Br J Psychiatry 110:478–488, 1964

Komaroff AL, Buchwald D: Symptoms and signs of chronic fatigue syndrome. Rev Infect Dis 13 (suppl 1):8–11, 1991

Koranyi EK: Morbidity and rate of undiagnosed physical illnesses in a psychiatric clinic population. Arch Gen Psychiatry 36:414–419, 1979

Lazarus A, Cotterell KP: SPECT scan reveals abnormality in somatization disorder patient (letter). J Clin Psychiatry 50:475–476, 1989

Lilienfeld SO, VanValkenburg C, Larntz K, et al: The relationship of histrionic personality disorder to antisocial personality and somatization disorders. Am J Psychiatry 143:718–722, 1986

Lipowski ZJ: Somatization: the concept and its clinical application. Am J Psychiatry 145:1358–1368, 1988

Lipsitt DR: Medical and psychological characteristics of "crocks." Psychiatric Medicine 1:15–25, 1970

Mai GM, Merskey H: Briquet's Treatise on Hysteria. Arch Gen Psychiatry 37:1401–1405, 1980

Maxmen G: Essential Psychopathology. New York, WW Norton, 1986

Meissner WW: Theories of personality and psychopathology: classical psychoanalysis, in Comprehensive Textbook of Psychiatry/IV, 4th Edition, Vol 1. Edited by Kaplan HI, Sadock BJ. Baltimore, MD, Williams & Wilkins, 1985, pp 337–418

Merskey H: Conversion disorders, in Treatments of Psychiatric Disorders, Vol 3. Washington, DC, American Psychiatric Association, 1989, pp 2152–2158

Meyer RG: The Clinician's Handbook: Psychopathology of Adulthood and Late Adolescence. Boston, MA, Allyn & Bacon, 1983

Moldofsky H, Tullis C, Lue FA, et al: Sleep-related myoclonus in rheumatic pain modulation disorder (fibrositis syndrome) and in excessive daytime somnolence. Psychosom Med 46:145–151, 1984

Monroe RR: Episodic behavioral disorders: an unclassified syndrome, in American Handbook of Psychiatry, 2nd Edition, Vol 3. Edited by Arieti S. New York, Basic Books, 1974, pp 238–254

Morrison JR: Early birth order in Briquet's syndrome. Am J Psychiatry 140:1596–1598, 1983

Morrison J: Childhood sexual histories of women with somatization disorder. Am J Psychiatry 146:239–241, 1989

Murphy GE: The clinical management of hysteria. JAMA 247:2559–2563, 1982

Nemiah JC: Somatoform disorders, in Comprehensive Textbook of Psychiatry/IV, 4th Edition, Vol 1. Edited by Kaplan HI, Sadock BJ. Baltimore, MD, Williams & Wilkins, 1985, pp 924–941

Newmark CS: Major Psychological Assessment Instruments. Boston, MA, Allyn & Bacon, 1985

Orenstein H, Raskind MA, Wyllie D, et al: Polysymptomatic complaints and Briquet's syndrome in polycystic ovary disease. Am J Psychiatry

143:768–771, 1986

Oxman TE, Rosenberg SD, Schnurr PP, et al: Linguistic dimensions of affect and thought in somatization disorder. Am J Psychiatry 142:1150–1155, 1985

Perley MJ, Guze SB: Hysteria: the stability and usefulness of clinical criteria. N Engl J Med 266:421–426, 1962

Phillips KA: Body dysmorphic disorder: the distress of imagined ugliness. Am J Psychiatry 148:1138–1149, 1991

Pies RW: Atypical depression, in Handbook of Clinical Psychopharmacology, 2nd Edition. Northvale, NJ, Jason Aronson, 1988, pp 329–356

Pritchard PB, Wannamaker BB, Sagel J, et al: Serum prolactin and cortisol levels in evaluation of pseudoepileptic seizures. Ann Neurol 18:87–89, 1985

Raskin NH: Pathogenesis of migraine, in The Migraine Dilemma. Foundation for Research in Head Pain and Related Disorders [undated monograph]

Roueche B: Medical mystery: could this really be "hysterical" neurosis. Medical Economics, October 11, 1982

Shader RI: Dissociative, somatoform and paranoid disorders, in Manual of Psychiatric Therapeutics, 2nd Edition. Boston, MA, Little, Brown, 1994, pp 15–23

Shimoda Y: The clinical and electroencephalographic study of the primary diencephalic epilepsy or epilepsy of the brain stem. Acta Neurovegetativa 23:181, 1961

Smith GR, Monson RA, Ray DC: Psychiatric consultation in somatization disorder. N Engl J Med 314:1407–1413, 1986

Spierings C, Poels PJ, Sijben N, et al: Conversion disorders in childhood: a retrospective follow-up study of 84 inpatients. Dev Med Child Neurol 32:865–871, 1990

Stevens CB: Lorazepam in the treatment of acute conversion disorder. Hosp Community Psychiatry 41:1255–1257, 1990

Strassberg D, Reimherr F, Ward M, et al: The MMPI and chronic pain. J Consult Clin Psychol 49:220–226, 1981

Susman EJ, Inoff-Germain G, Nottelmann ED: Hormones, emotional dispositions, and aggressive attributes in young adolescents. Child Dev 58:1114–1134, 1987

Valko RJ: Group therapy for patients with hysteria (Briquet's disorder). Diseases of the Nervous System 37:484–487, 1976

Weatherhead AD: Psychogenic headache. Headache 20:47–54, 1980

Weddington WW: Psychiatric aspects of chronic abdominal pain. Drug Therapy, February 1982, pp 45–51

8

Dissociative Disorders

> With amnesia, one forgets what's painful; with
> fugue, one runs away from it; with multiple
> personality, one displaces it onto a new identity;
> with depersonalization, one abandons it.
>
> Jerrold Maxmen

> What people call insincerity is simply a method
> by which we can multiply our personalities.
>
> Oscar Wilde

Popular portrayals of dissociative disorders—such as in the movie *The Three Faces of Eve*—have given the general public more "information" than they have received about much more common conditions. Indeed, even though some of the dissociative disorders may be more prevalent than once believed, they are still quite rare in comparison to schizophrenic, anxiety, and mood disorders. Nevertheless, the dissociative disorders present us with an intriguing puzzle and may offer us a "window" overlooking the borderland between a variety of organic and functional disorders.

The essential feature of all the dissociative disorders is "a disturbance or alteration in the normally integrative functions of identity, memory, or consciousness" (American Psychiatric Association 1987, p. 269). In effect, the individual's sense of self is radically altered, without, however, the total loss of reality testing seen in the psychoses. Four basic types of dissociative disorder are recognized: dissociative identity disorder (historically and popularly known as multiple personality disorder); dissociative ("psychogenic") fugue; dissociative ("psychogenic") amnesia; and depersonalization disorder. A fifth category, dissociative disorder NOS (not otherwise specified), covers more exotic syndromes, such as certain trance states.

Dissociation as a defense mechanism appears to operate in a variety of conditions, including certain personality disorders. We have already discussed it in relation to posttraumatic stress disorder (PTSD). It seems likely that dissociation may occur along a continuum of severity, with more or less complete fragmentation of identity, memory, or consciousness. On the more "benign" end of the continuum, we see dissociation as a normal mechanism of consciousness—for example, when you are driving for several hours on a long stretch of highway, you may find yourself somewhere without any recollection of "how" precisely you got there. On the more pathological end of the continuum, we find virtually complete fragmentation of the self for long periods of time, resulting in, for example, multiple personality disorder. We will begin our discussion with the relatively more benign conditions and work our way across to the more pervasive and incapacitating disorders.

Depersonalization Disorder

The Central Concept

Vignette

Chris was a 23-year-old college student who complained to a physician at the student health service that "it's weird . . . I feel spaced out all the time . . . like I can't tell what's real and what's a dream. Sometimes I feel like a zombie or something. And sometimes it's like I'm floating outside my body, just looking down and watching myself. It's real spooky. I see things funny sometimes, too—like the edges of tables are fuzzy or bent. Lately, I can't even get through class. My sleep and appetite are pretty bad, too. I know it sounds crazy . . . I don't know, am I a psycho or something?"

The answer is, probably not. In fact, brief periods of depersonalization may be seen in up to 70% of young adults (American Psychiatric Association 1987). In depersonalization disorder, however, the condition must be severe enough to cause marked distress or dysfunction. Commonly associated features include dizziness, depression, rumination, somatic concerns, sensory anesthesia, anxiety, fear of going "crazy," and a subjective sense of time distortion. The episodes of depersonalization usually begin rapidly, but disappear gradually. "Derealization" (i.e., the sense that the external world is somehow strange or altered) is often present. The use of psychoactive drugs (such as marijuana) may precipitate depersonalization experiences or may follow as a complication of the full-blown disorder.

Historical Development of the Disorder

In the golden age of neurosis, depersonalization disorder was termed "depersonalization neurosis" (Freedman et al. 1972). A number of workers—including Krishaber (1873) and Dugas (Dugas and Moutier 1898)—described syndromes involving feelings of "unreality" about oneself or one's surroundings. However, it was probably Mapother and Mayer-Gross in the early part of the 20th century who delineated the terms "depersonalization" and "derealization" in a manner recognizable to us. Eventually, the term "depersonalization" came to encompass the sense that one's self or one's surroundings were unreal, alien, or subtly altered. Depersonalization was thought to occur in virtually all of the psychoses and neuroses, and was conceived of as an early signal of mental illness (Freedman et al. 1972). Depersonalization was listed in DSM-I (American Psychiatric Association 1952) only as a symptom of "dissociative reaction," but attained full syndromal status in DSM-II (American Psychiatric Association 1968) and DSM-III (American Psychiatric Association 1980).

The Biopsychosocial Perspective

Biological Factors

The "biology" of depersonalization—if there is anything so homogeneous—remains obscure. As a symptom, depersonalization may be seen in a variety of neurological and physiological disorders (see discussion of the differential diagnosis). With respect to the "functional" disorder per se, we know very little about the pathophysiology. Depersonalization phenomena can be produced by electrical stimulation of the temporal lobes (during neurosurgery), and it is plausible to hypothesize that these brain regions are involved in depersonalization disorder (Lishman 1987). However, as yet, no convincing data have demonstrated such an involvement. Because, as we shall see, anxiety can precipitate depersonalization phenomena, we might hypothesize a pathophysiology similar to that of, for example, panic disorder (see Chapter 6). Again, we have little evidence of this, beyond the fact that depersonalization symptoms may respond to anxiolytics. Hollander et al. (1989), noting the comorbidity of panic and depersonalization, have suggested that serotonergic mechanisms may be involved in both conditions. We will discuss these issues later in this section.

Finally, Cohen (1988) has hypothesized that "it is only the patient who is anxious and hyperventilating who develops depersonalization. In such patients the depersonalization would be the result of the changes in metabolism and cerebral blood flow produced by the hyperventilation" (p. 578). This is an intriguing suggestion, but one that Cohen himself has found difficult to substantiate.

Psychological Factors

Freud believed that the sense of sudden alienation and unreality associated with depersonalization arises from a twofold defensive process: first, repression is activated in order to fend off unacceptable impulses, but fails to do so; next, the unacceptable feelings are masked as "unreal" (Freedman et al. 1972). In the 1920s, Hermann Nunberg linked depersonalization with shifting libido (Nemiah 1985). He noted that depersonalization often occurs in the context of sudden object loss, and hypothesized that the sense of unreality arises from the shifting of libido from the object onto the ego.

To put the idea more colloquially, we can imagine a recently bereaved widow—still in a state of "shock" 2 days after her husband's death—attending to every ache and pain she might otherwise have ignored. You may have had the experience of repeating a particular word to yourself so many times that it ceases to have meaning—it becomes "unreal." Perhaps, then, the widow who "hyper-attends" to her own bodily processes begins to experience her very self as "unreal" or her body as somehow alien. Indeed, Schilder first called attention to the role of heightened self-observation in depersonalization (Nemiah 1985). Summing up the view of many modern authors, Nemiah states that "depersonalization is a primitive, highly pathological defense that is allied to denial and is employed as an emergency measure when the more usual mechanism of repression fails to control unacceptable impulses" (p. 954).

We might demur a bit from this view by noting that depersonalization is not always "highly pathological," and occurs transiently in most of us. Depersonalization, as Kaplan and Sadock (1988) note, "is a frequent event in children as they develop the capacity for self-awareness, and adults often undergo a temporary sense of unreality when they travel to new and strange places" (p. 348).

Finally, we should note that cognitive-behavioral factors may play a role in depersonalization disorder. As Meyer (1983) points out, "Many people are not really bothered by such [depersonalization] experiences, whereas others feel as if they are going crazy. In this latter situation, the sense of depersonalization can be conditioned to anticipatory anxiety, leading to a vicious cycle reinforcing the belief that they might indeed be going crazy" (p. 149).

Sociocultural Factors

We have already noted the role of "object loss" in depersonalization. Other interpersonal factors may include emotional censure by parents, hostility between parents, and "parental deceptiveness" (Freedman et al. 1972). Kolb (1959), while addressing the genesis of disturbed body image in schizophrenia, raised questions that may also apply to the interpersonal roots of depersonalization. Specifically, could some "disturbance" in the physical interaction between mother and infant lead to an unstable body image in the latter? For example, if the infant is not held or fondled sufficiently, could this lead to a failure of the cortex to integrate a stable body image, and to subsequent feelings of depersonalization? Arieti (1974) has noted that these intriguing questions have not been satisfactorily answered with respect to schizophrenia; the same must unfortunately be said with respect to depersonalization disorder.

In a study of dissociative disorders among a random population in Winnipeg, Ross et al. (1991) found no correlation between dissociative experiences and income, gender, education, religion, or household composition. (The absence of gender effect differs from other studies of multiple personality disorder, which seems to be more common in females, as will be discussed later in this chapter.)

Pitfalls in the Differential Diagnosis

Depersonalization disorder may be confused with a plethora of both "organic" and "functional" disorders (Table 8–1). Let's consider the following vignette.

Table 8–1. Conditions presenting with depersonalization

Organic	Other psychiatric disorders
Temporal lobe epilepsy or tumor	Schizophrenia
Nondominant parietal lobe lesion	Depression
	Mania
Cerebrovascular disease	Phobic anxiety depersonalization syndrome
Migraine	
Encephalitis	Other anxiety disorders (panic disorder, PTSD)
Alzheimer's disease	
Huntington's disease	Other dissociative disorders
Hypoglycemia	
Hypothyroidism	
Psychotomimetic drugs	
Hyperventilation	

Source. Extensively modified from Cummings 1985.

Vignette

A 60-year-old female was brought to the emergency room by her husband because she had complained for several weeks that "my arms and legs aren't real" and "I feel like I'm walking in a dream." The patient had no psychiatric history, and family history was non-contributory. The patient showed no evidence of thought process disorder, and she denied auditory hallucinations. However, she did wonder whether people on the street could read her thoughts. She also felt that "I keep repeating the same scene over and over . . . it's like, I've been in this emergency room before." Neurological examination was grossly within normal limits, except for a possible left visual field defect. A computed tomography (CT) scan of the brain revealed a probable glioblastoma in the right temporal lobe.

This vignette demonstrates the importance of the temporal lobes in the diagnosis of depersonalization phenomena. The tipoffs in the case are the patient's age (depersonalization disorder rarely begins after age 40) and the contralateral visual field defect. Indeed, Lishman (1987) notes that "the most reliable neurological sign of deep temporal lobe lesions is a contralateral homonymous upper quadratic visual field defect, caused by interruption of the visual radiation in the central white matter" (p. 18). Although our patient's neurological examination was otherwise normal, deep temporal lesions may also result in a mild contralateral hemiparesis or sensory loss (Lishman 1987). Temporal lobe seizures may produce a variety of altered perceptual experiences as part of their "aura." Feelings of depersonalization or derealization are common, as are feelings of déjà vu or jamais vu (Lishman 1987). A clue to the presence of temporal lobe epilepsy (as opposed to depersonalization disorder) would be the presence of, for example, olfactory or gustatory hallucinations, and automatisms (features that are rarely seen in depersonalization disorder). By the way, patients with right-sided parietal lobe lesions may show so-called hemidepersonalization, in which they experience one side of the body as unreal, belonging to someone else, or distorted in size or shape (Cummings 1985).

As noted above, depersonalization disorder may be confused with a variety of related and unrelated "psychiatric" disorders (Table 8–1). Let's consider the following vignette.

Vignette

A 22-year-old man presented to the university health center with the complaint of "feeling unreal . . . sort of like my body is shrunk. Sometimes I feel like I have the face of a girl, or an animal." The patient had no formal psychiatric history but gave a history of "always feeling like I was different." He showed no formal thought process disorder, and he denied auditory or other hallucinations (other than the above-noted visual distortions). There was no history of psychotomimetic drug use. The patient was told he was suffering from a "stress reaction" and was given some relaxation exercises to do. One month later, the patient required hospitalization because of paranoid delusions concerning "the electrical implant in my face and brain." A preliminary diagnosis of schizophreniform disorder, r/o paranoid schizophrenia" was entertained.

This case points out that "depersonalization" is a symptom, not a diagnosis. It is often seen in schizophrenia (Arieti 1974) and may represent an intermediate or early stage of the illness (Arieti 1974; Cummings 1985). Depersonalization may also be seen in patients described by Roth (1959) as suffering from "phobic-anxiety-depersonalization syndrome." These individuals usually show premorbid traits of anxiety, oversensitivity, self-consciousness, and low self-esteem. Their illness presents as agoraphobia complicated by brief, self-limited bouts of schizophreniform symptoms, usually occurring when the individual is under severe stress. Though this condition is not found in American nosology, it does overlap with borderline personality disorder (Pies 1988), in which stress-related depersonalization may sometimes occur.

Depersonalization in the context of anxiety disorders and other dissociative disorders is discussed in the appropriate subsections below (see also Chapter 6).

Adjunctive Testing

Very little research exists on the neuroendocrine, electrophysiological, and radiographic aspects of depersonalization disorder. Of course, the electroencephalography and brain electrical activity mapping (BEAM) may be quite helpful in picking up cases of temporal lobe dysfunction.

On the Minnesota Multiphasic Personality Inventory (MMPI), patients with depersonalization disorder typically show elevations on scales 3, 7, and F, reflecting both anxious and histrionic traits (Meyer 1983). Anxiety and identity confusion may also lead to an elevated scale 8 (schizophrenia), according to Meyer (1983).

Until quite recently, there was no standardized instrument designed to yield uniform diagnosis of dissociative disorders. However, a preliminary report by Steinberg et al. (1990) indicates good to excellent reliability and discriminant validity for the Structured Clinical Interview for DSM-III-R Dissociative Disorders (SCID-D). The SCID-D is a structured clinical interview containing 200 items designed to assess five different symptom areas: amnesia, depersonalization, derealization, identity confusion, and identity alteration. More recently, Ross et al. (1991) utilized a 28-item Dissociative Experiences Scale (DES; Bernstein and Putnam 1986) to assess dissociative experiences in a random sample of 1,055 individuals in Winnipeg. DSM-III-R dissociative disorders (including depersonalization disorder) were correlated with two principal "factors," termed "activities of dissociated states" and "depersonalization-derealization." The first factor may help differentiate multiple personality disorder from other dissociative disorders (Ross et al. 1991). The individual components of these principal factors, shown in Table 8–2, may aid you in making a diagnosis of depersonalization and other related disorders.

Notice that the complaint "voices inside one's head" raises the sometimes difficult distinction between schizophrenia and dissociative disorders. Ross et al. (1991) suggest that "an auditory hallucination can be thought of as a depersonalized thought or as an exaggerated form of a normal internal dialogue" (p. 299). Of course, in schizophrenia, you will probably see a "delusional elaboration" around the internal stimuli.

Treatment Directions and Goals

Somatic Approaches

There is no specific pharmacological approach to depersonalization disorder, although anecdotal evidence points to the efficacy of anxiolytics and antidepressants. Cattell and Cattell (1974) stated that a combination of dextroamphetamine and Amytal "tends to neutralize the depersonalization experience in many instances" (p. 796), but controlled studies are lacking. More recently, Hollander et al. (1989) reported on the pharmacological dissection of panic and depersonalization, with fluoxetine proving effective in treating one patient's depersonalization/derealization symptoms. For the patient with Roth's "phobic-anxiety-depersonalization syndrome," phenelzine or other monoamine oxidase inhibitors (MAOIs) may be useful. Hollender and Ban (1979) reported a positive response in one patient with this syndrome who had failed to respond to psychotherapy, biofeedback, imipramine, diazepam, and two antipsychotics. As you can see, much of the information in this area is limited to single-case reports or uncontrolled studies.

Psychosocial Approaches

A variety of psychosocial approaches have been suggested for the patient with depersonalization disorder, ranging from psychoanalysis to psychodrama (Meyer 1983). As Meyer (1983) conceives it, "Any

Table 8–2.   Activities of dissociated states

Finding oneself in a place but being unaware how one got there.

Finding oneself dressed in clothes that one can't remember putting on.

Finding unfamiliar things among one's belongings.

Not recognizing friends or family members.

Experiencing depersonalization-derealization.

Not recognizing one's reflection in a mirror.

Having a sense that other people and objects do not seem real.

Feeling as though one's body is not one's own.

Hearing voices inside one's head.

Looking at the world through a fog.

Note.   Extensively modified from Ross et al. 1991.

technique useful for getting in touch with the less integrated aspects of the personality could be useful here." He further suggests that patients may be "trained to label experiences viewed as alien as actually an integral part of their personality and something to be dealt with in a confrontive and honest manner." However, there is little empirical evidence that such an approach is especially effective. Those who advocate psychotherapy or psychoanalysis state that a minimum of 5 years of treatment may be required (Shader and Scharfman 1989), perhaps because many patients with depersonalization disorder are quite obsessional. To the extent that a patient's presentation suggests an anxiety disorder, relaxation and other behavioral techniques might be useful. As yet, however, there is insufficient evidence pointing to any particular psychotherapeutic approach as the treatment of choice for depersonalization disorder.

Dissociative (Psychogenic) Amnesia

The Central Concept

Vignette

Ms. Mnemosyne, a recent immigrant to this country from Greece, upon arrival at the airport was involved in a terrible motor vehicle accident, in which her sister, Euterpe, was killed. Although she was only slightly injured, the patient had no recollection of anything that occurred in the 2 days following the accident; for example, she could not recall having been taken to the hospital, receiving a head CT scan (which was totally normal), and so forth. The patient's psychiatric history was remarkable for a recent, and probably unresolved, bout of depression and for a long history of vague somatic complaints (especially headaches) not explained by physical findings. After 1 week of hospitalization, during which the patient's family visited her frequently and assured her that she would get better, the patient's memory returned completely.

As our vignette suggests, dissociative amnesia entails the sudden inability to recall important personal information and goes beyond mere "forgetfulness." It is, by definition, not due to an organic factor, although Cummings (1985) notes "a high incidence of CNS [central nervous system] disorders among patients with psychogenic amnesia" (p. 40). Four types of dissociative amnesia are usually described. In localized dissociative amnesia—the most common type—there is failure to recall all events occurring during a circumscribed period of time, usually just following some traumatic event. In selective dissociative amnesia, the patient fails to recall some, but not all, of the events occurring during some specific time period. Less common is so-called generalized amnesia, in which the patient's inability to recall encompasses his or her entire life or identity; and continuous amnesia, in which the amnesia continues in anterograde fashion up to and including the present. Perplexity, disorientation, and "indifference" toward the memory loss may be associated features. And, as our vignette suggests, depression may precede the onset of dissociative amnesia (Cummings 1985).

Historical Development of the Disorder

Psychogenic amnesia as a concept has its origins in the broader notion of "hysterical neurosis." Prior to DSM-III, this category was divided into conversion- and dissociative-type neuroses. The dissociative type of hysterical neurosis included amnesic syndromes, fugue states, somnambulism, and multiple personality. One textbook glossary defined "hysterical neurosis" as "a neurosis that occurs in response to emotional stress and involves a sudden loss or impairment of function. It may be of the conversion type in which the senses of the voluntary nervous system are involved, or of the dissociative type in which the individual's state of consciousness is affected" (Freedman et al. 1972, p. 772).

The basic theory of dissociation originated with Charcot's theory that the stream of consciousness breaks up into diverse elements under certain pathogenic circumstances (see discussion of psychological factors). In the late 19th century, Janet noted amnesia as a part of fugue states and somnambulism (Freedman et al. 1972). Freud called attention to the very circumscribed (and usually temporary) form of amnesia manifested as the forgetting of familiar names (Fenichel 1945).

Freud associated this "parapraxis" with repression of some objectionable impulse. More recent thinking about psychogenic amnesia has emphasized the interaction of traumatic events with "psychodynamic factors that modify the clinical picture and ultimately determine the actual pattern of forgetting" (Linn 1989, p. 2186).

In DSM-IV (American Psychiatric Association 1994), the term "psychogenic amnesia" was changed to "dissociative amnesia," but, thankfully, significant changes in the criteria were not made. Because virtually all the existing literature uses the term "psychogenic amnesia," we shall occasionally interchange this term with its new (DSM-IV) counterpart.

The Biopsychosocial Perspective

Biological Factors

It may seem paradoxical to speak of "biological" factors in a syndrome that is, by its very designation, not "organic." But the paradox is no more compelling here than in any of the other so-called functional psychiatric disorders. As Lishman (1987) puts it, "It may fairly be presumed that a pathophysiology of some kind accompanies psychogenic amnesia, just as there must be a physiological basis for the influence of emotional and motivational factors on the normal processes of remembering and forgetting" (p. 36). And even if we were to conceive of a "pure," nonorganic form of dissociative amnesia, we very likely would find it associated with known organic factors in a large number of cases. As early as 1911, Janet noted that hysterical aphasia, mutism, or word blindness was often accompanied by right-sided sensorimotor symptoms (Flor-Henry 1983). Lishman (1987), summarizing the investigation of Kennedy and Neville (1957), notes that in 41% of cases involving abrupt failure of memory, psychogenic and organic factors together were implicated: "Sometimes organic brain disease was present along with an obvious psychological precipitant, and neither aetiology precluded the other. . . . Kennedy and Neville suggested that brain damage appeared to predispose to the development of primitive mental mechanisms of escape, or lower the threshold at which stress would bring them out" (p. 408).

Psychogenic amnesia is one of more than 50 possible symptoms included in Perley and Guze's (1962) criteria for "hysteria," a syndrome that served as the forerunner of our present-day somatization disorder (see Chapter 7). In his investigation of such "hysterical" patients, Flor-Henry (1983) discovered evidence for dominant-hemisphere dysfunction. It is not clear that this finding, even if correct, is applicable to dissociative amnesia per se, but it does provide us with an intriguing heuristic hypothesis. In our subsection on differential diagnosis, we shall examine some neurological conditions that may be confused with dissociative amnesia.

Psychological Factors

As adumbrated above, early psychoanalytic views of dissociative amnesia implicated repression as the chief etiological mechanism. There is, as Abse (1974) has noted, "a need to repress associated thoughts which would otherwise result in anxiety or other dysphoric emotion" (p. 159). Specifically, Abse points out that "in a circumscribed amnesia . . . these [forgotten] events may have been either directly evocative of painful feelings, or, paradoxically, involved at the time with pleasurable ones which would now, however, evoke either a sense of guilt or a painful sense of loss" (p. 159). In this light, let's consider the following vignette, based on a case described by Linn (1989):

A 30-year-old married man was found by a police officer, sitting in his parked car at the edge of the highway. The man appeared confused and disoriented and was taken to a hospital ER, where a thorough medical and neurological examination yielded no organic pathology. On psychiatric interview, the man had no recollection of his name, address, or occupation, nor any memory of how he had wound up in his car. He demonstrated full recollection of personal events prior to 1970 (age 10), but none for events since that time. Upon amobarbital interview, the patient revealed that, just prior to his being found by the police, he had had a stormy argument with his wife. It had ended with her "kicking me out of the apartment," which was in her name. It further emerged—in the course of psychotherapy—that a similar event had befallen the patient at age 10, when his alcoholic mother had abandoned him.

You can see how the peculiar pattern of "forgetting" relates symbolically to previous psychic trauma. It could be said that in dissociative amnesia, dissociation is the primary defense mechanism, with repression and denial functioning as secondary defenses (Kaplan and Sadock 1988). That is, the person primarily alters consciousness as a way of coping with a profound conflict or stressor. Secondarily, disturbing impulses are blocked from consciousness, and some aspect of external reality is ignored by the conscious mind.

Having said all this, we should take careful note of Lishman's (1987) point, that "it is possible . . . that certain cases of psychogenic amnesia may depend, at least in part, on failure in the initial processing of experience, rather than on a process of forgetting or repression" (p. 36). Thus, certain states of high emotional arousal may interfere with the registration or encoding of information, with the resulting amnesia having little or nothing to do with the dynamic mechanisms posited by psychoanalytic theory (Lishman 1987).

Sociocultural Factors

It is, of course, impossible to separate early familial experiences (i.e., "social" factors) from the developing individual's "psychology." This caveat aside, there is growing evidence that family-related traumata play an important role in the dissociative disorders (Sanders and Giolas 1991). Thus, in their study of dissociation and childhood trauma in psychologically disturbed adolescents, Sanders and Giolas (1991) found that the degree of dissociation was directly related to five factors in childhood: physical abuse or punishment, sexual abuse, psychological abuse, neglect, and "negative home atmosphere." In the questionnaire used to assess these adolescents, the following items seem pertinent to our "social" perspective:

- As a child, did you feel unwanted or emotionally neglected?
- As a child, did you have to take care of yourself before you were old enough?
- Did your parents verbally abuse each other?
- Did you ever think you wanted to leave your family and live with another family?

As we will see when we discuss dissociative identity disorder (multiple personality disorder), the degree of childhood abuse and neglect seems directly correlated with the extremity of the dissociative phenomena. The Sanders and Giolas study did not specifically address psychogenic amnesia, but it is reasonable to infer that this type of amnesia is correlated with similar childhood antecedents.

There is little research pertaining specifically to sociocultural factors in dissociative amnesia. We do know that dissociative amnesia is more common during periods of war or during natural disasters (Kaplan and Sadock 1988), so we might expect to find a high incidence of dissociative amnesia in regions prone to such events. If we regard dissociative amnesia as part of "hysterical" disorders in general, we can make a few observations regarding sociocultural influences. Hollingshead and Redlich (1958) found that hysterical reactions, unlike other "neurotic" disorders, occur more frequently in lower socioeconomic classes. There are numerous culture-bound syndromes that seem to be hysteriform in nature—for example, the "trance" states seen in some Haitian Voodoo cults, or the ataque seen commonly in Puerto Rican women. Whether these states are etiologically related to dissociative amnesia is not known.

Pitfalls in the Differential Diagnosis

Organic Disorders

A large number of "organic" conditions may be associated with amnesia, as Cummings (1985) has detailed (Table 8–3). Before offering some general principles of differential diagnosis applicable to these disorders, let's consider the following vignette.

Vignette

A 23-year-old man with a known history of paranoid schizophrenia was found wandering around a firehouse at 1 A.M. and was brought by ambulance to a psychiatric ER. There he proved to be disoriented to time and place. He appeared irritable and restless. When asked what he was doing outside the firehouse, he replied, "The firemen wanted me to burn down City Hall." The resident in the ER suspected an acute psychotic episode but, on physical examination, discovered a contusion near the right temporal region. A CT scan of the brain was normal, but an electroencephalogram (EEG) revealed localized suppression of alpha rhythm in both the right and left temporal regions. A more careful history, taken after the patient's initial disorientation had cleared, revealed that he had been riding in a taxi shortly before his being discovered outside the firehouse. He could not recall the final minutes of the cab ride, nor the hour or two he had spent wandering outside the firehouse. His first clear recollection was of seeing the lights of the firehouse. A check with the police revealed that an individual fitting the patient's description had hailed a taxi at about 10 P.M. on the night in question. The taxi was involved in a relatively minor collision, during which the passenger had struck the right side of his head against the rear passenger-side window. He had suffered, according to the cab driver's report to the police, "a blackout for about 30 seconds." Before the driver could stop him, the passenger had bolted from the car, shouting, "They're gonna get my brain!"

Aside from demonstrating the perils of premature diagnosis, this vignette presents a fairly typical picture of "posttraumatic" amnesia (not to be confused with the meaning of "postttraumatic" in PTSD). Traumatic brain injuries are probably the most common cause of

Table 8–3. Some organic conditions associated with amnesia

Condition	Clinical features
Wernicke-Korsakoff syndrome	Nystagmus, ataxia, neuropathy
Head trauma	Frontotemporal lobe dysfunction
Hippocampal infarction	Homonymous hemianopsia
Cerebral anoxia	History of cardiopulmonary arrest
Transient global amnesia	History of cerebrovascular disease
Cerebral tumor	Headache, hemiparesis
Herpes encephalitis	Aphasia, seizures

Source. Extensively modified from Cummings 1985.

amnesia seen in clinical practice (Cummings 1985). The bony housing of the temporal lobes renders them peculiarly susceptible to contusions from both coup and contrecoup injuries (i.e., both at the site of impact and at the opposite pole). The amnesia induced by head injury typically includes a period of retrograde memory loss (i.e., for events prior to the injury), memory loss associated with actual unconsciousness, and a period of anterograde memory loss (i.e., for events following the injury). Often, there is "shrinkage" of both the anterograde and retrograde amnesic periods as the patient recovers (Cummings 1985). In contrast, psychogenic amnesia almost always shows anterograde amnesia (American Psychiatric Association 1987); however, in rare cases, retrograde memory loss does occur. In such cases, ancillary testing may be necessary to ascertain the diagnosis.

Transient global amnesia, another "organic" cause of memory loss, presents with features similar to those of head injury. In transient global amnesia, as in posttraumatic amnesia, there is retrograde memory loss, usually of a few weeks' duration. There is also anterograde amnesia, but it is "ongoing"—that is, it continues to impair the acquisition of new information for a period of several hours. Most patients suffer only a single attack of transient global amnesia, but those with underlying cerebrovascular disease may have repeated attacks (Cummings 1985).

Unlike dissociative amnesia, transient global amnesia almost never entails a loss of personal identity. Moreover, in transient global amnesia, the pattern of memory loss shows a "temporal gradient"—that is, there is relative preservation of remote memory as one moves chronologically "behind" the retrograde amnesia. In dissociative amnesia, there is no gradient, and the patient often shows a "quirky" pattern of memory loss—that is, certain affectively charged memories may be lost, while others from around the same period are retained.

Cummings (1985) and Dubovsky (1988) have summarized the factors that help distinguish dissociative amnesia from several types of "organic" amnesia, including amnesia associated with dysfunction of the hippocampus, hypothalamus, and thalamus (Table 8–4).

We should close this subsection by noting that temporal lobe epilepsy may lead to memory impairment and amnesia, but the accompanying signs and symptoms (aura, stereotypic movements, olfactory or gustatory hallucinations, etc.) usually distinguish temporal lobe epilepsy from dissociative amnesia. Finally, bear in mind that alcoholic persons who do not suffer from Wernicke-Korsakoff syndrome may still show amnesia due to alcohol intoxication per se—so-called blackouts.

Functional Disorders

It should not surprise you that virtually any of the other dissociative disorders may sometimes be confused with dissociative amnesia, since

Table 8–4. Differential diagnosis of dissociative (psychogenic) and "organic" amnesia

Dissociative amnesia	"Organic" amnesia
Personal identity often lost despite being oriented to time/place.	Personal identity retained.
Ability to learn new information preserved.	Inability to learn new information.
Memory loss often selective for personal/"charged" information.	Memory loss nonselective.
Temporal gradient absent.	Temporal gradient present.
Long- and short-term memory equally affected.	Short-term memory more impaired than long-term memory.
Indifferent to amnesia.	Distressed by amnesia.
More common between ages 20 and 40.	More common between ages 60 and 70.
Symptoms in some cases improved temporarily with tranquilizers.	Amnesia worsened with tranquilizers.
Amnesia, confusion develop in context of psychic trauma.	Amnesia, confusion develop in context of physical illness or psychoactive drug use.
Prompt/sudden return of memory.	Gradual return of memory.

Source. Extensively modified from Cummings 1985; Dubovsky 1988.

amnesia is such a nonspecific finding. Thus, patients with dissociative fugue or dissociative identity disorder (multiple personality disorder) may show varying degrees and types of memory loss; however, they have many other distinguishing features, which will be detailed later in this chapter. Malingering must also be considered in the differential diagnosis of dissociative amnesia, but the presence of clear secondary gain usually permits the distinction.

We saw in Chapter 6 that "psychogenic amnesia" may be part of PTSD—that is, important aspects of the trauma may be "forgotten." Because this amnesic phenomenon is often prominent in PTSD, some clinicians argue that PTSD ought to be included among the dissociative disorders.

Finally, in my experience, patients with various psychotic disorders (e.g., mania, schizophrenia) often show "spotty" memory deficits for events occurring during the most florid phase of their psychoses. For example, one bipolar patient of mine never recalled any of the sexually tinged comments she made during her manic episodes but retained memories of many other "neutral" events. One could consider this a form of dissociative amnesia, probably arising from selective repression and denial, but the diagnosis of bipolar disorder would supersede.

Adjunctive Testing

Psychological Testing

Meyer (1983) notes that "a high 3-4/4-3 pattern on the MMPI, particularly the 3-4 profile, means fertile ground for the development of dissociative experiences" (p. 145). (You will recall that scale 3 measures hysteria and scale 4 measures psychopathy and "immaturity.") If the patient is "gravitating toward a general loss of integrated decision making," scale 8 (schizophrenia) may be elevated (Meyer 1983).

Neuroendocrine and Imaging Techniques

While there are, as yet, no well-established neuroendocrine or imaging techniques that "demonstrate" the presence of dissociative amnesia, these techniques are of critical importance in ruling out serious organic brain syndromes. We saw, in our vignette about the patient with head trauma, how the EEG may aid in diagnosis. CT scanning and magnetic resonance imaging (MRI) are also helpful in cases of amnesia, particularly those due to tumor, vascular lesions, or brain hemorrhage.

Sodium Amobarbital Interview

Finally, the Amytal (sodium amobarbital) interview may be of great help in confirming the diagnosis of dissociative amnesia (Cummings 1985). This procedure often abruptly terminates the amnesia, as may hypnotic suggestion. The treatment implications of the Amytal interview are discussed in the next subsection.

Treatment Directions and Goals

Many cases of dissociative amnesia resolve spontaneously once the patient is removed from the precipitating stressor (Purcell 1988). When this is not the case, both somatic and psychosocial treatments may be helpful.

Somatic Approaches

The literature seems curiously devoid of pharmacological therapies for dissociative amnesia, other than the use of sodium amobarbital or pentobarbital (Linn 1989). For example, the use of benzodiazepines or antidepressants in this disorder seems virtually unexplored. Linn (1989) has discussed some of the steps of the standard Amytal interview as follows:

> [T]o titrate the dose for the interview, it is helpful to observe the patient's face. A skin flush is an important preliminary sign. The eyes may suddenly fill with tears, or, conversely, the patient may relax and make some jocular remark. These are delicate endpoints . . . thereafter [the interviewer] may enter actively into a psychodrama with the patient, encouraging the expression of all thoughts and feelings that have caused suffering. . . . the patient should abreact with relative spontaneity. Persistent interrogation of a somnolent, nonresponsive patient usually is not productive. (p. 2188)

Linn (1989) notes the possibility of "an underlying paranoid psychotic disorder" in the patient with psychogenic amnesia. In such cases, antipsychotic medication may be appropriate. Similarly, although there are few data in this area, it would be reasonable to treat an underlying major depression with antidepressant medication.

Psychosocial Approaches

Maxmen (1986) has noted that the literature on treating dissociative disorders in general is "scant, devoid of controlled studies, [and] mainly anecdotal" (p. 251). He nevertheless summarizes the treatment of psychogenic amnesia (and fugue states) as follows: 1) Evaluate the patient and allow a few days for spontaneous remission. If the patient doesn't recover, 2) provide discussion, support, and persuasion (i.e., "gently persuade [the patient] to keep after lost memories"); 3) have the patient free-associate to events surrounding the amnesia; and 4) hypnotize the patient and instruct him or her to give a running commentary of known past incidents—this usually leads to abreaction and eventual termination of the amnesia.

Linn (1989) and Myerson (1966) emphasize how important it is to consider the stressful, precipitating events in psychogenic amnesia and to reduce that stress. Otherwise, further amnesia and even dangerous acting out may occur. Purcell (1988) notes further that if the psychogenic amnesia patient is found to have some underlying psychiatric disorder after resolution of the amnesic episode, treatment of the underlying condition should ensue. In the case of underlying personality disorder, for example, long-term psychotherapy may be required.

Dissociative (Psychogenic) Fugue

The Central Concept

Vignette

Mr. Pete Corro, a 34-year-old police officer, discovered his wife in the company of another man. She confessed to her husband that she had been involved in this affair for over 2 years. Upon hearing this, Mr. Corro stormed out of his house and, according to a neighbor's report, "ran down the road like a bat out of hell." He was spotted 2 weeks later in a nearby town, where he was working as a bartender under the name "Pedro Coraje." He recalled nothing of his previous life, occupation, or marriage. Nor did he remember how he had arrived in town or what he had done prior to becoming a bartender. He stated that he was "confused" about his life and had invented a name for himself, hoping he would remember his identity. Upon psychiatric examination, the patient exhibited no evidence of organic brain pathology or psychosis. Subsequent interview with his family showed the patient to have been a rather temperamental child who, in his adolescence, had had several encounters with the police. In high school, he had "gotten into drinking a lot," but had managed to complete the 12th grade. After 1 week in the hospital, the patient suddenly and fully recovered his memory. He and his wife entered marital counseling and were doing well 6 months later.

Mr. Corro shows the classic features of dissociative fugue: sudden, unexpected travel from home, with inability to recall one's past; assumption of a new identity; and absence of organic factors that would account for the symptoms. Often, in dissociative fugue, the patient's new identity contrasts sharply with his or her "original" identity; for example, a quiet, socially withdrawn individual assumes the identity of a flamboyant bon vivant. However, most fugues are less elaborate, consisting of brief, apparently purposeful travel with only partial construction of a new identity. One report indicated that about half of all fugues last less than 24 hours (Abeles and Schilder 1935, cited in Ford 1989). Most patients have more than one fugue episode (Berrington et al. 1956). Ford (1989) points out that many patients with fugue states also have symptoms of multiple personality (discussed later in this chapter) or conversion disorder (see Chapter 7).

Rice and Fisher (1976) discuss four types of fugue state, which they view "in terms of a continuum of severity": 1) fugue with awareness of loss of personal identity, the most severe type; 2) fugue with "change of personal identity," such as assuming a false name associated with some unconscious fantasy; 3) fugue without loss or change of identity, but with "reversion to an earlier period of the subject's life, with retrograde amnesia for events subsequent to that period"; and 4) "simple fugue," in which there is circumscribed memory loss of some past event. (This last type clearly overlaps with our current category of dissociative amnesia.)

Historical Development of the Disorder

Nemiah (1980) has detailed the classic descriptions of fugue states found in the psychological literature of the 19th and early 20th centuries. We have, for example, William James's meticulous description of the Rev. Ansel Bourne—the "Missing Preacher"—who disappeared one day in 1887 and turned up 2 months later as "a man calling himself A. J. Brown, who had rented a small shop . . . stocked it with stationery, confectionery, fruit and small articles, and carried on his quiet trade without seeming to any one unnatural or eccentric" (p. 1544).

Fugue-like states were described by many 19th- and early-20th-century investigators, including Pierre Janet and—in this country—A. A. Brill (see below). Freud seems to have had little interest in fugue states per se, being more absorbed in the somatic manifestations of hysteria, such as conversion (Nemiah 1980). The general psychoanalytic view of fugue states (or "poriomania," from the Greek, *poreia,* a journey) was that they are a species of hysteria and related to the mechanisms of dissociation and repression (see subsection on psychological factors in our discussion of the biopsychosocial perspective).

In DSM-II, the distinction was drawn between hysterical neurosis, dissociative type (including fugue states) and conversion type. In DSM-III and DSM-III-R, the dissociative disorders achieved autonomy, with psychogenic fugue as a subcategory.

The Biopsychosocial Perspective

Biological Factors

The American psychoanalyst A. A. Brill described a fugue state in one of his patients. Brill's conceptualization of the man's problem was an early attempt at a biological understanding of fugue states:

> [I]n one of his attacks during the Boer War, he [the patient] ran away from Canada and went to London, where, seeing calls for volunteers, he enlisted and was sent to South Africa. He fought bravely and was promoted to sergeant in a few weeks. When he came to himself, he was quite surprised to find he was a soldier. He did not have the least idea how he got to South Africa. . . . I diagnosed him as a psychic epileptic. I decided that he suffered from a form of epilepsy which does not manifest itself in fits . . . but rather in peculiar psychic actions which may last for a few minutes or hours or perhaps for weeks, months, or years. (Brill 1921, pp. 50–51)

Probably few neurologists today would agree with Brill's diagnosis—nor, indeed, did his supervisor, who diagnosed the patient as suffering from "dementia praecox." But the notion that something "neurological" underlies fugue states is one that persists to this day. Lishman (1987) notes that the hippocampus and mammillary bodies are involved in the "integration between affective and cognitive aspects of experience," and speculated that in dissociative fugue states, perhaps "the total apparatus fails to function harmoniously" (p. 36). And reading Mesulam (1985) on ictal phenomena, you may come away feeling that Brill was right:

> Several patients with temporolimbic seizure foci have engaged in self-mutilation. One female patient had a paroxysmal illusion of being possessed by a demon, and during these episodes felt compelled to escape from her home or the hospital in order to have sexual relations with some unclean and unattractive stranger. . . . Prolonged confusional and fugue states . . . have also been associated with ongoing seizure activity. (p. 294–295)

We will return to this issue when we discuss differential diagnosis.

Rice and Fisher (1976) have pointed out the relationship between fugue states and various sleep phenomena. They described a case in which a patient actually underwent EEG studies during fugue-like episodes. These investigators found that the patient's "sleep-talking" episodes "appeared to be fugues without locomotion . . . identical in verbal content to some of the fugues with locomotion that occurred during the diurnal state" (p. 79). These authors posited "a psycho-physiological link between fugue-states and sleep-dream mechanisms" (p. 79), noting particularly the role of post-REM periods.

For now, we should bear in mind Lishman's (1987) point that "organic and psychogenic factors may often . . . be inextricably mixed, with epileptic clouding helping to release abnormal traits in the personality. Thus in some cases an initial brief automatism may become greatly prolonged thereafter as an episode of hysterical dissociation" (p. 224).

Finally, we are a long way from understanding what, if any, changes or abnormalities in neurotransmitter function underlie dissociative fugue. Most likely, there is no single abnormality; rather, any dysfunction in the neurotransmitter systems that underlie memory storage and mood regulation predisposes one to fugue states. Episodic increases in endogenous opioid activity—implicated in the apparent insensitivity to pain noted by some patients who injure themselves—could conceivably play a role in other dissociative phenomena, including fugue states (Winchel and Stanley 1991). And in closing this section, we should note the observation made in DSM-IV that heavy alcohol use may predispose the individual to dissociative fugue.

Psychological Factors

Psychological factors are the "meat and potatoes" of our traditional understanding of dissociative fugue. As a first approximation, we may be guided by Ford's (1989) comment that if a common thread exists in fugue states, "it is probably the trait of being highly suggestible and the capacity to use massive repression and escape as a coping style" (p. 2193). Ford adds to this the concept of "hysterical cognitive style." He describes the case of a 33-year-old married male who went for a walk late one night after a disagreement with his wife and was subsequently robbed at gunpoint. The victim "came to" 48 hours later in an urban rescue mission and professed a complete loss of memory for the past, his identity, and his family. He rapidly regained his past memories via Amytal interview. However, he repeatedly missed psychotherapy appointments and would, on occasion, "run home to his mother." Ford summarized that "this man had prominent passive-dependent and immature personality characteristics . . . his psychogenic fugues were consistent with these characterologic features . . . his assumption of the role of a rescue mission derelict was to place himself into a totally dependent position" (p. 2193).

Ford also points to psychopathic traits in individuals prone to fugue states (Berrington et al. 1956), and a history of prior fainting episodes or suicide attempts. Ford interprets these seemingly unrelated features as evidence of "a specific coping style" that utilizes "escape." However, the high frequency of suicidality also raises the issue of depression as a "fugogenic" disorder. Indeed, a "depressive setting" appears to be present in the majority of patients with fugue states (Ford 1989). We will say more about this when discussing the pitfalls of the differential diagnosis of dissociative fugue.

Fisher (1945; cited in Riether and Stoudemire 1988), in a study of military patients with fugue, found that immediately preceding the fugue state, many patients had felt powerless and out of control. Fisher hypothesized that the amnesia and fugue state were ways of deceiving the superego by concealing the ego identity and thus preventing depression and despair (Riether and Stoudemire 1988). In effect, the new ego (personality) says to the original superego, "If you can't recognize me, you can't make me feel guilty!"

Finally, object-relations models of fugue states (Geleerd 1956; Luparello 1970) emphasize regression to an early, undifferentiated phase of the mother-child relationship—a phase in which the very concept of "self" is not clear.

Sociocultural Factors

We have already implied in our vignettes that dissociative fugue often follows a severe psychosocial stressor, such as an assault or a marital quarrel. Abse (1974), discussing "hysteria" in general, notes that "the flight into [hysterical] illness may provide escape from an intolerable job or family situation, or from military service" (p. 175). Parent-child issues may also play a role in fugue states, as suggested by a case in the French literature (Kammerer et al. 1967), which involved the simultaneous hospitalization of a father and son, both in fugue states, using corresponding assumed names! According to Riether and Stoudemire

(1988), when family background is investigated in cases of fugue, "a long history of turmoil, separations, and deprivations is typical"; for example, repeated humiliation of the child by the parents may be a significant predisposing factor.

There are few data comparing the incidence of dissociative fugue in various socioeconomic, religious, or ethnic groups. Abse (1974), discussing "classical forms of hysteria," notes that they are "common in the more outlying rural areas of this country, and are quite highly visible in clinics in such areas as Puerto Rico" (p. 184). A systematic survey of mental disorders in Puerto Rico did not demonstrate higher rates of psychopathology than those seen in non-Hispanic North Americans (Canino et al. 1987). However, fugue states and dissociative disorders were not specifically studied. There are several culture-bound syndromes that have fugue states as part of their presentation. For example, latah, a syndrome first described in Malaysia, may involve violent fugue states and psychotic-like symptoms (Meth 1974).

Finally, DSM-IV notes that fugue states may be associated with military conflict and natural disaster. We will say more about this association when we discuss the differential diagnosis of fugue states versus PTSD.

Pitfalls in the Differential Diagnosis

Organic Conditions

We have already discussed seizure activity in temporolimbic regions as a possible component of fugue states or as a model for understanding fugue-like states (Mesulam 1985). Seizures affecting temporolimbic regions are also part of the differential diagnosis of fugue states. Mohan and Nagaswami (1975) reported a case of fugue states and hypersexuality in a 28-year-old female with EEG abnormalities in the limbic system; the patient showed dramatic improvement with anticonvulsant medication. Lishman (1987) relates the following case, attributed to an epileptic focus in the left temporal region: "A man of 48 set out for his work in Oxford at the normal time one morning and remembered nothing more until he found himself on the sea-front at Bournemouth . . . some 10 hours later. He had apparently travelled

by train, changing twice, and had eaten a meal and paid for it normally" (p. 224). Despite this report, Lishman notes that, in general,
"the longer-lasting the fugue, the more wary one will be of accepting
a basis in cerebral dysrhythmia alone" (p. 224). Similarly, the more
complex and integrated the behavior, the less likely it is due to the ictal
phase of temporal lobe epilepsy alone. Glaser (1975) states that a
fugue of longer duration than a few minutes "with the patient moving
some distance and with amnesia for the experience is more likely a
postictal automatism" (p. 326). Similarly, Cummings (1985) attributes most instances of "unrecallable prolonged ambulatory behavior" in epileptic patients to "a period of retrograde or postictal
amnesia" (p. 118) or to inter-ictal behavior.

How does one differentiate between epileptic and psychogenic
fugue states? Roy (1977), in a study comparing epilepsy and psychogenic fugue, found that fugue had a later onset, greater frequency, and
more frequent association with concurrent affective disorder than did
epilepsy (Cummings 1985). Akhtar and Brenner (1979) note that
fugues due to temporal lobe seizures are often preceded by olfactory,
abdominal, or cephalic auras; illusions; stereotypies; and anxiety—features not usually seen prior to psychogenic fugue. The EEG, of
course, may also be helpful in confirming temporal lobe epilepsy,
though this remains a clinical diagnosis.

We should note that we are using the word "fugue" rather loosely
in this neurological context. In order to meet the DSM-IV criteria for
dissociative fugue, there must be the assumption of a new identity, or
at least "confusion about personal identity," and not merely a period
of confused wandering and amnesia (American Psychiatric Association 1994). DSM-III-R was even more restrictive, requiring "assumption of a new identity (partial or complete)" (American Psychiatric
Association 1987, p. 273). This DSM-III-R criterion was criticized by
Riether and Stoudemire (1988) as "somewhat overly restrictive," in
that most fugue states reported in the literature do not involve the
assumption of a new identity.

Other organic conditions may produce fugue-like behaviors. Alcoholic blackouts may produce not only amnesia for events that
occurred during the drinking episode, but also travel to distant locales
with no recollection of the actual journey (Lishman 1987). Gifford et

al. (1976) reported a case of fugue-like episodes (including adoption of a second identity) in a man who was self-medicating with prednisone. It seems probable that many of the organic factors listed by Cummings (1985) as causes of amnesia (see Table 8–3) can also produce or facilitate fugue-like episodes. Riether and Stoudemire (1988) specifically mention "fugue states" associated with metabolic abnormalities, head trauma, drug intoxication, and carbon monoxide poisoning. In addition, Akhtar and Brenner (1979) note brain tumors, migraine, hypertensive encephalopathy, malaria, and dementia. In short, when you are faced with a patient in a fugue state, you are also confronting a broad differential diagnosis involving dozens of organic factors.

Functional Disorders

A number of other Axis I disorders may present with a fugue-like picture. Other dissociative disorders, such as multiple personality disorder and psychogenic amnesia, are discussed elsewhere in this chapter.

We have already alluded to the precipitation of psychogenic fugue by some overwhelming stressor; it should not surprise you that in PTSD (see Chapter 6), dissociative states may occasionally occur. These may last from seconds to days, during which the PTSD victim behaves as though he or she were experiencing the traumatic event. These states may in rare cases involve limited travel and the appearance of an altered personality, but not to the extent seen in psychogenic fugue. Rather, the PTSD victim experiences brief, intrusive recollections, or "flashbacks," without assumption of a new identity.

Ford (1989) notes that fugue states are often associated with a "depressive setting." While fugue is clearly distinguishable from, for example, major depressive episode, the latter should be considered as a possible comorbid condition in the patient with fugue states. Akhtar and Brenner (1979) point out that fugue states may also be seen in bipolar patients, schizophrenic patients, and patients with personality disorder. For this reason, Ford (1989) suggests that "psychogenic fugue is not a 'diagnosis' but rather a symptom of an underlying psychiatric disorder. . . . it is probably incorrect to speak of a symptom occurring in a wide variety of psychiatric illnesses as a distinct diagnosis" (p. 2191).

Finally, malingering may often present with fugue-like symptoms, including inability to recall one's identity. Careful questioning under hypnosis or Amytal interview may provide clues to the underlying "secondary gain" (see next subsection).

Adjunctive Testing

It is obvious that neuroimaging and electroencephalographic techniques are not easily applied to the patient in the midst of a dissociative fugue—though we have already noted the work of Rice and Fisher (1976), which suggests that sleep-dream mechanisms are involved in fugue states. Clearly, CT, EEG, and other techniques and tests to rule out organic causes of fugue states are essential. There are very few data on neuroendocrine measures in patients with psychogenic fugue, although one might infer from an abnormal dexamethasone suppression test (DST) the presence of a comorbid major depressive episode.

The most useful adjunctive test in diagnosing dissociative fugue is the Amytal interview, already described earlier in this chapter. As a rule, "lost" memories and repressed material would be expected to return when Amytal is administered if the patient is truly suffering from dissociative fugue. Akhtar and Brenner (1979) note that in schizophrenic and organic conditions, the Amytal interview usually worsens the mental status, with cognitive dysfunction or loose associations, respectively, becoming more pronounced. Epileptic fugue states might yield a "false positive" on the Amytal interview (i.e., improve the patient's level of consciousness) if the barbiturate actually ameliorates seizure activity. However, the amnesia of epileptic fugues is not reversed by barbiturates (Akhtar and Brenner 1979). Even if memory does return, we should recall Ford's (1989) comment that "the restoration of memory by [Amytal interview] must not be interpreted as prima facie evidence that the fugue state was entirely of psychogenic etiology" (p. 2196).

Psychological testing is not generally done while the individual is still in the midst of the fugue state; once recovery begins, fugue patients show a testing pattern similar to that seen in patients with psychogenic amnesia (Meyer 1983). Thus, on the MMPI, one would expect a high 3-4/4-3 pattern. In our discussion of depersonalization, we took note of two scales useful in the diagnosis of dissociative disorders: the SCID-D and the DES. The SCID-D contains items designed to assess identity confusion and alteration, while the DES includes components designed to pick up "finding oneself in a place but unaware how one got there" and similar fugue-related features. Thus, both instruments could be useful if psychogenic fugue is suspected.

Treatment Directions and Goals

As with psychogenic amnesia, recovery from psychogenic fugue may be rapid, spontaneous, and complete; no specific treatment other than supportive care may be needed (Goldman 1988). When the patient does require specific treatment, several approaches may be reasonable. As Ford (1989) notes, "The choice of a technique may be regarded as largely a matter of the therapist's preference" (p. 2195).

Somatic Approaches

By far the best described somatic treatment is the Amytal interview. Ford (1989) uses a 5% solution of Amytal Sodium, infused intravenously at a rate of no faster than 1 cc per minute (50 mg per minute). The interview begins when the patient's speech becomes slightly slurred or when sustained rapid lateral nystagmus is present. The therapist begins with emotionally neutral topics and then progresses to areas of suspected trauma and repression. If the patient becomes severely agitated in the process of abreacting, it may be necessary to terminate the interview. At the conclusion of the procedure, the therapist may suggest that "all will be remembered" or may administer enough additional Amytal to produced amnesia for the interview itself (Ford 1989). Contraindications to the Amytal interview include a history of porphyria, barbiturate allergy, concurrent intoxication, or severe hepatic, renal, or cardiac disease. Though cardiopulmonary complications are rare, CPR equipment should be nearby. Ford (1989) has reviewed the complex medicolegal issues arising from material obtained during the Amytal interview; the clinician is well advised to obtain legal counsel in cases involving criminal charges.

There is practically nothing in the literature regarding the use of psychotropic medications for the treatment of dissociative fugue. Of course, if an underlying schizophrenic or depressive disorder emerges, treatment of the primary condition with the appropriate agent is appropriate.

Psychosocial Approaches

Ford (1989) discusses two approaches to the patient with psychogenic fugue: hypnosis and the "psychotherapy-anamnesis." The first approach is aimed at retrieving repressed memory and facilitating emotional abreaction. The psychotherapy-anamnesis entails the patient's "free associating" around the events immediately preceding the fugue state. Ford states that "not only will this assist in the restoration of memory, but valuable psychodynamic material is often obtained, and the groundwork is built for further psychotherapy, if indicated" (p. 2195). In addition, Goldman (1988) notes that "depending on the circumstances, environmental manipulation or supportive psychotherapy might play a role in ameliorating factors related to stress, or in helping the patient adapt to stress in the future" (p. 378). Despite the supposed dynamic underpinnings of dissociative fugue, a long-term psychoanalytic form of therapy is rarely recommended—perhaps in part because dissociative fugue usually resolves rapidly and completely on its own.

Dissociative Identity Disorder (Multiple Personality Disorder)

The Central Concept

Multiple personality disorder (MPD) is, of course, not a personality disorder and is thus not one of the Axis II conditions. Perhaps a better name for MPD would be "personality fragmentation disorder," because there is often a great deal of chaos among the supposedly well defined "personalities" of the MPD patient. DSM-IV settled on the term "dissociative identity disorder." But because the entire literature on this topic for the past 30 years has used the term "multiple personality disorder," we shall often use this term (i.e., MPD) interchangeably with the newer designation. Let's explore the basic concept through the following vignette, which we will relate largely in the patient's own words.

Vignette

The patient—Ms. Janet Prettifield—was a 23-year-old accountant who had been in treatment with a psychiatrist for nearly 1 year. Her initial presenting complaint was "feeling real depressed at times, and at other times, kind of crazy." She had given a history of significant physical abuse by her father when the patient was "very young," but she could not recall any details. At times, she experienced "muffled noises and weird words in my head . . . like someone is trying to talk to me." There was no delusional ideation surrounding these internal stimuli.

The psychiatrist's initial diagnosis was "posttraumatic stress disorder; r/o mixed personality disorder; r/o cyclothymia." The following excerpts are from the most recent session:

Well, Doctor, I . . . I'm beginning to think I may be schizophrenic or something. The voices . . . they've been with me for a long time, but lately, I'm losing track of things . . . missing pieces of time, like somehow I forget who I am or where I've been. I know that sounds crazy . . . maybe I am! But I do O.K. at work—I mean, I've been doing accounting for 5 years. Oh, I miss work now and then—if the voices get bad or if I wind up somewhere and can't figure out how I got there. Things got worse a couple of months ago when I couldn't keep up my condo payments and I had to move back in with my folks. I mean, my Mom's O.K., but my Dad . . . well, you'd have to meet him to understand. He can be a real pain. I mean, since I moved in, he's always on my case—"Do this. Don't do that. Come over here!" You know. Then the other day something really weird happened—I found this prescription . . . God, this is embarrassing! This prescription for birth control pills—and I had no idea where it came from or whose it was. I mean, the name said "Sally Morton," and I have no idea who . . . well, I shouldn't say that, exactly. See, when I was a kid, I used to have—you know, this friend. Her name was Sally, and whenever I felt like being naughty, Sally would come to visit. If I got in trouble, I used to blame Sally. Or if I had to be around my dad. I mean, he used to drink a lot and get really angry with me and Mom. I don't remember much but—

At this point in the narrative, Ms. Prettifield's expression changed markedly. She smiled broadly, and assumed a posture the psychiatrist described as "seductive." Her voice grew deeper and somewhat husky. Her narrative continued as follows:

Is that loser gone? I mean, really! Get a life, Janet! Hey, Doc, what did she tell you about me? Nothing bad, I hope. 'Cause believe me, I'm good—very good! Hey, you're not laughing, Doc! That was a joke. Geez, are all you shrinks so sobered-out? Lighten up! Hey, you don't wanna end up like poor old Janet do you—typing away on some word processor, crunching numbers for a living? Not me! I'm gonna live a little! Oh—and don't believe that bull about Daddy—he's a sweetheart. Little Janet just can't handle him the way ol' Sally can. I mean, the girl is depressed! Me, I like to enjoy life—do a little dope, have a few drinks. Not sweet little Janet. I don't know how I got stuck with her.

Later in the session, at the suggestion of the psychiatrist, Sally let Janet "return." Ms. Prettifield had no recollection of the transformation and no detailed knowledge of Sally, except as the name of her childhood "friend."

In this admittedly histrionic vignette, I've tried to capture many of the central features of multiple personality. In general, MPD entails the existence, within the patient, of two or more distinct personalities or personality states, each with its own distinctive and enduring traits. At least two of these personalities recurrently take control of the patient's behavior from time to time. (DSM-IV avoids the terminology "distinct personalities," referring instead to "distinct *identities* or personality states"; we will not be quite so punctilious in our discussion.) As the case of Ms. Prettifield suggests, personality A may be aware of personality B, without B being aware of A, or, at most, with B having only fragmentary knowledge of A. The number of alternate personalities ranges from 1 to 60, with the mean somewhere around 13. Most commonly, the personality that seeks treatment is unaware of the other personalities. Around 80% of MPD patients report having had "imaginary companions" as children; it seems likely that these may become the "nidus" for later pathological personalities. The transition between personalities is usually sudden and is often triggered by stress, environmental cues, or—as in our vignette—"suggestion."

Sometimes, one personality may "listen in on" or influence the thinking of another. As our vignette shows, one personality is often strikingly different from another; in some instances, two personalities may reflect popular cultural or religious stereotypes (e.g., the "madonna-whore" dichotomy). In some instances, one personality is the "protector" of the others. As Putnam et al. (1986) note, MPD often presents with a misleading and pleomorphic picture: the dramatic "appearance" of a personality ("alter") is unusual and may not occur for months or even years during therapy. Affective symptoms are very common, with depression observed in nearly 90% of cases. In declining order of frequency, associated features include mood swings, suicidality, insomnia, amnesic episodes, sexual dysfunction, conversion symptoms, fugue states (as Janet reported), panic attacks, depersonalization, substance abuse (as Sally reported), phobias, and auditory or visual hallucinations. Many MPD patients go out of their way to conceal evidence of their disorder and may initially deny experiencing amnesic episodes, "losing time," and so forth. As we will see in our discussion of the differential diagnosis, the presence of "voices" in the clinical picture often raises the question of schizophrenia. Note, by the way, that MPD often incorporates features of the other dissociative disorders we discussed.

Historical Development of the Disorder

Greaves (1993) cites a case documented by Gmelin, in 1791, as one of the earliest reports of MPD, involving a young woman with at least two identities. The popular concept of a dual or multiple personality goes back at least as far as 1886, with the appearance of Stevenson's *Dr. Jekyll and Mr. Hyde*. In the following year, we find the curious case of Felida X, as reported by Etienne Azam and commented on by the great J.-M. Charcot (Abse 1983). Felida was a troubled young woman who evinced a "drab personality" and a more vibrant, outgoing one, with each personality amnesic for the other. Transitions between states usually followed a period of fainting and "clouding of consciousness." Freud and Breuer were very interested in what Azam had termed *une condition seconde* ("a second psychic state"), and they utilized the concept in their later work on hypnoid states. But it was really Morton Prince, in 1905, who introduced us to the concept of "multiple alternating personality." He investigated the case of one Miss Beauchamp, who exhibited at various times three fragmentary personalities (christened, "the Saint, the Devil, the Woman" by Prince). A self-righteous, masochistic personality was dominant and alternated with a strongly aggressive ambitious character. Under hypnosis, a third personality fragment ("Sally") emerged, who seemed a kind of "impish child" (Abse 1974). Similar cases have been made famous by Thigpen and Cleckley (*The Three Faces of Eve*) and Schreiber (*Sybil*). Incidentally, Miss Beauchamp's "chief complaint" upon seeking therapy was "headaches, insomnia, bodily pains, persistent fatigue, and poor nutrition" (Nemiah 1980)—hardly the stuff of severe pathology, and a reminder that MPD may be "the great pretender" of psychopathology.

The Biopsychosocial Perspective

Biological Factors

The biology of MPD remains a "black hole," with only a few rays of escaping light. There is, first of all, some evidence suggesting familial factors in the transmission of MPD—which is not to say that genetic factors are necessarily at work. Several studies have demonstrated, however, that MPD is more common in first-degree biological relatives of MPD patients than in the general population (American Psychiatric Association 1987). In a study by Dell and Eisenhower

(1990) examining 11 adolescents with MPD, the disorder was present in 36% of the mothers of the subjects. But as we will see below, psychosocial factors may be a more plausible explanation for this finding than is genetic loading.

We keep returning to the temporal lobes in discussing the dissociative disorders, and with MPD we do so again. As far back as 1892, Charcot suggested a link between MPD and epilepsy (Putnam 1984). Cummings (1985), summarizing the literature, states that epilepsy has been noted in up to 25% of patients with multiple personality and that an even larger percentage have a history of brain injury. Schenk and Bear (1981) noted that 13 of 40 patients with temporal lobe epilepsy showed dissociative phenomena, including classic MPD symptoms. Spiers and his colleagues (1985) have seen patients with "temporolimbic epilepsy" and associated multiple personality. They speculate that there may be "a subgroup of patients . . . in whom the epilepsy influences the clinical course and perhaps the genesis of the psychiatric disorder" (Spiers et al. 1985, p. 299). This group of investigators further speculates that "electrical instability of temporolimbic areas could lead to an enhancement of affect-laden sensory limbic associations." As a result, "external stimuli begin to take on great importance." Could this partly explain the rapidity with which MPD patients "switch" into a new personality state, as if they have been "seized"? At present, this is still informed speculation. Nevertheless, there is evidence that nondominant temporal lobe dysfunction may be associated with autonomous dissociative states (Mesulam 1981). The observation that changes in "handedness" occur across alternate personality states in MPD raises another question: Could MPD have some link with shifts in hemispheric dominance? (Putnam 1984). When evoked potentials of MPD patients are compared with those of control subjects feigning alternate personalities, the MPD patients show stable differences from personality to personality—differences that apparently cannot be duplicated by the control subjects. Moreover, once "integration" of the patient's personalities has occurred, evoked potentials may show differences from those obtained prior to integration. Spectral EEG studies also reveal differences among the MPD patient's various personalities. At this point, we still don't know whether all these findings reflect some genuine physiological concomitant of MPD or merely a consistent "artifact" of differing states of alertness or tension.

We know practically nothing about the neurochemistry of MPD, but some clues from pharmacological treatment may be emerging (see discussion of treatment directions and goals). Kluft (1984) noted some improvement in MPD patients treated with antidepressants, for example, but this may be true primarily of patients with MPD and comorbid major depression.

Psychological Factors

The capacity to "call up" a variety of ego states is not in itself pathological. Fenichel (1945) noted that

> many children try to solve conflicts by isolating certain spheres of their lives from one another, such as school from home. . . . one of the two isolated spheres usually represents instinctual freedom and the other good behavior. They even split their personality and state that they are two children with different names, a good one and a bad one, and deny the good one's responsibility for the bad one's deeds. (p. 157)

In a similar vein, Abse (1983), discussing the work of Jeanne Lampl–De Groot (1981), points to several instances of adaptive utilization of "something normatively like multiple personality"; for example, "a mother, nursing her baby, is able to revive the experiential world of her own infancy" (p. 341). But in the more pathological forms of dissociation, the individual loses the "flexibility" of this hypothetical mother, who, quickly enough, can leave the world of her own infancy. The MPD patient, as Abse notes, "switches from one fixed pattern of personality . . . to another without later adequate progressive integration of these patterns" (p. 341).

Kaplan and Sadock (1990) have admirably summarized the putative psychodynamics of MPD. They note that severe psychological or physical abuse in childhood leads to a compensatory distancing of the self from horror and pain. This need to distance leads to a "splitting off" of different aspects of the original personality, with each sub-personality expressing some necessary emotion or quality. In essence, the dissociated selves become, over time, an ingrained method of self-protection from perceived emotional threats (Kaplan and Sadock 1990).

Ross (1990), seeking to correct some "cognitive errors" in our thinking about MPD, has drawn the important distinction between personalities and dissociated ego states of a single personality. As he puts it, "Alter personalities are dissociated components of a single personality. They are stylized embodiments of conflicted memories, feelings, thoughts, and drives. The patient's mind is no more host to numerous distinct personalities than his or her body is to different people" (p. 349). (For convenience, we shall use the terms "personal-ities" or "alters" when referring to the various dissociated ego states of the MPD patient, even though the former term suggests a more stable and developed entity.)

Finally, we should note the hypothesis of Bliss (1980) that relates MPD to "the subject's unrecognized abuse of self-hypnosis" (p. 1395). Bliss argues, in effect, that MPD patients may actually create their own subpersonalities via a process akin to hypnotic induc-tion. For example, one patient "creates personalities by blocking everything from her head, mentally relaxes, concentrates very hard, and wishes" (p. 1395). How widespread this mechanism is can't really be ascertained from the 14 patients studied by Bliss.

Sociocultural Factors

The mother-daughter "dyad" may be of great importance in the etiology of MPD, as Schreiber's case of Sybil brings out. Sybil's mother was apparently "afflicted with a psychotic character disorder and behaved cruelly toward her daughter" (Abse 1983, p. 356). More generally, Abse (1983) points to disturbances of the "separation-individuation phase" of infant development as important in the etiol-ogy of MPD.

Wilbur and Kluft (1989) point out that "MPD is often the reflection of and sequel to severe family pathology" (p. 2201). More specifically, they note that "an increased awareness of the prevalence of child abuse . . . and a sensitization to the mistreatment and exploita-tion of women have led to heightened interest in a condition associated with 97 percent incidence of child abuse . . . and a 4:1 . . . to 9:1 predominance of women among its sufferers" (p. 2199).

"Non-abuse" etiologies rooted in social interaction have been noted by Kluft (1987):

> One young girl was sitting on her grandfather's lap, chanting in the language of his native land, when he suddenly died of a heart attack and fell over on her. She split off a personality that spoke in the grandfather's native language and grieved for him." (p. 366)

There are few data on the cross-cultural prevalence of MPD based on strict diagnostic criteria. Early (19th-century) reports by Janet and others certainly suggest that MPD exists on both sides of the Atlantic. Recently, a study by Takahashi (1990) looked at diagnosis in 489 Japanese psychiatric inpatients. Although 7 were diagnosed as having a dissociative disorder (using DSM-III criteria), none had MPD. This is a far lower frequency than seen in the United States, if Ross (1990) is correct in stating that MPD "is about as common in the general population as schizophrenia, affecting 1–2 percent of the general population" (p. 351). (Skodol [1989] notes that some clinicians report MPD occurring in as many as one in every seven hospital admissions.)

The results from the Takahashi study may mean that the prevalence of MPD varies between cultures, or such variance may represent an artifact of differences in diagnostic methods. It is interesting to note that the rate of child abuse appears to be far lower in Japan than in the United States; it is also intriguing to wonder, as Dr. Takahashi does, whether something in Japanese culture guards against personality fragmentation.

Pitfalls in the Differential Diagnosis

Organic Disorders

We have already discussed the association between MPD-like symptoms and temporal lobe dysfunction. Clearly, any patient with suspected MPD must be evaluated for a possible seizure disorder. Because amnesia is a prominent part of MPD, you should also remember that a variety of lesions may be associated with amnesia (e.g., hippocampal infarction, cerebral tumor, and herpes encephalitis) (Cummings 1985). (By the way, Putnam [1989] points out that a careful physical examination may also reveal sites of self-mutilation in MPD that are often hidden from casual inspection.)

Other Psychiatric Disorders

The difficulties in diagnosing MPD may be appreciated by reviewing a case reported by Putnam et al. (1984). The patient, a woman in her early 30s, had been variously diagnosed as having a rapid-cycling bipolar disorder, "pseudoneurotic schizophrenia," acute schizophrenic reaction, unipolar depression, and schizoaffective disorder! The pitfalls in the differential diagnosis of this disorder originate because of both the pleomorphic picture presented by the MPD patient and the "cognitive set" of the clinician (Ross 1990): if you don't believe MPD exists, you certainly will not diagnose it.

In Putnam et al.'s case, for instance, the patient underwent "mood swings" over periods of seconds to minutes; these ultimately proved to be the rapid switching from personality to personality and are hardly characteristic of true bipolar disorder. To appreciate the broad differential diagnosis of MPD, let's consider the following vignette, extensively modified from cases reported by Torem (1990).

Vignette

Theresa was a 30-year-old female admitted to the inpatient psychiatric unit for treatment of "severe eating disorder." She gave a 12-year history of repeated binge eating, followed by self-induced vomiting and laxative abuse. At one stage during her college years, Theresa had lost nearly 20 pounds and had been treated at the college mental health clinic for "anorexia." On careful interviewing, Theresa revealed that many of her binge-purge episodes were ego-alien; as she described the experience, "It's like someone has just taken over." During the interview, Theresa often used the words "she" and "we" when discussing herself. She acknowledged periods of amnesia not related to the use of drugs or alcohol. Examination of a diary that she had kept for years revealed marked and sudden changes in both the style and the substance of the entries, with the use of several different female names for the writer. Under hypnosis, Theresa revealed an alter personality named Maxine, who expressed a fear that when the host personality (Theresa) "grows up," she (Maxine) will be abandoned. This appeared to reflect the actual abandonment of Theresa by her mother when Theresa was 4 years old. Maxine expressed the view that "if Theresa doesn't eat, she won't grow up and leave me."

The vignette demonstrates MPD's chameleon-like quality and its tendency to incorporate features of other psychiatric disorders. As we will see, treatment of MPD requires that it be considered the hierarchically "dominant" condition.

Some of the many conditions that may be confused with MPD, or that mistakenly appear as diagnoses instead of MPD, are listed in Table 8–5. Some of the key differences are also indicated (see Solomon and Solomon 1982 for further details).

Given the many conditions that may be confused with MPD, what are some clinical clues that may help you make the diagnosis? A synopsis of the most important ones is provided in Table 8–6. In addition, Putnam (1989) notes the following clues on mental status examination: dramatic changes in style of dress from session to session; rapid fluctuations in rate, pitch, and accent of speech; rapid blinking or eyelid fluttering accompanying altered personality; "voices" from within the patient's head; rapid fluctuations in judgment occurring along an "age dimension" (e.g., from child to adult state); and "marked inability to learn from past experiences."

We should note, in closing, the importance of amnesic symptoms in the differential diagnosis of MPD, as emphasized by Spiegel and Cardeña (1991). They point out that DSM-III-R did not include the amnesia criterion, despite the abundant clinical data showing that amnesic symptoms are present in virtually all MPD patients (Ross 1989). Spiegel and Rosenfeld (1984) note that patients with MPD frequently have "asymmetrical amnesia"—that is, the second personality is often aware of what goes on when the primary personality is "out," but the converse is not the case. Rather, the primary personality may be mystified by its own lapses in attention or memory gaps

Table 8–5.   Differential diagnosis of dissociative identity disorder (MPD)

Condition confused with or diagnosed instead of MPD	Differential features
Dissociative fugue/ dissociative amnesia	Usually limited to single episode; lack of shift from one identity to another.
Schizophrenia	More pervasive psychosocial dysfunction and thought process disorder; flat or inappropriate affect (in MPD, affect appropriate for particular subpersonality). "Voices" in schizoprenia usually external, vs. internal in MPD. Reality testing more likely preserved in MPD within given "alter."
Borderline personality disorder	Identity confusion/diffusion rather than clear alternation; dissociation, if present, usually in response to stress, not suggestion. Anger, loneliness, boredom more pervasive in BPD.
Mood disorder (esp. bipolar) with psychotic features	No evidence of rapidly shifting identities; even manic states tend to be more gradual in onset, with preservation of some baseline personality traits. Delusions tend to be mood-congruent (grandiose or nihilistic) rather than bizarre (e.g., "I'm possessed") as in MPD.
Conversion disorder or other somatoform disorder	Symptom emerges in context of significant stressor (e.g., paralysis of legs after rape). In MPD, conversion symptom often accompanies sudden personality change.
Posttraumatic stress disorder	Other signs (hypervigilance, affective blunting) present; no alternation of identities, but flashbacks may be accompanied by unusual behaviors; dissociative episodes, if present, usually brief, without organized assumption of new identity, voice, etc.
Malingering	Typical external clues missing (e.g., no reports from friends or family that patient shows marked changes in behavior; clear secondary gain (e.g., pending legal charges) present in malingering.

resulting from the second personality's manifestation. Spiegel and Rosenfeld contrast this type of amnesia with the relatively "spared" recall seen in patients showing so-called age regression (i.e., reliving the past in the present, with age-appropriate vocabulary, mental content, and affect). This sort of regression may be seen in highly hypnotizable individuals and—in my experience—in regressed borderline personality disorder patients with comorbid PTSD. Such patients often do recall their "age regression" periods and perceive themselves as adults who have relived some earlier, often traumatic, experience (Spiegel and Rosenfeld 1984).

Adjunctive Testing

Neurophysiological Techniques

Although we don't have a neurophysiological "test" for MPD, some interesting physiological correlates exist that may help distinguish MPD from, say, malingering. Cummings (1985) notes that the alternate personalities of the MPD patient may show differing degrees of

Table 8–6. Clues to the presence of dissociative identity disorder (multiple personality disorder)

---

1. Time distortions, lapses, or other problems with memory.
2. Being told by others of behaviors the patient doesn't remember.
3. Use of "we" or "she" in referring to self.
4. Discovery of writing, possessions, and so forth, that the patient cannot recall or recognize.
5. Severe headaches that do not seem to respond to conventional treatments.
6. Hearing inner voices, sometimes commenting on patient's actions.
7. History of persisting "imaginary companions."
8. History of traumatic or abusive episodes during childhood.
9. Being addressed by unfamiliar names or in a familiar manner by persons who are not known to the patient.
10. History of autohypnotic experiences.

Source. Extensively modified from Greaves 1980; Kluft 1984.

pain sensitivity, galvanic skin response, and—as noted earlier—EEG patterns, evoked potential patterns, and handedness. To repeat, the EEG alterations may reflect changes in alertness, arousal, concentration, and muscle tension (Coons et al. 1982; Cummings 1985). As Coons et al. (1982) tersely put it, "It is not as if each personality is a different individual with a different brain. Instead, to put it simply, the EEG changes reflect changes in emotional state" (p. 825). Thus, it is not altogether surprising that one study of regional cerebral blood flow showed temporal lobe hyperperfusion in one of the sub-personalities of an MPD patient but not in the main personality (Kaplan and Sadock 1988).

Hypnosis

Hypnosis is certainly the most widely used ancillary procedure in the diagnosis of MPD, if clinical observation and interviewing do not permit diagnosis. (As we will see below, hypnosis also has therapeutic applications.) Braun (1984) advises withholding hypnosis even as a diagnostic tool until "extra time in observation and building rapport" have been given a chance. Braun adds, "Since these patients have often been abused, I do not want to do something abruptly or early on that might be perceived as another assault" (p. 35). Once hypnosis has been decided upon, "merely inducing hypnosis and observing often suffices to yield the material needed to make the diagnosis" (Braun 1984, p. 35). A specialized technique called "talking through" may be useful; this entails utilizing the host personality as a kind of pipeline into the underlying personalities, who are presumed to be listening. One pays careful attention to shifts in facial expression, posture, voice, and so forth, in order to perceive the emergence of alternate personalities. Braun is careful to point out that "the injudicious use of hypnosis (via pressure, shaping responses, and insensitivity . . .) may create a fragment or elicit an ego state which can be misinterpreted as a personality" (p. 35).

Psychological Testing and Related Techniques

Putnam et al. (1984) has noted that, despite apparently severe amnesic periods, "neuropsychological functioning generally remains normal in

MPD" (p. 174), thus distinguishing MPD from the "organic" amnesias. Meyer (1983), discussing the MMPI, notes that "since the personalities in a multiple personality [patient] will vary markedly, depending on what facets of that individual they are expressing, no particular patterns could be expected" (p. 148). However, a 3-8/8-3 MMPI code is commonly described in dissociative reactions.

We have already discussed the Dissociative Experiences Scale, which has been shown to discriminate patients with MPD from patients with nondissociative conditions and normal subjects (Sanders and Giolas 1991). Recently, Loewenstein et al. (1987) described a technique called "experiential sampling" in the diagnosis of MPD. This technique involves the use, at random intervals, of a rating instrument that assesses variations in mood, behavior, and motivation. Loewenstein et al. found that an MPD patient's alternate personalities tend to fill out this questionnaire in differing ways, but that any given alternate tends to be internally consistent—for example, one alternate usually circled the items, whereas another typically marked through them.

Treatment Directions and Goals

The overarching goals of treatment include securing the safety of the patient, providing him or her with empathic understanding, and gradually facilitating integration of the various personalities (Wilbur and Kluft 1989). Symptomatic relief of anxiety, insomnia, and depression is also important, even if core MPD pathology is unaffected.

Somatic Approaches

Kluft (1984) has written extensively on what he calls "the practical psychopharmacology of MPD" (p. 53). Like most clinicians, Kluft acknowledges that medications generally do not affect the core psychopathology of MPD but that they can alleviate some of the distressing symptoms of the disorder—even if only in a specific subpersonality. Treatment is, unfortunately, "empirical and informed by anecdotal experience rather than controlled studies" (Kluft 1984, p. 53). Moreover, a given medication may affect the personalities differently—even with respect to allergic reactions! Several classes of psychotropics may be utilized in MPD, including tricyclics, MAOIs, sedative-hypnotics, anticonvulsants, and antipsychotics. Kluft (1984) described a patient with MPD and depression who became euthymic on imipramine but continued to dissociate. Hypnotherapy plus imipramine, however, seemed to help with both mood and personality integration. MAOIs may be helpful in MPD patients with symptoms of "hysteroid dysphoria" (see Chapter 7) or atypical depression. Interestingly—despite the superficial similarity between "switching" personalities and the mood shifts of bipolar disorder, lithium has not been found to be especially helpful in MPD. And despite the hypothesized association between MPD and seizure disorders, anticonvulsants do not seem consistently beneficial either (Kluft 1984). Antipsychotics and "minor tranquilizers" (e.g., benzodiazepines) may be useful as general sedative agents when a patient is in crisis, but—once again— they do not affect MPD's core pathology. Moreover, antipsychotics sometimes adversely affect personality integration and pose the risk of tardive dyskinesia.

Given all this pessimism, it is no wonder that Kline and Angst (1979, p. 70) summed up the pharmacological treatment of MPD with the words "not indicated." Nevertheless, Ross and Gahan (1988) note that "concurrent depression, anxiety, or other disorders [in MPD] may require medication in their own right" (p. 46). These authors add an important guideline: that "disorders affecting all alters [alternate personalities] are probably more likely to respond to medication than ones isolated to single alters" (p. 46). In a recent review of MPD, Greaves (1993) concluded that the treatment of choice for MPD is intensive psychotherapy, facilitated with hypnosis, combined with "the judicious use of ancillary chemotherapy, mainly . . . anxiolytics and occasionally antidepressants" (p. 377).

Finally, DeVito (1993) has summarized the usefulness of Amytal interviews (amobarbital) as an alternative to hypnosis in treating complex MPD patients.

Psychosocial Approaches

Extensive reviews of the psychosocial approaches to MPD have been presented by Wilbur and Kluft (1989) and Ross and Gahan (1988).

Excellent discussions also appear in Kluft and Fine's (1993) book. Despite this literature, treatment approaches to MPD have not been subject to rigorous empirical evaluation. Based mainly on clinical and anecdotal experience, the essence of the psychosocial approach to MPD entails the following principles and practices: 1) helping the patient to perceive, abreact, and work through the reasons for each alter (Wilbur and Kluft 1989); 2) facilitating the intrapsychic forces that counteract dissociation, long before there is any reduction in the number of personalities; and 3) facilitating the actual fusion or "coming together" of personalities, after an adequate therapeutic foundation has been laid. The ultimate goal of "fusion" has been defined by Wilbur and Kluft (1989) as including (among other things) 3 months of 1) continuity of contemporary memory, 2) absence of overt behavioral signs of multiplicity, 3) subjective sense of unity, and 4) absence of alter personalities upon hypnosis.

Given these general goals, what are the psychosocial techniques used to treat MPD? Psychoanalytically oriented therapy is widely used, with or without facilitation by hypnosis. (Ross [1990] points out that hypnosis is a "useful but not an essential adjuvant technique" [p. 353].) Behavioral approaches have also been used, though Wilbur and Kluft (1989) believe that "many MPD patients experience behavioral protocols as punitive and respond poorly" (p. 2201).

Hypnosis is a facilitator of treatment or an adjunct to treatment, not a treatment per se. When integrated into a broader therapeutic framework, hypnosis can help one gain access to personalities, encourage abreaction, breach amnestic barriers, and promote personality integration (Wilbur and Kluft 1989).

Ross and Gahan (1988) have helped us bridge the gaps between diverse therapeutic approaches by enumerating techniques used in every case of MPD. Essentially, these are as follows:

1. Effecting education and discussion, in which the patient's host personality and alters are given information about MPD.
2. Stating the goals of cooperation among alters and of ultimate integration.
3. "Mapping the system" (i.e., getting to know all the alters and laying out their various relationships before the patient).

4. Dismantling amnesic barriers by encouraging internal communication among alters.
5. Encouraging or mitigating abreaction, depending on how traumatic the recollection.
6. Negotiating, in which the therapist tries to "mediate" the often conflicting demands of the patient's alters.
7. Reaching "contracts" with the patient's personalities so that suicidal or violent impulses can be managed appropriately.

Integrated Case History

A 21-year-old woman who presented herself as a Ms. Ellen Berger sought help in an outpatient psychiatric clinic. The patient's chief complaint was that "sometimes I wind up with cuts and I don't know how I get them." She gave a long history of "losing track of time," going back at least to age 5 or 6. She had been evaluated 4 years ago, during her senior year in high school, and had been given a diagnosis of "borderline personality disorder" by a school psychologist. The patient related long-standing problems with interpersonal relationships; frequent bouts of depression; episodic self-injurious acts (which she could recall only occasionally); and "sometimes hearing noises, like someone calling me from inside a well." Her personal/family history was notable for significant physical and sexual abuse by her mother, who died when the patient was 12. The history of abuse was not related by the patient, but by her older sister, who had herself been sexually molested by her mother and father. The patient's sister also related "some weird things that go on with Ellen . . . sometimes she goes by another name, 'Roxanne' . . . she dresses real, well . . . flashy, and goes out a lot." In contrast, the patient's sister described "Ellen" as "pretty shy, and sort of a bookworm." The patient gave a history of poor appetite, early morning awakening, and decreased concentration over the past month or two, adding, "I'm not really too clear on the time business."

On mental status examination, the patient appeared to be somewhat unkempt and was dressed in very dark colors. Her affect appeared blunted and at times tearful. She was oriented to day and date and recalled three items at 3 minutes with no difficulty.

At times during the interview, her attention seemed to wander, and the patient would often respond to a question with, "What . . . I'm sorry." There were no overt delusional beliefs elicited. The patient did express the belief that "I'm not always the person I think I am or that I'm supposed to be."

A physical examination was completely normal, except for many superficial lacerations and small, healed scars on the patient's forearms. A sleep-deprived EEG showed "no epileptiform activity, but some minor dysrhythmias in the right temporal region, suggestive of old trauma." Psychological testing showed a 3-8/8-3 pattern on the MMPI and a markedly elevated score on the DES.

A provisional diagnosis of "dissociative identity disorder (multiple personality disorder) r/o superimposed major depressive episode" was made. The patient entered twice-weekly outpatient psychotherapy with a psychiatrist and was also started on nortriptyline 50 mg at hs. In the first phase of treatment, the therapist's goal was simply to establish a sense of trust and rapport. After several sessions, the patient asked the question, "So what's the matter with me . . . am I wacko or something?" At that point, the therapist assured her that she was not "crazy" but that she appeared to have a problem with her identity. The therapist announced that he hoped to get "better acquainted with the different sides" of the patient, and hoped that he could soon hear from them. This prompted some anxiety on the patient's part, and she needed to break off the session. However, at the next session, the patient spontaneously presented with a wholly different demeanor, voice, and style of dress, consistent with an alternate identity. The therapist listened to "Roxanne" for most of the session, then said, "I hope you'll be talking soon with Ellen . . . I'd like to see the two of you on better terms." Although "Roxanne" at first disparaged this idea, she ended the session by saying, "Ellen is kind of a nerd, but maybe I'll find something nice to say to her." Therapy over the ensuing year focused on exploring other, less fully formed identities (of which three were identified) and on facilitating "communication" between the two principal identities. The antidepressant was tapered off after 6 months, at which time neither Ellen nor "Roxanne" voiced any depressive complaints.

Subsequent therapy focused on "mediating" between the often

conflicting demands of the very conservative Ellen and those of the more disinhibited "Roxanne." Several sessions also encouraged abreaction of some traumatic memories—mainly involving sexual abuse by the patient's mother—that seemed integral to the formation of "Roxanne." Gradually, the patient came to see "Roxanne" as serving a defensive function in her psychic life; that is, as the outgoing and sexually provocative identity, "Roxanne" had enabled the more passive Ellen to escape from her sense of victimization.

Conclusion

Psychologically induced loss of memory, consciousness, or identity is the thread that runs through the dissociative disorders. Nevertheless, we still lack a unifying biopsychosocial model to explain these phenomena. It is also unclear where the boundaries of dissociative disorders begin and those of related conditions end—PTSD being a prime example. On the whole, the biology of dissociative disorders remains obscure and the pharmacological treatment of these disorders disappointing. In contrast, our psychosocial understanding of these conditions has been refined in recent years. But while there is growing evidence that physical or sexual abuse plays a causal role in some of these disorders, it is not clear why such traumata lead to MPD in some cases and to PTSD or borderline personality disorder in others. However sophisticated the DSM-IV classification may be, it will probably not resolve these thorny questions.

References

Abeles M, Schilder P: Psychogenic loss of personal identity. Arch Neurol 34:587–604, 1935

Abse DW: Hysterical conversion and dissociative syndromes and the hysterical character, in American Handbook of Psychiatry, 2nd Edition, Vol 3. Edited by Arieti S. New York, Basic Books, 1974, pp 155–194

Abse DW: Multiple personality, in New Psychiatric Syndromes: DSM-III and Beyond. Edited by Akhtar S. New York, Jason Aronson, 1983, pp 339–361

Akhtar S, Brenner I: Differential diagnosis of fugue-like states. J Clin Psychiatry 40:381–385, 1979

American Psychiatric Association: Diagnostic and Statistical Manual of Mental Disorders. Washington, DC, American Psychiatric Association, 1952

American Psychiatric Association: Diagnostic and Statistical Manual of Mental Disorders, 2nd Edition. Washington, DC, American Psychiatric Association, 1968

American Psychiatric Association: Diagnostic and Statistical Manual of Mental Disorders, 3rd Edition. Washington, DC, American Psychiatric Association, 1980

American Psychiatric Association: Diagnostic and Statistical Manual of Mental Disorders, 3rd Edition, Revised. Washington, DC, American Psychiatric Association, 1987

American Psychiatric Association: Diagnostic and Statistical Manual of Mental Disorders, 4th Edition. Washington, DC, American Psychiatric Association, 1994

Arieti S: Interpretation of Schizophrenia. New York, Basic Books, 1974

Bernstein KF, Putnam FW: Development, reliability and validity of a dissociation scale. J Nerv Ment Dis 174:727–735, 1986

Berrington WP, Liddell DW, Foulds GA: A re-evaluation of the fugue. Journal of Mental Science 102:280–286, 1956

Bliss EL: Multiple personalities. Arch Gen Psychiatry 37:1388–1400, 1980

Braun BG: Uses of hypnosis with multiple personality. Psychiatric Annals 14:34–40, 1984

Brill AA: Basic Principles of Psychoanalysis. New York, Washington Square Press, 1921

Canino GJ, Bird HR, Shrout PE, et al: The prevalence of specific psychiatric disorders in Puerto Rico. Arch Gen Psychiatry 44:727–735, 1987

Cattell JP, Cattell JS: Depersonalization: psychological and social perspectives, in American Handbook of Psychiatry, Vol 3. Edited by Arieti S. New York, Basic Books, 1974, pp 766–799

Cohen SI: The pathogenesis of depersonalization: a hypothesis (letter). Br J Psychiatry 152:578, 1988

Coons PM, Milstein V, Marley C: EEG studies of two multiple personalities and a control. Arch Gen Psychiatry 39:823–825, 1982

Cummings JL: Clinical Neuropsychiatry. Orlando, FL, Grune & Stratton, 1985

Dell PF, Eisenhower JW: Adolescent multiple personality disorder: a preliminary study of eleven cases. J Am Acad Child Adolesc Psychiatry 29:359–366, 1990

DeVito RA: The use of Amytal interviews in the treatment of an exceptionally complex case of multiple personality disorder, in Clinical Perspectives on Multiple Personality Disorders. Edited by Kluft RP, Fine CG. Washington, DC, American Psychiatric Press, 1993, pp 227–240

Dubovsky SL: Concise Guide to Clinical Psychiatry. Washington, DC, American Psychiatric Press, 1988

Dugas L, Moutier F: La depersonnalisation. Paris, Alcan, 1898

Fenichel O: The Psychoanalytic Theory of Neurosis. New York, WW Norton, 1945

Fisher C: Amnesic states in war neuroses: the psychogenesis of fugues. Psychoanal Q 14:437–468, 1945

Flor-Henry P: Cerebral Basis of Psychopathology. Boston, MA, John Wright, 1983

Ford C: Psychogenic fugue, in Treatments of Psychiatric Disorders, Vol 3. Washington, DC, American Psychiatric Press, 1989, pp 2190–2196

Freedman AM, Kaplan HI, Sadock BJ: Modern Synopsis of the Comprehensive Textbook of Psychiatry. Baltimore, MD, Williams & Wilkins, 1972

Geleerd ER: Clinical contribution to the problem of the early mother-child relationship. Psychoanal Study Child 11:336–351, 1956

Gifford S, Murawski BJ, Kline NS, et al: An unusual adverse reaction to self-medication with prednisone: an irrational crime during a fugue state. Int J Psychiatry Med 7:97–122, 1976

Glaser GH: Epilepsy: neuropsychological aspects, in American Handbook of Psychiatry, Vol 4. Edited by Arieti S, Reiser MF. New York, Basic Books, 1975, pp 314–355

Greaves GB: Multiple personality: 165 years after Mary Reynolds. J Nerv Ment Dis 168:577–596, 1980

Greaves GB: A history of multiple personality disorder, in Clinical Perspectives on Multiple Personality Disorders. Edited by Kluft RP, Fine CG. Washington, DC, American Psychiatric Press, 1993, pp 355–380

Hollander E, Fairbanks J, Decaria C, et al: Pharmacological dissection of panic and depersonalization (letter). Am J Psychiatry 146:402, 1989

Hollender MH, Ban TA: Ejaculatio retarda due to phenelzine. Psychiatr J Univ Ottawa 4:233–234, 1979

Hollingshead AB, Redlich FC: Social Class and Mental Illness. New York, Wiley, 1958

Janet P: L'Automatisme Psychologique. Paris, Alcan, 1889

Kammerer T, Gurfin L, Durand De Bousingen R: Autogenic training and the structure of hysteria. Clinical study. Remarks on the psychopathology.(apropos of 20 cases treated at the Strasbourg Psychiatric Clinic). Rev Med Psychosom Psychol Med 9:117–126, 1967

Kennedy A, Neville J: Sudden loss of memory. BMJ 7:428–433, 1957

Kaplan HI, Sadock BJ: Synopsis of Psychiatry, 5th Edition. Baltimore, MD, Williams & Wilkins, 1988

Kaplan HI, Sadock BJ: Synopsis of Psychiatry, 6th Edition. Baltimore, MD, Williams & Wilkins, 1990

Kline NS, Angst J: Psychiatric Syndromes and Drug Treatment. New York, Jason Aronson, 1979

Kluft RP: Aspects of the treatment of multiple personality disorder. Psychiatric Annals 14:51–55, 1984

Kluft RP: An update on multiple personality disorder. Hosp Community Psychiatry 38:363–373, 1987

Kluft RP, Fine CG (eds): Clinical Perspectives on Multiple Personality Disorder. Washington, DC, American Psychiatric Press, 1993

Kolb LC: The body image in the schizophrenic reaction, in Schizophrenia: An Integrated Approach. Edited by Auerback A. New York, Ronald Press, 1959, pp 87–97

Krishaber M: De la nevropathie cerebro-cardiaque. Paris, Masson, 1873

Lampl-De Groot J: Notes on multiple personality. Psychoanal Q 50:614–624, 1981

Linn L: Psychogenic amnesia, in Treatments of Psychiatric Disorders, Vol 3. Washington, DC, American Psychiatric Press, 1989, pp 2186–2189

Lishman WA: Organic Psychiatry, 2nd Edition. Oxford, UK, Blackwell Scientific, 1987

Loewenstein RJ, Hamilton J, Alagna S, et al: Experiential sampling in the study of multiple personality disorder. Am J Psychiatry 144:19–21, 1987

Luparello TJ: Features of fugue: a unified hypothesis of regression. J Am Psychoanal Assoc 18:379–398, 1970

Maxmen G: Essential Psychopathology. New York, WW Norton, 1986

Mesulam M-M: Dissociative states with abnormal temporal lobe EEG: multiple personality and the illusion of possession. Arch Neurol 38:178–181, 1981

Mesulam M-M: Principles of Behavior Neurology. Philadelphia, PA, FA Davis, 1985

Meth JM: Exotic psychiatric syndromes, in American Handbook of Psychiatry, Vol 3. Edited by Arieti S. New York, Basic Books, 1974, pp 723–739

Meyer RG. The Clinician's Handbook of Psychopathology of Adulthood and Late Adolescence. Boston, MA, Allyn & Bacon, 1983

Mohan KJ, Nagaswami S: A case of limbic system dysfunction with hypersexuality and fugue state. Diseases of the Nervous System 36:621–624, 1975

Myerson AT: Amnesia for homicide. Arch Gen Psychiatry 14:509, 1966

Nemiah JC: Dissociative disorders, in Comprehensive Textbook of Psychiatry/III, 3rd Edition, Vol 2. Edited by Kaplan HI, Freedman AM, Sadock BJ. Baltimore, MD, Williams & Wilkins, 1980, pp 1544–1561

Nemiah JC: Dissociative disorders (hysterical neurosis, dissociative type), in Comprehensive Textbook of Psychiatry/IV, 4th Edition, Vol 1. Edited by Kaplan HI, Sadock BJ. Baltimore, MD, Williams & Wilkins, 1985, pp 942–957

Perley MJ, Guze SB: Hysteria: the stability and usefulness of clinical criteria. N Engl J Med 266:421–426, 1962

Pies RW: Atypical depression, in Handbook of Clinical Psychopharmacology, 2nd Edition. Northvale, NJ, Jason Aronson, 1988, pp 329–356

Purcell SD: Dissociative disorders, in Review of General Psychiatry, 2nd Edition. Edited by Goldman HH. Norwalk, CT, Appleton & Lange, 1988, pp 374–380

Putnam FW: The psychophysiological investigation of multiple personality disorder: a review. Psychiatr Clin North Am 7:31–40, 1984

Putnam FW: Diagnosis and Treatment of Multiple Personality Disorder. New York, Guilford, 1989

Putnam FW, Loewenstein RJ, Silberman EK, et al: Multiple personality in a hospital setting. J Clin Psychiatry 45:172–175, 1984

Putnam FW, Guroff JJ, Silberman EK, et al: The clinical phenomenology of multiple personality disorder: review of 100 cases. J Clin Psychiatry 47:285–293, 1986

Rice E, Fisher C: Fugue states in sleep and wakefulness: a psychopharmacological study. J Nerv Ment Dis 163:79–88, 1976

Riether AM, Stoudemire A: Psychogenic fugue states: a review. South Med J 81:568–571, 1988

Ross CA: Multiple Personality Disorder: Diagnosis, Clinical Features, and Treatment. New York, Wiley, 1989

Ross CA: Twelve cognitive errors about multiple personality disorder. Am J Psychother 44:348–356, 1990

Ross CA, Gahan P: Techniques in the treatment of multiple personality disorder. Am J Psychother 42:40–52, 1988

Ross CA, Joshi S, Currie R: Dissociative experiences in the general population: a factor analysis. Hosp Community Psychiatry 42:297–301, 1991

Roth M. The phobic anxiety–depersonalization syndrome. Proc Royal Soc Med 52:587–595, 1959

Roy A: Nonconvulsive psychogenic attacks investigated for temporal lobe epilepsy. Compr Psychiatry 18:591–593, 1977

Sanders B, Giolas M: Dissociation and childhood trauma in psychologically disturbed adolescents. Am J Psychiatry 148:50–61, 1991

Schenk L, Bear D: Multiple personality and related dissociative phenomena in patients with temporal lobe epilepsy. Am J Psychiatry 138:1311–1316, 1981

Shader RI, Scharfman EL: Depersonalization disorder, in Treatments of Psychiatric Disorders, Vol 3. Washington, DC, American Psychiatric Association, 1989, pp 2217–2221

Skodol AE: Problems in Differential Diagnosis. Washington, DC, American Psychiatric Press, 1989

Solomon R, Solomon V: Differential diagnosis of multiple personality. Psychol Rep 51:1187–1194, 1982

Spiegel D, Cardeña E: Disintegrated experience: the dissociative disorders revisited. J Abnorm Psychol 100:366–379, 1991

Spiegel D, Rosenfeld A: Spontaneous hypnotic age regression: case report. J Clin Psychiatry 45:522–524, 1984

Spiers MA, Schomer DL, Blume, HW, et al: Temporolimbic epilepsy and behavior, in Principles of Behavior Neurology. Edited by Mesulum M-M. Philadelphia, PA, FA Davis, 1985, pp 289–326

Steinberg M, Rounsaville B, Ciccheti D: The Structured Clinical Interview for DSM-III-R Dissociative Disorders: preliminary report on a new diagnostic instrument. Am J Psychiatry 147:76–82, 1990

Takahashi Y: Is multiple personality disorder really rare in Japan? Dissociation 3:57–59, 1990

Torem MS: Covert multiple personality underlying eating disorders. Am J Psychother 45:357–368, 1990

Wilbur CB, Kluft RP: Multiple personality disorder, in Treatments of Psychiatric Disorders, Vol 3. Washington, DC, American Psychiatric Association, 1989, pp 2197–2216

Winchel RM, Stanley M: Self-injurious behavior: a review of the behavior and biology of self-multilation. Am J Psychiatry 148:306–317, 1991

9

Personality Disorders

A paranoid is a man who knows a little of what's going on.

William Burroughs

Personality disorders are pervasive, persistent, usually life-long patterns of maladaptive behavior that are not attributable to Axis I disorders, specific organic factors, or cultural role difficulties (Kaplan and Sadock 1988). Having given this rather tidy definition, we should quickly add that the act of "carving out" particular personality disorders has the potential for being somewhat arbitrary. After all, if we point to individuals with maladaptive traits A, B, and C, and then to other individuals with maladaptive traits D, E, and F, we have not necssarily identified two "disorders" in any objective sense. We might find, for example, that neither cluster of traits allows us to predict anything at all about the family history, clinical course, prognosis, response to treatment, or biochemical features of individuals with these traits. Furthermore, we might find that by combining traits A, E, and F into a "new" disorder, we are able to make accurate predictions in all the aforementioned spheres. Thus, the validity of a putative personality disorder—as with all noso-logic terms in medicine—ultimately depends on the utility of the category and on how closely it corresponds to certain observ-able patterns in the "real world." It is this premise that underlies the seminal work of Siever and Davis (1991), to which we shall return many times. These and other researchers are trying to identify the

431

various components or "dimensions" of personality disorders and the underlying biological correlates. In this chapter, we examine the three main clusters of personality disorders identified in DSM-IV (American Psychiatric Association 1994), using our customary biopsychosocial approach. However, building on the work of Siever and others, we also examine personality disorders from a "dimensional" perspective that will allow us to link the personality disorders to various Axis I disorders.

Before undertaking this task, we should begin with a more general question: What features tend to characterize the individual with any personality disorder? D. Adler (1990), in discussing what he calls the "nonpsychotic chronic patient," has nicely summarized the "domains of malfunctioning" common to virtually all the personality disorders. These domains are shown in condensed form in Table 9–1.

Keep in mind that these domains are not pathognomonic of the personality disorders; for example, the domains are also seen in more severe conditions such as schizophrenia. However, as Adler's terminology suggests, the personality disorder patient rarely becomes psy-

Table 9–1.   Domains of malfunctioning in personality disorders

Psychosocial dysfunction: poor functioning in both social and occupational roles.

Behavioral problems: "immature" traits such as manipulative, entitled, inconsistent, oppositional, or destructive behaviors.

Cognitive impairments: defective sense of reality (occasionally of psychotic proportions), worsening under stress.

Affective impairments: inability to modulate affect; unstable intensity and range of affect.

Immature intrapsychic coping mechanisms: use of primitive but nonpsychotic defenses, such as splitting, acting out, passive aggression, projection.

Source.   Extensively modified from D. Adler 1990.

chotic for more than a few hours or days (see subsection on differential diagnosis later in this chapter).

In addition to the domains listed above, the personality disorder patient typically lacks empathy for others and tends to "externalize" blame. (Thus, the old joke about the narcissistic person's retort to his therapist: "What do you mean I'm grandiose? If I were, do you think I'd choose a loser like you for a therapist?") The individual with a personality disorder typically shows a certain rigidity of function. No matter how many times the "old ways" of behaving have failed, the individual resists changing them. It is usually pressure from family, spouse, or employer that brings the individual into treatment. (Speaking of spouse or employer: if ever a patient failed Freud's "test" of mental health—the ability to love and to work—it is the patient with severe personality disorder.) This brings up the ego-syntonic quality of most personality disorders: it is usually someone else, not the identified patient, who is "bothered" by the behaviors in question and must endure them. In the classical psychoanalytic formulation, personality disorder patients were contrasted to "neurotic" patients in the realm of anxiety: the personality disorder patient was said to lack anxiety, the neurotic patient, to wallow in it. To some degree, this formulation holds up. For example, the classic sociopathic individual is not "anxious" about forging checks, but rather about getting caught at it. (Compare this person with the obsessive-compulsive "neurotic" person, who is usually quite anxious about his or her ritualistic behavior, even though those same behaviors may temporarily reduce anxiety.) But the "ego-syntonic/ego-alien" distinction proves a bit facile. For beneath the personality disorder patient's "character armor" (to borrow Wilhelm Reich's term), one often finds the very anxiety that seems lacking on the surface. Indeed, D. Adler (1990), drawing on the work of G. Adler, Kernberg, and others, believes that most personality disorders may be understood in terms of two concepts: aloneness and worthlessness. He argues that "all individuals with personality disorder suffer from both these feelings. A sense of aloneness, leading to annihilatory panic, may obscure issues of worth, but both gnaw at the individual's sense of self-integration" (p. 19). We will explore these ideas further in discussing the specific personality disorder clusters.

The Odd/Eccentric Cluster (Cluster A): Paranoid, Schizoid, and Schizotypal Personality Disorders

The Central Concept

Vignette

Mr. Dion A. Rap, a 37-year-old certified public accountant, came to the mental health clinic at the insistence of his fiancée, Charlene, who felt that "Dion just can't take life as it comes. He's always assuming the worst about me and everyone else. Some of the things he's accused me of . . . I can't even talk about them!" The patient described himself as "kind of a loner my whole life," with few if any close friends. He had done well academically and graduated with a business degree from a major university. Even in college, however, the patient "always felt that the faculty had it in for me . . . like they were making things just a little harder for me than for everyone else." Mr. Rap had lived alone until 1 year prior to evaluation, when he moved in with his (then) girlfriend. He found the move "pretty rough . . . I was used to doing things my way . . . sometimes I felt . . . and still feel that Charlene is deliberately trying to get my hackles up. You know, like by leaving the caps off bottles and things. A few weeks ago, she started coming home late from work, and I kinda of accused her of fooling around with somebody. I don't know, even though she denies it, I just can't help thinking it's true." At interview, Mr. Rap showed a "cool, detached" affect and no signs of thought process disorder. There were no fixed delusional beliefs, beyond the suspiciousness noted, and no hallucinations. Provisional diagnosis was "personality disorder NOS [not otherwise specified] ('Mixed'), with predominantly paranoid and some schizoid features."

Indeed, Mr. Rap shows the suspiciousness, sense of being exploited or wronged, restricted affect, oversensitivity to imagined slights, and ideas of suspected infidelity typical of paranoid personality disorder (PPD). In addition, his history of social isolation and lack of close friends suggest some "schizoid" traits. Mr. Rap does not show many traits of the third personality disorder in the "odd" cluster, schizotypal personality disorder, which is characterized by ideas of reference (not of delusional proportions); "magical thinking" (e.g., preoccupation with telepathy or clairvoyance); odd, idiosyncratic speech without formal thought process disorder; and unusual perceptual experiences, such as sensing the presence of an "unknown force" in the room. Schizotypal patients share with schizoid patients a history of social isolation and constricted affect.

Historical Development of the Concept

Our modern understanding of the generic term "paranoia" has its roots in Freud's description of projection—arguably the chief defense mechanism in most paranoid states. However, Adolf Meyer is usually credited with introducing the diagnosis of the "paranoid character" into psychiatry (Vaillant and Perry 1980). The basic construct has been codified in DSM-II through DSM-IV (American Psychiatric Association 1968, 1980, 1987, 1994).

The history of schizoid personality disorder has been reviewed in detail by Akhtar (1987). As early as 1908, Bleuler had described the "schizoid personality" as quiet, suspicious, "comfortably dull," and yet "sensitive." At about the same time, Hoch described the "shut-in" personality as one characterized by secretiveness, an inclination toward mystical pursuits, shyness, sensitivity, and excessive daydreaming. Note that some of these features overlap with our modern construct of schizotypal personality disorder. Indeed, Akhtar (1987) points out that in DSM-III, "[w]hat had customarily been understood as schizoid personality was . . . broken down into three separate syndromes: the schizoid, the avoidant, and the schizotypal" (p. 507).

DSM-III-R, in Akhtar's (1987) view, provided a richer description of schizoid personality disorder that softened "the rigid separation of the schizoid and avoidant types" (p. 509). The difference between DSM-III and DSM-III-R lay partly in the latter's recognition that things are not always as they seem; specifically, that "the indifference and withdrawal . . . in schizoid personality may be more apparent than real" (Akhtar 1987, p. 509), allowing for some overlap with avoidant personality disorder (see subsection on differential diagnosis).

In a sense, schizotypal personality disorder arose from the confluence of two forces: the need to subsume a variety of pathological types left over from DSM-II, and the tendency to view "schizotypy" as a trait along a continuum, which includes schizophrenia at the "far end." DSM-II contained three categories that, when taken together, could be considered the "forerunners" of schizotypal personality disorder: "latent schizophrenia," "simple schizophrenia," and "schizoid personality." Latent schizophrenia was regarded as a "prepsychotic" state, sometimes termed "borderline" or "pseudoneurotic" schizophrenia (Freedman et al. 1972). Simple schizophrenia also lacked frank psychotic features and was characterized by gradual loss of drive, social withdrawal, and vocational deterioration. Schizoid personality in DSM-II was characterized by avoidance of close or prolonged relationships; a limited range of responses to social cues; seclusiveness; "eccentricity"; autistic thinking; an inability to express hostility; and "excessive daydreaming" (Freedman et al. 1972). Each of these three categories has contributed a "piece" of our current diagnosis, schizotypal personality disorder.

The other force behind the validation of schizotypal personality disorder is the considerable family research on "schizotypy" as a trait. Numerous family and adoption studies suggest that schizotypal personality traits are more common in the biological relatives of chronic schizophrenic patients than in control subjects. Siever and Davis (1991) have reviewed the biological studies demonstrating a genetic association between schizophrenia and schizophrenia-related personality traits ("schizotypy") (see next subsection). As Vaillant and Perry (1985) note, "The proposed separation of schizoid and schizotypal personality disorders rests on tentative evidence that the former disorder occurs less often in the relatives of schizophrenics than does schizotypal personality disorder" (p. 971).

The Biopsychosocial Perspective

Biological Factors

In their investigations of schizotypal personality disorder, Siever and Davis (1991) distinguish between "positive" and "negative" (or deficit) symptoms, as shown in the Table 9–2. With this dichotomy in mind, Siever and colleagues have gathered a wealth of data strongly suggesting that schizotypal features—both positive and negative—are associated with specific biological and neuropsychological abnormalities. As Siever and Davis (1991) summarize,

> Eye movement dysfunction has been demonstrated not only in patients with chronic schizophrenia, but also in schizotypal patients . . . [eye movement dysfunction] has been particularly associated with deficit symptoms in schizotypal patients. Performance on other tests of visual or auditory attention . . . has also been reported to be impaired in schizotypal subjects . . . as well as in schizophrenic patients. (p. 1649)

In contrast to the above findings, elevated levels of homovanillic acid (HVA) in schizotypal personality disorder patients (vs. control subjects) have been associated with the psychotic-like ("positive") symptoms of this disorder. Siever and Davis speculate that "dopaminergic activity could modulate the expression of an underlying genotype for the schizophrenia-related disorders toward or away from severe psychotic symptoms" (p. 1650).

There are very few data on the biological correlates of either PPD or schizoid personality disorder (Grant 1991), and little information on genetic or familial factors in these conditions (American Psychiatric Association 1987). Although Marmar (1988) makes the claim that "if

Table 9–2. Schizotypal symptoms

Positive symptoms	Negative symptoms
Magical thinking	Social isolation
Ideas of reference	Odd speech
Recurrent illusions	Inadequate rapport
	Undue social anxiety
	Suspiciousness

Source. Extensively modified from Siever and Davis 1991.

a patient has paranoid personality disorder, the chances are good that someone in the family has a paranoid disorder" (p. 403), no empirical evidence is cited. Vaillant and Perry (1985) note that PPD "occurs in the biological relatives of identified schizophrenic patients [and] is considered part of the schizophrenic spectrum" (p. 969). However, the gender and familial pattern are not known. Finally, the work of Kagan and colleagues (1987) on "behavior inhibition to the unfamiliar" may have relevance to schizoid personality disorder. Kagan et al. have found strong evidence that about 12% of children are born with a predisposition to be irritable as infants, shy and fearful as toddlers, and cautiously introverted as youngsters. A variety of physiological variables are correlated with these traits (e.g., pupillary dilation, elevated heart rate, and elevated urinary catecholamines). Rosenbaum and colleagues (1988) have shown a correlation between behavioral inhibition in childhood and adult anxiety disorders, and it is tempting to speculate on the possible additional association with schizoid personality disorder; however, to my knowledge, this issue has not been rigorously investigated.

Psychological Factors

D. Adler (1990) suggests that Cluster A (i.e., paranoid, schizoid, and schizotypal) patients "are individuals who seem to use fantasy as a framework for psychic survival and a sense of worth" (p. 19). Akhtar (1987), too, comments on "the rich fantasy life that underlies the apparent detachment of the schizoid individual" (p. 507). Other features of the schizoid personality emphasized by Akhtar—and not by DSM-IV—include overt aloofness but covert neediness and "hunger" for love; overt self-sufficiency but covert feelings of inner emptiness; and overt lack of sexual interest but covert "voyeuristic and pornographic interests." This "overt-covert" dichotomy, according to Akhtar, "emphasizes the centrality of splitting and identity diffusion in schizoid personality" (p. 510). Significantly, DSM-IV changed "is" indifferent to praise and criticism (as in DSM-III-R) to "appears" indifferent.

In their review of PPD, Vaillant and Perry (1985) discredit the early psychoanalytic view that PPD is caused by "an underlying conflict over homosexuality." Rather, "homosexuals . . . serve as foci for the paranoid's projected feelings and conflicts over dependency, passivity, and intimacy" (p. 969). PPD patients often believe themselves inadequate, and "to avoid humiliation, they blame others for wrongdoing" (Vaillant and Perry 1985, p. 969). Vaillant and Perry (1985)—in a formulation that parallels that of Akhtar—state that "paranoiac patients often fear love as much as hate. In manifestly rejecting intimacy, the paranoid character may exhibit an obsessive over-involvement with the enemy" (p. 969).

Schizotypal patients are rather straightforwardly described in DSM-IV with respect to their "external" behaviors and beliefs. But what of their inner emotional and psychic lives? How do schizotypal patients experience themselves and the world? Stone (1989b) describes five features of schizotypal personality disorder that illuminate these issues: sense of discontinuity, anhedonia, tendency to misinterpret, concreteness, and ego-boundary problems. In brief, schizotypal patients often experience "a disturbing sense of discontinuity with respect to time and person" (p. 2719); for example, it is hard for them to develop "an integrated and stable image" of themselves and others. (You will see this manifested quite dramatically when you inform the patient of your upcoming vacation; he or she may find it hard to believe that you will ever return!) With respect to anhedonia, schizotypal patients tend to be "impervious to the joys [of life]," but "exquisitely sensitive to conflict and unpleasantness" (p. 2720). Thus, close relationships, which are often associated with pain, are avoided. The schizotypal patient's tendency to misinterpret reality is linked with a responsiveness "to symbols, to possible meanings, rather than to facts" (p. 2721). For example, a patient concludes that his wife no longer loves him because she left a pack of cigarettes on the bed, 2 years after the patient had told her that he "hates it when she smokes." Such patients not only misinterpret reality but also fail to make ordinary and adaptive generalizations (Stone 1989b) (e.g., learning that people commonly smile in social situations and that this does not indicate derision of the patient). Schizotypal patients tend to be overly concrete (as are many schizophrenic patients) and often humorless; they have difficulty tuning in to the figurative meanings of conversation. Finally, schizotypal patients—like schizophrenic patients—have intense ego-boundary problems, though not as severe as those of schizophrenic patients. Sometimes it may be hard for the patient to know where he or she leaves off and the therapist begins (Stone 1989b).

Sociocultural Factors

Before focusing on Cluster A disorders, what can we say generally about personality disorders and sociocultural influences? As a rule, there is an increased prevalence of personality disorders in inner cities, prisons, and areas of social disintegration. Morover, personality disorders in general are three times as common in the lowest socioeconomic classes as in the highest (Grant 1991). Zimmerman and Coryell (1989) have shown that, compared with individuals without personality disorder, those with "any" personality disorder are more likely to be single, unmarried, or separated. Because personality disorders are usually evident quite early in life, we can regard most of these correlations as consequences of the personality disturbance, rather than as causal factors. Of course, the "arrow" of causality is sometimes turned around, as when an urban ghetto or prison setting exacerbates an individual's underlying sociopathy. It is also possible that early, pervasive, and destructive environmental influences do actually "shape" later character pathology (see discussion below on sociopathic personality disorder), but the evidence is equivocal. Regarding cultural factors and personality disorder, Vaillant and Perry (1985) offer the following useful observation:

> Denmark reveals a low incidence of murder and of anger turned outward, and a high incidence of suicide and anger turned against the self . . . characteristic of depressive and passive-aggressive personalities. Similarly . . . Burma reveals a very low rate of suicide and a high rate of homicide . . . characteristic of antisocial and paranoid personalities. (p. 962)

But despite "common sense and anecdotal evidence," as Vaillant and Perry note, "there are no firm data to link any psychiatric disorder with any specific culture" (p. 962).

With respect to Cluster A disorders, little is known about sociocultural determinants of—as distinct from cultural adaptations to—

these disorders. In discussing PPD, Vaillant and Perry (1985) note that "there is some evidence that persons who are the recipients of irrational and overwhelming parental rage identify with their parents and tend to project the rage onto others that they once experienced directed toward themselves" (p. 969).

Perhaps as a cultural adaptation to their disorder, many PPD patients wind up "among leaders of cults and other fringe groups" (American Psychiatric Association 1987, p. 338).

With respect to schizoid personality disorder, once again, little is known about sociocultural determinants. Stone (1989a)—apparently on the basis of clinical experience—points to the role of physical, sexual, or emotional abuse. After describing a schizoid woman who had been beaten throughout childhood by her mother, Stone (1989a) notes, "Many schizoid patients have endured such humiliation as children, and have, out of loyalty to the offending caretaker(s), developed a cripplingly low self-esteem . . . as though the abuse were somehow deserved" (p. 2714). (It is not clear, however, why such children would develop schizoid personality disorder as opposed to PTSD or multiple personality, for example.) Arguing along similar lines, and drawing on the work of Guntrip and Fairbairn, Rizzuto et al. (1981) have proposed a link between the "schizoid character structure" and anorexia nervosa. Specifically, they argue that "the specific cause of the schizoid development of the anorexic patient is the mother's real inability to see the child as itself . . . instead, the mother relates to the child as a physical body reality, perceived in a fixed manner . . . the child experiences utter isolation, and compensates with compliant behavior" (p. 475).

Arieti (1974) also looks to disturbed parent-child interactions in the genesis of the "schizoid personality." He describes the schizoid personality structure as "character armor" against "the distressing others who constitute the family and the world" (p. 103). Arieti sees the parents of the preschizophrenic individual as fostering the belief that "action does not pay" because "it provokes a storm of intense and threatening emotional responses in the surrounding adults" (p. 104).

But Vaillant and Perry (1985) note that while, retrospectively, clinicians often identify "bleak, cold, unempathic childhoods" in schizoid individuals, careful longitudinal studies are lacking. Moreover, these authors point out that "the effect of cold, aloof parenting itself may only produce a schizoid adult when it interacts with a shy, anxious, and introverted temperament in the child" (p. 971).

DSM-III-R noted that schizoid personality disorder patients are often seen "in jobs that involve little or no contact with others, or living in skid-row sections of cities" (American Psychiatric Association 1987, p. 339); presumably, these epidemiological features are consequences of or adaptations to schizoid personality disorder.

There is little in the published literature pertaining to sociocultural aspects of schizotypal personality disorder. Because there appears to be a genetic and phenomenological link between schizotypal personality disorder and schizophrenia, we might infer that the sociocultural determinants—or accompaniments—are also similar. Thus, we might predict that, like schizophrenic patients, schizotypal personality disorder patients cluster predominantly in lower socioeconomic levels. However, there seems to be little research bearing on this. Zimmerman and Coryell (1989), in a study of a large nonpatient sample, found that compared with individuals without any personality disorder, individuals with schizotypal personality disorder (not surprisingly) had a higher rate of marital separation. (This is true of the personality disorder group as a whole.) There appear to be some gender differences in the proportion of "positive" versus "negative" symptoms in schizotypal personality disorder, with women showing more positive features (e.g., ideas of reference, magical thinking, etc.). This might, of course, be a biologically based difference, but Raine (1992) hypothesizes that it "may in part reflect an exaggeration of normal sex differences in the general population" (p. 362), suggesting the possibility of sociocultural determinants.

We should close our discussion of the "biopsychosocial" perspective on Cluster A personality disorders by referring again to the work of Siever and Davis (1991), who have attempted to integrate the biological and psychosocial dimensions of personality disorder. To cite but one example: How might abnormalities in, say, attention or smooth pursuit eye movement (SPEM) affect the mother-infant bond with respect to later development of schizotypy? Siever and Davis (1991) hypothesize that "an altered capacity to respond smoothly and appropriately to maternal cues grounded in an underlying disturbance in cognitive/perceptual organization could easily impair the development of synchronous, mutually satisfying relationships . . . [and result in] less empathy and rapport, and erratically inappropriate or 'odd' behavior" (p. 1654).

In short, a dysfunctional brain leads to impaired "bonding" and, perhaps, to abnormal behavior.

Pitfalls in the Differential Diagnosis

Medical and "Organic" Disorders

Lishman (1987) points out that while intellectual impairment is the hallmark of chronic organic brain syndromes, "this may be manifest only indirectly by way of behavioural change" (p. 14). Following the work of Kurt Goldstein, Lishman gives the following description of what DSM-III-R called organic personality syndrome. (Keep in mind, as you read, the Cluster A disorders we've just discussed.)

> There is often restlessness, with purposeless overactivity. Typically this occurs within a progressively diminishing sphere of interests and activities . . . when taxed beyond his ability, [the individual] may become evasive and sullen . . . social interaction is often marked by lack of concern or callousness towards others, stubborn egocentricity, or withdrawal from social contact. (p. 14)

A full discussion of each disorder that can produce such behavioral changes would take a chapter in itself; the organic conditions commonly associated with personality changes in general are summarized in Table 9–3. Welch and Bear (1990) have provided a thorough

Table 9–3. Etiological factors in organic personality syndrome

Frontal lobe neoplasm	Temporal lobe epilepsy
Head trauma	Multiple sclerosis
Cerebrovascular disease	Huntington's disease

Source. Extensively modified from American Psychiatric Association 1987.

review of this area. With respect to Cluster A disorders, Cummings (1985) notes that paranoid personality features have followed brain damage to either hemisphere. Bear et al. (1982), in describing the interictal personality changes of temporal lobe epileptics, note the appearance of circumstantiality, hyposexuality, and hyperreligiosity. Such features, in my experience, may be seen in some schizotypal personality disorder patients, and lack of interest in sexual relations is a common finding in schizoid personality disorder. The emotional constriction of the schizoid individual may also resemble the "apathy" observed in patients with damage to the medial frontal lobes (Cummings 1992).

Psychiatric Disorders

The first diagnostic difficulty in facing the Cluster A patient is that there is significant overlap of symptoms within the cluster itself—not to mention the apparent comorbidity of Cluster A disorders with those in Clusters B and C (Zimmerman and Coryell 1989). With respect to overlap within Cluster A, keep in mind that DSM-III-R "permitted" the same patient to receive diagnoses of both schizoid and schizotypal personality disorders, since the exclusion criteria for the former did not preclude features of the latter! If all that leaves you a bit confused, it may be helpful to heed the observation of Widiger et al. (1988): "Little new information may be provided by a schizoid personality disorder diagnosis, in addition to the schizotypal diagnosis. Schizoid and schizotypal personality disorders may be but slightly different variants of a single personality disorder, or different points along a schizophrenic spectrum" (p. 792).

In practice, I find it useful to focus on "eccentricities" of thinking and behavior in reaching the diagnosis of schizotypal personality disorder. A patient of mine, for example, once described an experience of "being in bed" with her deceased nephew. She "knew" this because she "could feel his elbow against me and smelled his hair." She retained enough reality testing to say, "I know you're scientific and don't believe in these things, Doctor . . . but spirits do exist!" This relative intactness of reality testing also helps distinguish the schizotypal personality disorder patient from the schizophrenic patient—though the line between fixed delusion and eccentric belief is often very fine. The schizotypal personality disorder patient also shows far less thought process disorder than the patient with schizophrenia and may converse quite normally until you hit some "trigger" topic such as telepathy, clairvoyance, and so forth. At that point, there may be some mild "loosening" of associations and eccentricities of word usage. Although schizophrenia of the "residual" type may resemble schizotypal or schizoid personality disorder, there is usually a discernible "active phase" (hallucinations, frank delusions, etc.) in the history of the schizophrenic patient.

With respect to PPD, the differential diagnosis is usually easier. Whereas the schizoid and schizotypal patients are, respectively, "aloof" and "eccentric," the PPD patient usually comes across as quite hostile: within a few minutes, you may feel your muscles tightening ever so slightly and a certain defensiveness creeping into your replies. More "objectively," the PPD patient usually has more social relations than the schizoid individual, though these are almost always tinged with suspiciousness and ambivalent hostility/dependency. The PPD patient usually lacks the "spacey" thought content of the schizotypal patient (e.g., preoccupation with ESP, spirits, etc.). It is sometimes difficult to distinguish PPD from paranoid schizophrenia, but the latter typically entails far more social and occupational dysfunction, thought process disorder, and abnormalities of affect.

Other personality disorders show considerable overlap with those in Cluster A. Avoidant personality disorder and borderline personality disorder (BPD), as we will discuss, are especially easy to confuse with Cluster A disorders. Specifically, it is often hard to distinguish avoidant personality disorder from schizoid personality disorder, because social withdrawal is common to both. It may help you to know that avoidant personality disorder is actually much more prevalent in clinical settings than is schizoid personality disorder (Widiger et al. 1988). As Widiger et al. (1988) put it, "Many more persons appear to be socially withdrawn because of an anxious insecurity than because of an apathetic indifference" (p. 790). (Indeed, if Akhtar [1987] is right, even the schizoid individual is not "indifferent" to social connectedness.) Another clue is that the avoidant personality disorder patient is more likely to focus on embarrassment in social situations than is the schizoid individual, who will generally profess lack of interest. (Now all you have to do is distinguish avoidant personality disorder from social phobia!) Schizotypal patients share with avoidant personality disorder patients "excessive social anxiety"; but whereas avoidant patients usually express fear of criticism in social situations, schizotypal patients usually express paranoid fears (American Psychiatric Association 1994).

Borderline personality disorder, discussed in detail under Cluster B personality disorders, is very likely a "heterogeneous hodgepodge," to borrow a phrase from Widiger et al. (1988). BPD patients certainly can become transiently "paranoid," and thus their diagnosis can be confused with PPD. They can also relate unusual experiences of the "self," including marked identity diffusion, and thus resemble some schizotypal patients. BPD patients, finally, can sometimes appear quite socially withdrawn or even "indifferent" to others, thus appearing (albeit transiently) somewhat "schizoid." However, in my experience, BPD patients are ultimately distinguishable from Cluster A patients along a dimension I am tempted to call "enmeshed retaliatory impotence"—I am alluding, of course, to how the therapist often feels when dealing with the shifting, hostile-dependent, idealizing-devaluing aspects of the borderline patient. PPD patients often evoke hostility and withdrawal in therapists but (in my experience) rarely "suck in" the therapist in the way one often experiences with BPD patients, as we will discuss further. Aside from such countertransferential clues, BPD patients usually have a more prominent history of self-destructive acts, substance abuse, and unstable (as opposed to remote or hostile) relationships than do Cluster A individuals.

Adjunctive Testing

Neuroimaging and Neuroendocrine Testing

We do not have a specific and sensitive biological "test" for the Cluster A personality disorder—or, for that matter, for any of the personality disorders. However, we have already noted a number of physiological correlates or "markers" for schizotypal personality disorder—for example, elevated cerebrospinal fluid and plasma HVA, and abnormal

SPEMs (Siever and Davis 1991). Siever (1992) has recently presented data showing that in comparison with other personality disorder patients and normal control subjects, schizotypal personality disorder patients show a larger ventricle-brain ratio (VBR) in the region of the frontal horn. He has also shown a correlation between poor SPEMs and conceptual disorganization in schizotypal personality disorder, as well as between abnormal SPEMs and a number of psychosocial problems (e.g., sexual dissatisfaction, social incompetence or introversion, social isolation). Unfortunately, to my knowledge, this sort of integrated research approach has not been applied to the other Cluster A disorders.

Neuropsychiatric Testing

Once again, much of the work here has come out of Siever et al.'s investigations of schizotypal personality disorder. For example, these patients often show impairment on neuropsychiatric tests of prefrontal lobe function, such as the Wisconsin Card Sort (WCS) Test. (You may recall that schizophrenic patients also show abnormalities of frontal lobe function.) These prefrontal abnormalities associated with schizotypal personality disorder appear to be correlated with the "deficit" symptoms of the disorder listed earlier (Siever 1992). In nonclinical populations screened for "schizotypy" (but without formal diagnoses of schizotypal personality disorder), it is more difficult to demonstrate the perceptual organization deficits seen in some schizophrenic patients (Silverstein et al. 1992). However, Chapin et al. (1987) provide an interesting confirmation of both the borderline/schizotypal personality disorder distinction and the schizotypal personality disorder/schizophrenia "link." In a test of reaction time to a visual stimulus (light), these workers found that schizophrenic and schizotypal patients had a similar deficit and that this deficit was not observed in hospitalized BPD patients.

Results for Cluster A personality disorders on more "classical" tests are summarized in Table 9–4. Of special interest is the "approach" taken by the PPD patient to the Minnesota Multiphasic Personality Inventory (MMPI) and other structured tests. As Meyer (1983) notes,

It might be expected that the paranoid personality will be high on scale 6 [paranoia]. However, . . . this is not always the case, as such individuals are hyperalert about being perceived as paranoid and may guard against this. . . . the paranoid personality will occasionally use some kind of random or devious scheme with the MMPI. . . . they are easily irritated at the forced choice format. . . . they also become irritated at the significant self-disclosure required. (p. 182)

The MMPI profile of the paranoid personality, Meyer further notes, "reflects the use of denial and projection, the inclination to focus on

Table 9–4.   Psychological testing for Cluster A personality disorders

Personality disorder	MMPI	WAIS	Rorschach
Paranoid	Elevation of scales 3, 6, 1, and K common.	Rigidity and suspiciousness may bring down comprehension; best score on similarities.	F% and F+% are high; few M or color responses.
Schizoid	Often normal when patient is not stressed; high 0 scale (social introversion).	Verbal scale may be lowered by interpersonal problems; lower picture arrangement and completion scores.	High % animal and few color-based responses.
Schizotypal	2-7-8 code often seen in "preschizophrenic" patients; scale 0 raised; scales F and 4 also high.	Similar to pattern noted with schizophrenic patients.	Similar to pattern noted with schizophrenic patients.

Note. MMPI = Minnesota Multiphasic Personality Inventory; WAIS = Wechsler Adult Intelligence Scale.
Source. Extensively modified from Meyer 1983.

physiological concerns . . . and the need to present a facade of adequacy" (p. 182).

With regard to schizoid and schizotypal personality disorder, Meyer (1983) notes that, although there are some similarities between them on testing, in many respects "the schizotypals are closer to the schizophrenic, particularly in their performance on tests such as the revised Wechsler Adult Intelligence Scale (WAIS-R) and Rorschach" (p. 187) (see Table 9–4). This finding is consistent with the familial and biological affinities we have already discussed.

Treatment Directions and Goals

Somatic Approaches

Your first, intuitive inclination may be to use antipsychotic medication for patients with this group of disorders; however, there is little systematic research to support this approach (Liebowitz 1989). In one placebo-controlled study by Goldberg et al. (1986), thiothixene did not have a clearly beneficial effect on the schizotypal trait cluster, as assessed by structured interview and the Global Assessment Scale (GAS). However, the authors did find that "there are some patients with [borderline and schizotypal personality disorders] who do respond to thiothixene. . . . they are the ones who were more severely ill at baseline with regard to illusions, ideas of reference, psychoticism, phobic anxiety, and obsessive-compulsivity" (p. 685). Stone (1989b) also recommends the use of anxiolytics in schizotypal personality disorder patients "during times of crisis." I have had good results treating one schizotypal woman (with marked depressive features) using fluoxetine 20–40 mg/day; antipsychotic medication has not been necessary.

In an excellent review of personality disorders, Gorten and Akhtar (1990) conclude that "transitory psychotic states or symptoms," "cognitive distortions, and "paranoia" may respond to low-dose antipsychotic medication. Similarly, Ellison and Adler (1990) note that "often the neuroleptic dosage can be lower and the time course of treatment briefer with psychosis in personality disorders than . . . in patients with schizophrenia or bipolar disorder" (p. 48). With respect to PPD, Meissner (1989), while acknowledging the occasional utility of low-dose antipsychotics, minor tranquilizers, or antidepressants for "specific target symptoms," offers the following cautionary note:

> One of the difficulties . . . is that [PPD patients] are often extremely resistant to taking medications of any kind, frequently seeing them in terms of issues of control, powerlessness, and loss of autonomy. . . . the gains from insisting on the patient's taking the medication can be minor, whereas the negative implications for the patient's overall therapy may prove to be major. (p. 2711)

Stone (1989a) takes an even more negative view of medication for schizoid personality disorder patients, stating that their "fundamental temperamental traits of aloofness, oversensitivity, and uncommunicativeness are . . . resistant to [psychotropic] drugs—which, therefore, have little place in the treatment of schizoid personality" (p. 2718).

Psychosocial Approaches

Before recommending specific psychotherapeutic approaches for each of the Cluster A disorders, what can we say generally about the treatment of personality disorder patients? First off, there simply is no body of systematic research on the optimal treatment of any personality disorder (Gorten and Akhtar 1990). Thus, most of what I will recommend comes from the clinical experience of myself and others and from a few large-scale, controlled studies. With respect to personality disorders in general, the basic components of psychotherapy are summarized in Table 9–5. You may feel that these guidelines are so general as to apply to the treatment of any patient—and there is truth to that. It may be fair to say that the personality disorder patient needs the same "right ingredients" of psychotherapy as do "neurotic" patients—only more so. On the other hand, most personality disorder patients will not require the degree of therapeutic surveillance and control needed with frankly psychotic patients, although there are exceptions to this dictum.

With respect to the Cluster A disorders, the essentials of psychotherapeutic treatment are summarized in Table 9–6 (see Stone

[1989a, 1989b] and Meissner [1989] for a detailed discussion of these issues).

In working with Cluster A personality disorder patients, one of the most vexing questions facing the therapist involves the issue of reality testing. Many residents ask me, "How should I handle it when my patient talks about these weird out-of-body experiences, ideas of reference, and so on?" The temptation for us—as "ambassadors of reality"—is to come at the "content" of the patient's statements directly. This rarely succeeds and may only alienate the patient—particularly the paranoid or schizotypal patient. Rather, you should approach the affect directly, and the content only indirectly. How does this work in practice? Let's look at a prototypical dialogue between a therapist and a patient with mixed schizotypal and PPD features. This is an excerpt from their fifth session:

Patient: I had this experience last night . . . you probably think I'm nuts, but I felt, well—a presence in my bedroom.
Therapist: What sort of presence?

Table 9–5. Key elements of psychotherapy with personality disorder patients

Understand and address the core issues of aloneness and low self-esteem.

Keep therapeutic expectations in line with adaptive defects; work *with*, not *on*, the patient.

Don't underestimate the power of the relationship, even though the patient may act "as if you are not in the room."

Attend to your countertransference.

Establish a "safe holding environment."

Try to reach agreement as to the therapeutic tasks.

Establish an empathic relationship.

Help the patient perceive and gradually change self-defeating behaviors.

Utilize "supportive" as well as "insight-oriented" approaches (e.g., social skills groups).

Source. Extensively modified from D. Adler 1990.

Table 9–6.   Psychotherapy and Cluster A personality disorders

Paranoid personality disorder

Help the patient develop meaningful trust in the therapist via empathic responsiveness to patient's idiosyncratic needs.

Resolve the depressive elements contained in the patient's sense of self as "victim"; work through underlying feelings of weakness, impotence, and vulnerability.

Respect and maximize patient's autonomy (e.g., vis-à-vis use of medication).

Avoid directly "challenging" projective defenses and perceptions; focus on patient's feelings and gently test alternatives to paranoid stance.

Carefully monitor countertransference—for example, unconscious need to play aggressor to patient's victim, or feeling helpless, worthless, etc. (playing out role of victim).

Deal with litigiousness, if possible, by mending breaches in alliance; refer to other clinician if legal threats escalate.

Schizoid personality disorder

Usually limit visits to 1 to 2 times per week; avoid evoking anxiety over too much intimacy.

Be relatively "active"; for example, make empathic opening remark rather than wait for patient to "begin."

Try to understand latent/symbolic content of seemingly concrete remarks.

Respect the patient's need for emotional distance.

Avoid "rushing" the patient into self-disclosure.

Use educative measures to help patient become more assertive/less self-conscious.

Schizotypal personality disorder

Provide consistency and punctuality in order to foster stable and integrated image of therapist (and, by extension, of patient).

Use "boredom" in sessions constructively (e.g., as index of what patient is suffering or concealing).

Maintain firm ego boundaries, set appropriate limits, and clarify transference distortion (e.g., "You seem to see me as . . . ").

Remember that education and direct advice giving may be more helpful than interpretation of dreams, unconscious drives, and so forth.

Realize that it's not so much "the words" as "the music"; that is, the schizotypal patient places great value on interaction with an empathic therapist and may not need (or even "hear") sophisticated interpretations.

Source.   Extensively modified from Meissner 1989; Stone 1989a, 1989b.

P.: I don't know—like, something evil. Like a dark force. That sounds like something from *Star Wars,* doesn't it?

T.: It sounds pretty scary to me.

P.: It was! I almost called the police but I figured they'd laugh.

T.: Can you remember what was going on that night? Had anything unusual or stressful happened?

P.: Oh, I know you! You're gonna explain it all away! Look, I've told you, there are real things out there, life-forces and energies that people can't see!

T.: Well, I know it's upsetting to you when I suggest other possibilities. I try to keep an open mind about the sort of experience you had, because lots of people report similar experiences.

P.: They do?

T.: Sure. Many people have unusual experiences from time to time. But what happened to you sounded pretty frightening.

P.: Yeah, it was.

T.: And I doubt it helped that you were all alone at the time.

P.: It's always that way. I never have someone around when I need them, and when someone is around, I start pulling back.

Although the dialogue above could be part of a psychodynamically oriented approach, I tend to "titrate" the amount of interpretation and exploration of unconscious material very carefully; typically, a more here-and-now, directive approach is more useful with the Cluster A individual. A variety of approaches and formats have been described for working with this kind of patient (Meissner 1989; Stone 1989a, 1989b). Behavioral methods, originally developed by R. P. Liberman for schizophrenic patients, may be modified for use with schizoid and schizotypal patients. Although there is little systematic research on the use of group therapy for Cluster A patients, clinical evidence suggests this approach may be useful in some cases. In general, the approach should be more "supportive" than "psychoanalytic," because some Cluster A patients are prone to decompensation when exploratory techniques are perceived as intrusive. Family therapy may also be appropriate if the identified patient is living at home or if family members are struggling with the patient's pathology.

The Dramatic/Erratic Cluster (Cluster B): Antisocial, Borderline, Histrionic, and Narcissistic Personality Disorders

The Central Concept

So much has been written about Cluster B personality disorder that the best we can hope for in this discussion is an intelligible overview; for more detailed information, you are encouraged to read the numerous references cited. Let's at least look at the opening kickoff.

Vignette

Mr. E. M. Rorrim, a single, 42-year-old editor at a major publishing house, sought psychotherapy "in order to enhance my approach to the idiots I have to work with." The patient gave a history of superior academic performance throughout high school and college. His literary talents as an editor had secured him an excellent position in his late 20s, and he had done "very well" in his field. However, he had actually held a number of editing jobs over the years, owing to—as he put it—"the inability of certain people to make good use of my talents." He acknowledged "some difficulties" in his personal relationships, having just come through "a mega-messed-up relationship with a real bitch." The patient acknowledged that "people generally find it hard to take me . . . I think most of it is envy, but I can be something of an SOB." The patient denied any history of involvement with the law, but acknowledged that "in college, I got into trouble for this computer scam I set up; actually, I still think it was pretty neat." The "scam" involved a "phony computer dating service that basically just generated credit card numbers. I never got to use any of them, though," he added, smiling. The patient denied active substance abuse, but had, over the years, "gotten into just about everything. In the 60s, I dropped a little acid. In the 70s, pot. In the 80s, coke. But lately, all I do is a little pot now and then." He had had no psychiatric hospitalizations, but "in college, they thought I was pretty messed up, so I saw the university shrink for a month or so. I thought, hey, this guy couldn't cure ham. I mean, all he did was point out my so-called problems. So I more or less blew him off."

The patient acknowledged that on three occasions—most recently, 2 months prior to evaluation—he had made ambivalent suicide attempts. In the latest attempt, he had "taken a bottle of Tylenol, but I got to the ER fast and they pumped me out." He acknowledged "mood swings" for most of his life but gave no history consistent with bipolar disorder. He described himself as "kind of the golden boy on the outside, but its like, fool's gold. Inside, I think there's just a lot of hot air." Throughout the interview, the patient showed a superficial, smiling (or as the resident put it, "sneering") affect.

Mr. Rorrim's case represents a kind of characterological pastiche: he shows a combination of narcissistic, antisocial, and borderline traits. Predominantly, however, he shows the features of narcissistic personality disorder. These include oversensitivity to criticism, interpersonal exploitativeness, a grandiose sense of self-importance, preoccupation with fantasies of unlimited success, an inordinate sense of entitlement, a constant need for admiration, and a distinct lack of empathy. Sociopathic (antisocial) personality disorder typically involves evidence of conduct disorder prior to age 15 (e.g., truancy, fighting, cruelty to animals, fire setting) and a pattern of irresponsible, antisocial behavior since age 15. The pattern usually includes unstable work history; failure to conform to social norms; irritability or aggression; failure to honor financial obligations; repeated lying to or "conning" of others; and disregard for the safety of self or others. Borderline personality disorder tends to be the least stable of the three disorders mentioned. The hallmarks of BPD include a pattern of intense and unstable relationships; impulsive or self-destructive acts; affective instability; inappropriate, intense anger; "identity disturbance" (e.g., regarding sexual orientation); chronic feelings of emptiness or boredom; and frantic efforts to avoid "abandonment." DSM-IV has added the additional feature of "transient, stress-related paranoid ideation or severe dissociative symptoms" (American Psychiatric Association 1994).

The Cluster B disorder not exemplified in our vignette—histrionic personality disorder—is sometimes quite difficult to distinguish from narcissistic personality disorder. It is characterized by constant demands for approval, attention, or praise; inappropriate seductiveness; excessive concern with appearance; emotional "incontinence"; shallow, rapidly shifting affect; extreme self-centeredness; and an "impressionistic" style of speech.

Historical Development of the Concept

The Cluster B disorders have traveled a "long and winding road" to their present diagnostic homes. Narcissistic personality disorder (NPD) is the relative newcomer in the DSMs, appearing as a disorder only in 1980 in DSM-III. Meissner (1985) has provided an excellent review of the psychoanalytic concept of "narcissism" as it developed from Freud to Hartmann to Kohut. We will discuss some of these views below. Antisocial personality disorder (APD) was first described in something close to its present form by Cleckley in 1938, in his book *The Mask of Sanity* (Cleckley 1964). Cleckley noted that in APD, unlike most other psychiatric disorders, overt anxiety and depression are not common (Vaillant and Perry 1985). In the 1950s, DSM-I (American Psychiatric Association 1952) used the term "sociopathic personality disturbance" as an umbrella concept, embracing drug addiction, sexual deviation, and various antisocial behaviors. Later work by Glueck and Glueck (1968) refined the concept and demonstrated the roots of APD in childhood conduct disorder. Histrionic personality disorder (HPD) is the offspring of that hoary concept hysteria. Chodoff and Lyons, in 1958, pointed out that the term "hysteria" had at least five historical usages: a personality type; a conversion reaction; a "neurotic" disorder characterized by phobias and anxiety; a particular pattern of psychopathology; and a term of disapproval (Vaillant and Perry 1985). Brody and Sata, in 1967, first coined the term "histrionic personality disorder," and by 1972, a description of "hysterical" or histrionic personality disorder similar to our present one had coalesced (Freedman et al. 1972).

Because we will devote most of our discussion to BPD, it may help to take a slightly more detailed look at the history of this concept. Cowdry (1987) provides us with an excellent synopsis:

> The early formulations of the borderline syndrome identified a group of persons with chronic marginal functioning, polymorphic symptoms, and idiosyncratic thought processes who were felt to show a mild form of schizophrenia, variously referred to as pseudoneurotic schizophrenia, psychotic character, or "latent" schizophrenia. These formulations were developed at a time when the American concept of schizophrenia cast a broad net and included persons who would probably now be characterized as having brief reactive psychoses, bipolar affective disorder, or schizoid or schizotypal illness. As the concept of schizophrenia has narrowed . . . the border of schizophrenia identified by the "borderline" diagnosis now appears farther from the core concept of schizophrenia. (p. 15)

Indeed, as the concept of BPD moved away from that of schizophrenia, it veered toward the affective disorders—to paraphrase one psychiatrist writing in the 1980s, "borderline personality disorder equals depression plus obnoxious behavior." It turns out that this appealingly simple formulation is probably wrong, too, and that BPD is very likely a "heterogeneous hodgepodge" with several etiologies.

The Biopsychosocial Perspective

Biological Factors

Most of the biological research in the Cluster B spectrum has involved BPD and APD. With respect to BPD, Andrulonis et al. (1981) found that a small percentage (less than 10%) of borderline patients had histories of overt central nervous system (CNS) injury or dysfunction (e.g., seizures or head trauma). Other studies have suggested low threshold for "excitability" in the limbic system or deficiencies in central serotonin metabolism of BPD patients; these abnormalities could underlie the impulsivity and mood lability of the borderline patient (Gunderson and Zanarini 1987). Coccaro et al. (1989) found a blunted prolactin response to the serotonin-releasing agent fenfluramine in BPD patients, suggesting diminished serotonergic function. And, despite the recent deemphasis of BPD as some variant of schizophrenia, one study of auditory evoked potentials suggests an affinity between these disorders (Kutcher et al. 1987). Patients with BPD or schizophrenia—but not patients with other personality disorders—showed a prolonged P300 latency, suggesting dysfunction of auditory neurointegration. (Interestingly, the presence or absence of comorbid schizotypal personality disorder did not affect outcome.) Hyperresponsiveness of the cholinergic and noradrenergic systems may also be present in BPD (Siever and Davis, 1991); we will say more about this in our subsection on adjunctive testing.

Siever and Davis (1991) have summarized the biological correlates of the personality dimension they term "impulsivity/aggression." With respect to "sociopathic" individuals—not all of whom met the DSM-III-R criteria for APD—Siever and Davis noted the following findings: less inhibition of motor responses, weaker sympathetic responsiveness, and more rapid habituation in skin conductance response than in other patient types. The authors interpret these data to mean that "impulsive or sociopathic individuals are more likely to respond to important environmental stimuli by motor responses than by an evaluative delay characterized by cortical activation, sympathetic arousal, and an inhibtion of motor output" (p. 1651). In short, sociopathic individuals act first and think later. More aggressive or violent sociopathic individuals may also show abnormalities in serotonergic function; for example, diminished serotonergic tone has been correlated with aggression toward both self and others (Siever and Davis 1991). Interaction between serotonergic and noradrenergic systems may be an important determinant of whether violence is directed at "self" or "other." The XYY chromosomal pattern was once thought to be correlated with APD, but reexamination of the data does not support this conclusion; the vast majority of XYY men are not antisocial (Grant 1991). Nonetheless, there is ample evidence of a familial and/or genetic factor in APD. For example, APD has been found to be more frequent in men whose close biological relatives had antisocial behavior problems (Cadoret et al. 1985). We have already mentioned (see Chapter 7) the association between APD and somatization disorder (Briquet's syndrome) and the possibility that a common biogenetic substrate underlies these disorders.

Psychological Factors

The most efficient approach to a psychodynamic understanding of the Cluster B disorders is via the concepts developed by G. Adler (1981) regarding the borderline-narcissistic personality disorder continuum. To a more limited degree, these concepts are applicable to APD and HPD. The seminal contributions of Kernberg, Masterson, Kohut, and others are simply beyond the scope of our summary, but you will find it well worth your time to peruse the references cited (Kernberg 1975; Kohut 1977; Masterson 1976).

G. Adler (1981) points to three key elements in understanding the psychopathology of the borderline-narcissistic continuum: 1) the capacity to maintain a cohesive self, 2) the capacity to form stable self-object transferences, and 3) the achievement of "mature aloneness." (Because of the special vocabulary adopted by Adler and others, I will sometimes use somewhat different terminology in elucidating their views.) Patients who lie along the borderline-narcissistic continuum typically suffer from a sense of inner "fragmentation"; they often complain of "not feeling real, or of feeling "empty" and depleted. Under various types of stress, the feelings of inner emptiness and depletion may evolve into feelings of depersonalization or even "annihilation" (G. Adler 1981). Psychotic experiences can occur, though this happens more commonly in BPD than in NPD patients.

Individuals on the borderline-narcissistic continuum, according to Adler, have difficulty maintaining a stable, internalized image of significant people in their lives (e.g., lovers, parents, and therapists). Instead, these individuals usually go through a stereotyped series of reactions in their relationships. The "other" may at first be idealized or "placed on a pedestal," but disappointment, anger, and fears of abandonment soon follow. The patient may utilize primitive defenses such as "splitting" and "projective identification"—that is, seeing others as either "all good" or "all bad" (splitting), or attributing to others one's own feelings and then "inducing" the other to behave congruently with this projection (a very rough and condensed description of projective identification). These concepts may become a bit more clear through a brief vignette:

Vignette

The patient, a 24-year-old single woman, had been in dynamically oriented therapy with the therapist for 2 months. While, at first, the patient had told her therapist, "You're the best . . . you're an artist!," she had an extremely strong reaction to his announcement that he would be taking a brief vacation. She told him, "You're just like all the rest, you phony! You string me along, then you take off! You're worthless! Why don't you just admit you hate my guts? Why don't you admit you want to get rid of me?" The patient proceeded to throw the therapist's antique ashtray at his office window. After calling security and having the patient bodily removed from his office, the therapist informed the patient by letter that "under the circumstances," he could no longer treat her.

Finally, individuals on the borderline-narcissistic continuum have great difficulty with what Adler (1981) calls "the achievement of mature aloneness." The patient experiences separation from significant others in three ways: 1) the patient feels "totally bereft of any image, memory, or fantasy" of the absent person as a "holding or sustaining person"; 2) the patient remembers only destructive or angry images of the absent person; and 3) the patient experiences his or her anger as "actively destroying" positive images of the absent person. The therapeutic implications of these dynamics are discussed in our subsection on treatment.

With respect to HPD and APD (which may be two phenotypic sides of the same genotypic coin), some of the dynamics discussed previously are applicable. For example, Helene Deutsch's description of the "as if" personality, which we now view as a forerunner of BPD, also fits some aspects of HPD. As Chodoff (1989) notes, "In the absence or weakness of a 'central core,' the histrionic personality seems to consist simply of a number of different exteriors—almost like a kind of chameleon in which the uncovering of each layer serves only to reveal another layer with a different emotional coloration, in compliance with the perceived requirements of the interpersonal environment" (p. 2728). In addition, the HPD patient displays a cognitive style of "imprecision and exaggeration" and a mode of information processing "that is global and diffuse rather than detailed and consecutive" (Chodoff 1989, p. 2728).

The APD patient, while superficially characterized by a certain wreckless bravado, actually partakes of the same basic "weaknesses" we've described in borderline and narcissistic patients. As Reid and Burke (1989) note, the APD patient demonstrates "very primitive defenses against loss, at the level of basic trust, expressed through the hostility of grievance . . . and the protecting of oneself from abuse or leaving by others . . . externalization and avoidance of . . . one's inner life lead to ego splits reminiscent of narcissistic or borderline personality, but 'riddled with rage and sadism.'" (p. 2743).

Sociocultural Factors

As we have seen repeatedly, it is almost impossible to separate psychological from "social" factors when the latter includes early parent-child interactions. G. Adler (1981) notes that the feeling of borderline aloneness may be related to failures at certain developmental stages in early childhood and, specifically, to dysfunctional mother-child interactions during Mahler's "rapprochement subphase" (roughly, 16 to 24 months of age). If the mother (or "mothering figure," to be fair) is either overly "engulfing" or insufficiently nurturing during this phase, the infant (it is posited) may develop pathology in the narcissistic-borderline continuum. Similar dynamics have been hypothesized for HPD but with a "twist." As Chodoff (1989) puts it, "A serious interference in the [histrionic] patient's early relationship with her mother turns the little girl to her father for fulfillment of her needs for nurture. . . . consequently, she tends to go through life attempting to seduce men into serving as substitute mothers" (p. 2728).

The HPD individual thus embarks on what Chodoff (1989) aptly terms "a career of pseudosexuality in the service of dependency" (p. 2729). Cultural factors are also at work in the female predominance of HPD. Chodoff (1989) points out that HPD

> is a diagnosis predominantly applied to women. . . . This may be related to the historical subordination of women to men . . . women have had to come to terms with a world in which the dominant values have always been set by men. When combined with certain

more specific genetic and psychodynamic determinants, this cultural tradition and the attitudes that result lead to the caricature of femininity called the HPD. (p. 2728)

Nigg et al. (1991) make the case that "a high prevalence of reported childhood trauma, particularly sexual abuse" (p. 846), is seen in patients with BPD. These authors have shown that a history of childhood sexual abuse in BPD patients may be correlated with "extremely malevolent representations" in the earliest memories of these patients—once again revealing the nexus between psychological and social factors. The research literature suggests that sexual abuse in BPD occurs across economic classes and ethnic groups (Nigg et al. 1991). Also, Herman et al. (1989) found that sexual or physical abuse discriminates BPD patients from those with other Axis II disorders or (Axis I) major mood disorders.

The sociocultural factors involved in APD are a matter of some controversy. The traditional view that APD arises from "maternal deprivation" in the first 5 years of life now appears to be a gross oversimplification, at best (Vaillant and Perry 1985). Thus, Robins (1966) examined the interaction of heredity and environment in the genesis of antisocial personality among 524 children referred to a child guidance clinic. Robins found that having a sociopathic or alcoholic father strongly predicted a child's developing an antisocial personality, regardless of whether the child was reared in the presence of the biological father. Nevertheless, "adequate and strict discipline . . . statistically diminished the risk of delinquency in children who had delinquent parents" (Vaillant and Perry 1985, p. 977). Supporting the role of environmental and maternal factors is the work of Glueck and Glueck (1968), which showed that an incohesive home, lack of consistent maternal discipline, and lack of maternal affection allowed prospective identification of children who would be seriously delinquent by age 18. Finally, DSM-III-R noted that APD "is more common in lower-class populations, partly because it is associated with impaired earning capacity, and partly because fathers of those with the disorder frequently have the disorder themselves, and consequently, their children often grow up in impoverished homes" (American Psychiatric Association 1987, p. 343).

Finally, we should note Christopher Lasch's (1979) thesis (put forth in his book *The Culture of Narcissism*) that "narcissism" is a growing sociocultural phenomenon in Western society, related to a breakdown in the traditional structure of family and society:

> Instead of guiding the child, the older generation now struggles to "keep up with the kids," to master their incomprehensible jargon, and even to imitate their dress and manners. . . . these changes, which are inseparable from the whole development of modern industry, have made it more and more difficult for children to form strong psychological identifications with their parents. (p. 291)

Pitfalls in the Differential Diagnosis

Organic Disorders

As we have noted, patients who "look borderline" may have a history of "minimal brain dysfunction," head injury, or other cerebral insult, such as intraoperative anoxia (Andrulonis et al. 1981).

Psychiatric Disorders

As you might expect, it's not always easy to distinguish among the four Cluster B personality disorders, and there appears to be signficant comorbidity within this cluster. Zimmerman and Coryell (1989), using structured interviews based on DSM-III criteria in a nonpatient sample, found that 3 of 13 persons with BPD met the criteria for HPD and that 4 of the 13 met the criteria for APD. Similarly, antisocial individuals scored very high on dimensions of narcissistic and borderline pathology. Nevertheless, Zimmerman and Coryell found that BPD individuals are distinguished from individuals with other personality disorders by their high rates of alcohol and tobacco use, suicide attempts, and comorbid diagnosis of schizophrenia. This last factor is particularly interesting, since Gunderson and Singer (1985) view brief psychotic episodes as an integral part of BPD—contrary to the criteria in DSM-III-R, but consistent with those in DSM-IV. While observable traits like alcohol abuse may be useful in distinguishing among the Cluster B disorders, my own experience suggests that psychodynamic factors may be more helpful. For example, you will probably find less frequent use of splitting and projective identification in HPD and APD patients than in BPD and severely disturbed NPD patients. With respect to distinguishing between patients with NPD and those with BPD, I find that the former are less likely to "unravel" under stress and are more likely to view the therapist in a consistent manner. This is not to say that the NPD patient is stable or predictable; but he or she is less likely to become transiently psychotic and is less likely to idealize you in one session and flay you alive in the next than is the BPD patient. G. Adler (1981) notes that "patients with a narcissistic personality disorder do not experience the feelings of aloneness experienced by borderline patients" (p. 48). Ironically, the item "intolerance of being alone" was deleted from the BPD criteria when DSM-III blossomed into DSM-III-R, in order to avoid overlap with the criteria for dependent personality disorder. Instead, DSM-III-R emphasized the borderline patient's "frantic efforts to avoid real or imagined abandonment" (American Psychiatric Association 1987, p. 347). In practical terms, the NPD patient is likely to call you during your office hours and complain that you are doing a terrible job, whereas the BPD patient is more likely to call you sobbing at three in the morning, complaining of having "nothing inside."

There is also significant overlap between the Cluster B disorders and the personality disorders in other clusters. Thus, borderline and schizotypal patients show significant symptomatic overlap, as noted earlier in this chapter. I find it useful to examine my own countertransference in distinguishing these two types. With BPD patients I usually feel a bit anxious and "threatened." With schizotypal personality disorder patients, my reaction is more one of "bewildered beneficence"—that is, I am puzzled and somewhat alienated by the patient's peculiarities of thinking, but my caregiving capacities are firmly engaged.

Finally, the Cluster B disorders show significant overlap with numerous Axis I disorders. We have already noted the comorbidity between BPD and schizophrenia found in the Zimmerman and Coryell (1989) study; these authors also found significant comorbidity between APD and Axis I alcohol or drug abuse/dependence. BPD has often been seen as a variant form of mood disorder, and there is reasonable evidence to support this view (see Stone 1992 for a complete review). Beeber and colleagues (1984) find significant overlap between BPD and Liebowitz and Klein's (1981) concept of "hysteroid dysphoria," a syndrome of marked affective instability and rejection sensitivity. Similarly, Akiskal (1992) and his group emphasize the overlap—if not a common "neuropharmacologic substrate"—between BPD and various "subaffective" disorders.

Thus, it is often very hard to distinguish BPD from dysthymic disorder or (especially) cyclothymic disorder, based solely on symptomatic criteria. Once again, I find the dynamic perspective helpful here: although the "pure" cyclothymic individual shows considerable mood instability, he or she rarely uses such primitive defenses as splitting or projective identification, and virtually never "crosses over" into psychosis when faced with separation or loss. Of course, it is quite possible for an individual to be both cyclothymic and "borderline"!

Adjunctive Testing

Neuroimaging and Neuroendocrine Testing

Once again, most of the available data involve patients with BPD, and most of the summary that follows is drawn from the excellent review by Cowdry (1992). There is very little evidence of structural brain abnormalities in BPD patients. However, there is some evidence of abnormal SPEMs in BPD patients, similar to abnormalities seen in schizotypal and schizophrenic patients. BPD patients, like many major depression patients, may also show abnormalities of REM sleep, such as shorter REM latency or enhanced reduction of REM latency in response to the muscarinic agonist arecoline. Siever and Davis (1991) suggest that BPD and other patients with the dimension of "affective instability" may have "greater cholinergic responsiveness" than do control subjects. In contrast, although some studies have shown a high prevalence of nonsuppression on the dexamethasone suppression test (DST) in BPD patients, the DST has generally failed to distinguish BPD patients from patients with other personality disorders or major affective disorder. There are a few studies suggesting that thyroid-stimulating hormone (TSH) response to thyroid-releasing hormone (TRH) stimulation is blunted in BPD patients and that this abnormality is not correlated with the presence of major depression (Cowdry 1992). In contrast to many patients with major depression, patients with BPD—especially those with schizotypal features—may be hyperresponsive to catecholamine-releasing agents, such as amphetamines (Schulz et al. 1988).

With respect to APD, Cummings (1985) reviewed 14 electroencephalographic studies (1944–1978) of individuals with antisocial personality or those incarcerated for various types of crime. He found that, with the exception of two studies, between 24% and 78% of subjects showed various electroencephalogram (EEG) abnormalities. However, Marmar (1988) suggests that many of these EEG abnormalities may have been secondary to adolescent substance abuse.

There are few data on structural or neuroendocrine abnormalities in HPD or NPD.

Psychological Testing

Typical MMPI, Wechsler Adult Intelligence Scale (WAIS), and Rorschach patterns for the Cluster B disorders are summarized in Table 9–7. As a broad generalization, Cluster B individuals show elevation on scale 4 (psychopathic deviant) of the MMPI; do poorly on WAIS subtests requiring sustained effort (reflecting the impulsivity of these individuals); and show a low percentage of F, W, and M responses on the Rorschach (signifying poor reality testing, problem solving, and organizational abilities). Of particular interest is the resemblance of BPD and "remitted" schizophrenic patients on the Rorschach (see Siever and Klar 1986 for summary). Also useful in the diagnosis of BPD is the Diagnostic Interview for Borderlines (DIB), developed by Gunderson and colleagues (1981).

Treatment Directions and Goals

Liebowitz et al. (1986b) have provided an excellent review of the somatic and psychosocial treatment of the personality disorders. Clearly, the psychodynamic approach to the borderline patient alone could fill several volumes; what follows is necessarily a mere sketch of treatment.

Somatic Approaches

Most of the psychopharmacological literature relating to Cluster B disorders has focused on the treatment of BPD (Cowdry 1987). Cowdry has approached this issue in a manner that I have found

Table 9–7. Psychological testing for Cluster B personality disorders

Personality disorder	MMPI	WAIS	Rorschach
Antisocial	4-9/9-4 is "classic"; elevated scales 8, 6, 4 are seen in violent APD patients.	Low scores in verbal subtests reflect poor school history.	F+% is low; there is a high number of popular and animal responses; "weapons" (i.e., shapes perceived as guns, knives, etc.) are common; there is a low number of M and W responses.
Borderline	Scales 3, 4, 7 are elevated; if patient is deteriorating, scale 8 is elevated.	Results are noncontributory.	There are poor form level; contaminations; and self-references; similar to those in remitted schizophrenic patient.
Histrionic	2-3/3-2 is typical; in crisis, scale 2 is elevated above 70 T.	Verbal score is less than performance score, with low scores on information and arithmetic.	Cards are seen as "ugly" and "scary," but patient denies dysphoria; sexualized responses; low number of W and M responses relative to IQ.
Narcissistic	Low score on scale 0 (superficial relationships); scale 4 is elevated.	There is poor performance on tasks requiring persistence and detailed responses.	There is an emphasis on CF and pure C responses; F+% is not high.

Note. MMPI = Minnesota Multiphasic Personality Inventory; WAIS = Wechsler Adult Intelligence Scale.
Source. Extensively modified from Meyer 1983; Siever and Klar 1986.

useful: he attempts to identify treatable "co-morbid states" and "critical target symptoms." Thus, some patients with BPD may show prominent social isolation, mild thought disorder, or paranoid thinking. These individuals "may warrant a trial of maintenance antipsychotic medication in low doses" (Cowdry 1987, p. 16). The presence of clear-cut major depression in a BPD individual intuitively suggests a role for classical antidepressants; however, there is little evidence from controlled studies to support this strategy, and there is some evidence that it may "backfire." For example, Soloff et al. (1986) failed to find any association between response to amitriptyline in BPD and the presence or absence of major depression; moreover, some patients taking amitriptyline showed an increase in behavioral dyscontrol. Interestingly, haloperidol had significant positive effects on anxiety, hostility, depression, and schizotypal symptoms. This report, and early work by Brinkley and colleagues (1979), suggest that antipsychotics may exert a "broad spectrum" effect in BPD. Of course, any decision to use antipsychotics, particularly in this population, must be weighed against the risk of tardive dyskinesia and carefully discussed with the patient. The medications that have proved useful in some studies of BPD include carbamazepine, monoamine oxidase inhibitors (MAOIs), or lithium (see Cowdry 1987 for discussion). A recent open-label study of five BPD patients refractory to phenelzine and antipsychotic therapy found that fluoxetine may be useful in reducing depression, suicidality, and impulsivity; hostility and psychotic symptoms did not change significantly (Cornelius et al. 1991).

With respect to the other Cluster B disorders, the research data are far more limited. The syndrome of "hysteroid dysphoria," as noted above, may overlap with HPD. Liebowitz et al. (1986a) note the utility of phenelzine in this type of patient. There are very few pharmacological studies of NPD as such. Given the vulnerability to rejection seen in NPD, Liebowitz et al. (1986b) suggest that MAOIs may be helpful. Similarly, pharmacological approaches to APD per se have not been rigorously studied. To the extent that APD patients show aggressive or violent tendencies, the use of lithium, carbamazepine, or serotonergic agents (such as trazodone) may be reasonable. Adults with residual symptoms of attention deficit/hyperactivity disorder

(ADHD) who appear to be "borderline" or "sociopathic" may benefit from methylphenidate; for example, Stringer and Joseph (1983) found methylphenidate useful in two patients with APD and childhood histories of attention-deficit disorder. (Keep in mind, however, that some patients with BPD may react dysphorically when given methylphenidate [see Lucas et al. 1987].)

Psychosocial Approaches

The psychodynamic and behavioral approach to the Cluster B disorders is summarized in Table 9–8. For further discussion of this topic see Liebowitz et al. 1986b; Chodoff 1989; Reid and Burke 1989; and Linehan 1992.

As a generalization, all these disorders require the utmost care in two critical respects: when dealing with the patient's rapidly shifting mood states and (possibly) consequently shifting object relations; and when dealing with your own, often quite strong, feelings toward the patient. These two elements are linked in a fairly obvious way: when a "borderline" patient sees you as the "horrible," "punishing" monster who will exploit or abandon him or her—and expresses this as "diffuse, primitive, rage"—you are likely to have a rather strong negative reaction (especially when the conversation takes place at three in the morning and ends with the patient's slamming down the receiver). It is astoundingly easy to call a halt to therapy under such circumstances, using a variety of self-justifying ploys (e.g., "I can no longer treat this patient because he/she is not really motivated to change"; "This patient needs long-term hospitalization at the Institute for Living"; etc.). In such cases, supervision or consultation with a colleague is critical. I have found another element of treatment to be critical in dealing with Cluster B patients: the setting of limits. This applies to both the limits of what the therapist will tolerate and the limits of what he or she can provide. If you allow a narcissistic patient to exploit you repeatedly by phoning 10 times a day, "dropping in" at odd hours, failing to show up for appointments, and so forth, and these behaviors are not confronted, two things will surely happen: the patient will remain ill, and you will remain angry. At the same time, retaliatory behaviors on the part of the therapist (such as terminating

Table 9–8.   Psychodynamic and behavioral approaches to Cluster B personality disorders

Personality disorder	Treatment approach	
	Psychodynamic	Behavioral
Histrionic	Identify, explore, and interpret maladaptive patterns of choosing intimate partners (e.g., "need to please," needs for nurturance). Balance therapeutic "responding" and "withholding" in face of patient's dependency needs.	Reinforce warmth and genuineness; modify emotional excesses and attention getting. "Harness" patient's need to please by reinforcing gradual abatement of histrionic behaviors.
Narcissistic	Balance empathy and confrontation; explore patient's oversensitivity to therapist's empathic failures; help patient heal incomplete sense of self, especially low self-esteem.	"Model" new, more adaptive behaviors via role playing; use "distraction" to reduce impulsivity.
Antisocial	Patient is very difficult to treat in one-to-one psychotherapy; countertransferance may make alliance impossible.	Consider group therapy in institutional setting; reinforce prosocial behaviors. It is not clear if aversive methods are effective long-term.
Borderline	Focus on fragile sense of identity and rapidly shifting feelings toward therapist and significant others; help patient identify feelings behind actions; attend carefully to countertransference; titrate limit setting and "here and now" supportive approach against exploration and interpretation.	Provide impulse-control training; provide social skills training via role playing and videos; help make self-destructive behaviors ungratifying; "target" specific behaviors for each session and work toward specific goals; help patient problem-solve specific maladaptive behaviors, such as self-injury in response to "rejection."

Source. Extensively modified from G. Adler 1981; Chodoff 1989; Reid and Burke 1989.

treatment) often lead to precisely the same results—except that the patient will remain ill outside of treatment, and you will remain angry with both the patient and yourself. The setting of limits thus requires a delicate balance of empathy and self-assertiveness on the therapist's part.

Consider the following vignette.

Vignette

A 24-year-old female with BPD had been in treatment with a psychodynamically oriented therapist for 3 months. The patient had a long history of mild, self-injurious behavior (e.g., episodic, superficial wrist cutting) that had been explored but "tolerated" by the therapist. Near the end of one session, the patient informed the therapist that she had "a neat little gun" at home and that from time to time, she thought about shooting herself. The therapist replied that work as an outpatient could not continue under that sort of threat and that two alternatives were available to the patient: enter an inpatient unit immediately or give up the gun.

The therapist further stipulated that "proof" would be necessary that the gun had been relinquished. At first, the patient reacted with sarcasm and anger (e.g., "You don't trust me, do you? You're looking for an excuse to dump me in some nut house"). The therapist replied that the main concern at this point was the patient's safety, and that no "trust" was possible if the patent were dead. The patient sullenly agreed to "get rid of the gun" and to call the therapist the next day to "check in." Five days later, the therapist received a letter from a friend of the patient, stating that she (the friend) had been given the gun and that she had disassembled it. Work in outpatient therapy continued.

I have found that the treatment of patients with Cluster B disorders—particularly BPD and NPD—benefits from the careful "titration" of so-called supportive and exploratory approaches. (This distinction is a bit misleading, since a properly timed interpretation can be very "supportive.") "Support" is a much-maligned and misunderstood term in the psychotherapy world. It is far from patting the patient on the shoulder and saying, "There, there. Things will get better. Buck up!" "Supportive" therapy, rather, has two main goals: to reinforce the "higher level" defenses and coping mechanisms available to the patient and to provide direction and guidance ("ego-lending") in certain critical situations (Pies 1991; Sifneos 1971). The previous case vignette illustrates how an initially alienating intervention by the therapist can cement the therapeutic alliance in the long run. Keep in mind that while the vignette focuses on individual psychotherapy, there is an abundant literature on the use of group or family therapy formats in the treatment of Cluster B (and other) personality disorders. This is not to say, however, that such formats are especially successful. Thus, both BPD and NPD patients may have great difficulty adapting to, and staying in, a group therapy format (G. Adler 1989; Gunderson 1989). In some cases, though—particularly with some BPD patients—I have found that a group setting can "diffuse" the intense (and threatening) transference reactions that often develop in "one-to-one" treatment.

Finally, a brief note on the treatment of APD. One infers from Table 9–8 a rather bleak view of treatment for these patients, and, unfortunately, that seems to be the experience of most clinicians (including the present writer). As Reid and Burke (1989) put it, "Many observers think that even where external controls exist, such as parole, prison, or hospital, individual psychotherapeutic relationships rarely change sociopaths' behavior" (p. 2745). On the other hand, many clinicians believe that sociopathy exists along a continuum of criminality and aggressiveness on the one hand, and essentially narcissistic vulnerability on the other. It may be that APD patients on the more "narcissistic" end of the spectrum can—within the context of long-term individual treatment—achieve some modest but permanent gains. In my experience, work with APD patients frequently requires the "adjunctive" use of support groups, parole officers, spouse, and family members, in order to "keep the patient in line." This is particularly true when substance abuse accompanies or exacerbates the sociopathy. In such cases, I make Alcoholics Anonymous (AA) or similar approaches a mandatory (and non-negotiable) part of treatment.

The Anxious/Fearful Cluster (Cluster C): Avoidant, Dependent, Obsessive-Compulsive (and Passive-Aggressive) Personality Disorders

The Central Concept

Vignette

Mr. Langsam Tsiser, a single, 43-year-old German-born engineer, was referred for psychotherapy by his employer. The patient presented with the statement, "I really do not understand these people at the office. Perhaps they have nothing better to do than to send me for therapy." While the patient had a solid academic record and was viewed as a "competent" engineer, he had a long history of difficulties with both teachers and employers. They typically regarded him as "a slow worker," albeit with "high standards of performance." Often, employers found the patient to be "defensive" when faced with constructive criticism. The patient typically responded by saying that "they expect me to work like a horse at that place. The fact is, I am probably the best one they have there." The patient would often get his work assignments in late, and, in one or two instances, appeared to do an intentionally poor job, given how easy it was. This pattern affected the productivity of the patient's entire office staff, which led to the current referral.

At the initial interview, the patient presented the evaluator with a detailed list of all the tasks he had successfully completed in the past year. He objected to the evaluator's open-ended questions, stating, "If you had prepared yourself a bit better for this, we could have accomplished the interview much more efficiently." His affect was generally tense and constricted. When it came time to decide on the date of a follow-up appointment, the patient took nearly 5 minutes, flipping through his appointment book and posing one objection after another to the proposed time.

Mr. Tsiser, as you may have surmised, combines personality traits from two DSM-III-R Cluster C disorders: passive-aggressive personality disorder (PAPD) and obsessive-compulsive personality disorder (OCPD). The evident traits of PAPD include procrastinating and feeling irritable when faced with unwanted chores; feeling that others make unreasonable demands, and that one is doing a much better job than others think he or she is doing; avoiding obligations by conveniently "forgetting" them; and obstructing the work of others by failing to do one's own share. Patients with OCPD also have difficulty completing tasks on time, but it is mainly their perfectionism and rigidity that reduce their efficiency. OCPD patients also show an unreasonable insistence that others "do things my way"; an excessive devotion to work or productivity; constricted emotional and personal lives; indecisiveness; preoccupation with "order," rules, and lists; a tendency to "hoard" worthless objects; and a reluctance to give of themselves in the absence of personal gain. Together, OCPD and PAPD have a prevalence of around 5% in the community (Zimmerman and Coryell 1989). Avoidant personality disorder (AVPD) and dependent personality disorder (DPD) appear to be less common. AVPD is characterized by a pervasive, long-standing pattern of social discomfort and fear of scrutiny or disapproval. Individuals with AVPD usually show great reluctance to form intimate relationships in the absence of "guaranteed," uncritical acceptance, which, as you might guess, dramatically cuts down on the number of one's close friends or confidant(e)s. Nevertheless, unlike schizoid individuals, AVPD individuals do desire social relationships.

Dependent personality disorder is characterized by a pervasive and long-standing pattern of "leaning on" others for making everyday decisions, and an excessive compliance with the opinions or demands of others, even when the individual believes they are wrong. DPD individuals rarely show personal initiative, often feel helpless or anxious when alone or "abandoned," and react to perceived criticism with excessive "hurt feelings."

It may not be easy to discern the common feature of the Cluster C disorders—namely, a deep and pervasive anxiety—because of the "character armor" worn by some affected individuals. Thus, the obsessive-compulsive individual may appear haughty and a bit tyrannical at times, apparently quite unlike the "timid" dependent personality. We will review evidence showing that the "surface structures" of these disorders may be misleading, and that their "deep structures" (to borrow Noam Chomsky's term) are actually quite similar. Nevertheless, as Siever and Klar (1986) note, "the rationale for including these disorders in one cluster is . . . less than compelling" (p. 303). These authors cite several studies showing that obsessive traits, for example, cluster distinctly from oral, dependent traits. DSM-IV decided to relegate passive-aggressive personality disorder to the dustbin of "Personality Disorders Not Otherwise Specified," perhaps in recognition that most PAPD individuals do not appear outwardly "anxious," unless someone else is hurrying them along.

Historical Development of the Concept

The individual Cluster C disorders grew out of disparate historical traditions (Vaillant and Perry 1985). Thus, the term "passive-aggressive" was first used by American miltary psychiatrists in World War II and was later solidified by Veterans Administration studies. (Our European counterparts are apparently not as convinced of the validity of this symptom cluster.) The DSM-II formulation of this disorder emphasized the psychoanalytic concept of the "oral-sadistic" character (Widiger et al. 1988).

In contrast, the term "obsessive-compulsive" grew out of Freud's work on the defense mechanisms that (he believed) underlie obsessions. In Europe, the term "anankastic personality" (from the Greek *anankastos,* meaning "forced") became roughly synonymous with OCPD. In DSM-II, the term "compulsive personality" was used to describe "a type of personality characterizd by rigidity, over-conscientiousness, extreme inhibition, and inability to relax" (Freedman et al. 1972). DSM-III continued to use the term "compulsive personality disorder," in order to avoid confusion with the Axis I condition, obsessive-compulsive disorder (OCD). However, DSM-III-R restored the "O-word," arguing that "important features of the [personality] disorder are captured by the term 'obsessive'" (American Psychiatric Association 1987, p. 429). As we will see, the personality disorder OCPD has far less to do with the Axis I "neurotic" disorder OCD than once was believed.

Dependent personality disorder has its roots in the concept of the "oral character," as developed by Abraham and Freud (discussed later in this section). Because dependent traits, self-doubt, and passivity occur in a variety of psychiatric disorders, it is not entirely clear that DPD is a disorder in its own right (Vaillant and Perry 1985).

Finally, AVPD, a newcomer to our nosology, first arose in DSM-III; prior to that classification, AVPD-type individuals probably would have been classified as "schizoid," "dependent," or "inadequate" personalities (Vaillant and Perry 1985). AVPD underwent some interesting transformations from DSM-III to DSM-III-R. As Widiger et al. (1988) note, "The DSM-III . . . criteria . . . may have focused too heavily on social inhibition. DSM-III-R includes additional features of the psychoanalytic concept of the inhibited phobic character, such as an exaggeration of the risks in everyday life and an inordinate fear of being embarrassed" (p. 790). The DSM-IV concept of AVPD is quite like that of DSM-III-R.

The Biopsychosocial Perspective

Biological Factors

We have far less familial, genetic, and biological information for the Cluster C disorders than for many of the other personality disorders we have discussed. DSM-III-R noted that OCPD "is apparently more common among first-degree biologic relatives of people with this disorder than among the general population" (American Psychiatric Association 1987, p. 355), but cited "no information" for the familial patterns of the other Cluster C disorders. There are data indicating that "submissiveness" is more likely to be concordant in monozygotic than in dizygotic twins, suggesting that DPD may have some genetic underpinnings (Vaillant and Perry 1985). There are also some interesting male-female differences in DPD and OCPD, which we will discuss below.

There appear to be very few neuroendocrine, electroencephalographic, or neuroimaging studies of the Cluster C disorders per se. Viewed dimensionally (see Siever and Davis 1991), "anxious/inhibited individuals" often show pathophysiological abnormalities (e.g., higher tonic levels of cortical and sympathetic arousal, lower sedation thresholds, decreased habituation to novel stimuli) when compared with various control groups.

Finally, some intriguing work was recently presented by Goldman and colleagues (1992), in which 55 patients with major depression underwent assessment of "perceptual asymmetry" on dichotic listening tests. Twenty-seven of these patients were also assessed via structured interviews for the presence of personality disorders. The study found that "Cluster C" traits were associated with less "left ear advantage" (LEA) for complex tones, reflecting diminished right-hemisphere activity. (In contrast, schizoid traits were associated with greater LEA.) The meaning of these findings is unclear, but they suggest that anxious, avoidant individuals may have peculiarities of cerebral dominance.

Psychological Factors

If forced to summarize the psychodynamics of the Cluster C disorders, you might say this: disappointment in others or fear of one's own impulses lead, respectively, to a pattern of defiance or avoidance. For example, in AVPD, the patient's timidity may stem from the fear "that his or her impulses will fly out of control and cause danger, guilt, or embarrassment. The avoidant behavior typically helps to maintain a denial of an unconscious wish or impulse" (Frances and Widiger 1989, p. 2760; see MacKinnon and Michels 1971 for further discussion). Similarly, in DPD, "when dependent needs are stimulated, passivity results because the individual finds these needs unacceptable" (Perry 1989a, p. 2765; see Whitman et al. 1954, for further discussion). Moreover, the dependent individual fears criticism (as does the APD individual) and tries to "smooth over" trouble with others rather than confront them. In a slight twist to this dynamic, the passive-aggressive individual "externalizes an internal conflict over hostility and dependency and therefore sees others as frustrating his or her dependent needs. The person then reacts with superficial compliance but covertly hostile behavior" (Perry 1989b, p. 2785).

Obsessive-compulsive personality disorder requires a bit of historical commentary. You probably know that early psychoanalytic formulations of this disorder emphasized the concept of "anality" and saw OCPD and OCD as lying along the same dynamic continuum. Even in the 1970s, one textbook made the following summary:

> [T]he period between the ages of 9 months and 2 years usually sees the initiation of parent-child struggles over toilet training, bedtime hours, and the control of hostile expression . . . problems related to strict toilet training are reflected in the so-called "anal character" who shows the triad of (1) parsimony, (2) excessive neatness, and (3) stubborness." (Freedman et al. 1972, p. 373)

Today, both pillars of this view have been shaken if not pulled down. There is little empirical evidence to support the link between OCPD and "toilet training" problems, or between OCPD and its near-namesake, OCD (Nemiah 1985; Vaillant and Perry 1985). For example, most people with OCPD do not develop the "neurosis" of OCD; conversely, many patients with OCD do not have premorbid "obsessional" character traits.

Nevertheless, struggles between child and parents during Erikson's stage of "autonomy vs. shame and doubt"—which does coincide with Freud's anal stage—may play a role in OCPD (Vaillant and Perry 1985). As Vaillant and Perry (1985) put it, "Attention to the details and minutiae of childhood tasks may become a major way for the child to avoid parental criticism and to win affection and attention" (p. 984). You can see how a behavioral model might explain the development of OCPD—in effect, as the consequence of parental reinforcement of obsessive traits. Similarly, cognitive theorists would point to the "self-defeating and irrational cognitions" of the individual with one of the Cluster C disorders—for example, the internalized notion that "I must do everything well and have the approval of others, or else I'm an incompetent jerk."

Sociocultural Factors

Familial, ethnic, and cultural influences undoubtedly affect the prevalence of Cluster C disorders, but the data in this regard are few. DPD is more often diagnosed in women than in men; it is also more common in the younger children of a sibship than in the older children (Vaillant and Perry 1985). In contrast, OCPD is more frequently diagnosed in males, and—based on anecdotal data—appears to be more common in the older children of a sibship. We did not discuss these gender- and sibship-related differences under our "biological" heading because there are so few biological studies of the Cluster C disorders; nevertheless, these male-female differences could have biological underpinnings. Most workers, however, favor a sociocultural explanation. For example, Kagan and Moss (1960) have suggested that American society punishes dependent behavior in males but rewards it in females (Perry 1989a). In contrast, the "obsessive" traits of punctuality, orderliness, and emotional restraint might be encouraged in men, because these traits are adaptive in highly industrialized, technological societies, in which men are preferentially employed. As Vaillant and Perry (1985) put it, "In Western societies, compulsive personality traits are heavily reinforced by the Northern European Protestant work ethic" (p. 984).

One could argue, of course, that a cultural bias toward inculcating "dependency" in females would not explain the high rate of diagnosed disorder (DPD) in females; after all, wouldn't the dependency-promoting culture sanction this trait in its female members and discourage "pathologizing" it? Conversely, if obsessive traits are valued in men, wouldn't diagnosis be biased against "seeing" this as a disorder in men? Perhaps this seeming contradiction may be resolved in this way: because of the divergent pressures on men and women in Western industrialized society, a subgroup within each gender acquires a clearly pathological version of the "acceptable" traits for that gender; that is, a certain number of women become "too dependent," while a certain percentage of men become "too obsessive." The particular individuals who make up these subgroups might very well be genetically predisposed (perhaps by virtue of their gender) to acquire these disabling traits. On the other hand, they could come from the most "stereotypic" families—that is, those that most forcefully inculcate gender-based differences.

With regard to sibship, "obsessive" traits might also be reinforced in the oldest children of a sibship, who are traditionally put in charge of their younger brothers and sisters. Conversely, the younger members of a sibship might be under subtle pressures to "go along and get along" with their older siblings, thus developing dependent traits.

Pitfalls in the Differential Diagnosis

Organic Disorders

The Cluster C traits of anxiety, avoidance, passivity, excessive dependency, and obsessionality are seen in a wide variety of "medical" disorders. Many of these have already been discussed in our chapter on anxiety disorders (Chapter 6), under differential diagnosis. Lishman (1987) notes that after head injury, the individual may appear tense, ruminative, and indecisive. Alternatively, the brain-injured patient may show "a passive and childish dependence . . . with petulant behavior" (Lishman 1987, p. 161). The "temporal lobe syndrome" described by Bear and Fedio (1977), although not supported as a distinct entity by some studies (Lishman 1987), may present with interictal traits of "hypermoralism," obsessionality, dependence, and restricted affect, all of which may be mistaken for OCPD. Clearly, the key to correct diagnosis is a good, longitudinal history—remember that personality disorders are usually lifelong disturbances. Any marked change in personality, especially after age 40, should initiate a thorough search for organic causes.

Psychiatric Disorders

Conditions that may be confused with specific Cluster C personality disorders are summarized in Table 9–9.

We have already discussed the differential diagnosis of AVPD versus schizoid personality disorder. A more vexing issue is the overlap between AVPD and social phobia. Liebowitz et al. (1986a), noting that "many individuals with pervasive social anxiety are classified . . . as having avoidant personality disorder," argue that "the belief that personality disorder can always be distinguished from chronic affective or anxiety dysregulation requires reconsideration" (p. 96). We will examine the pharmacological implications of this point in our treatment section. For now, you should bear in mind that AVPD is often more pervasive than social phobia, since the latter may be limited to, for example, public-speaking anxiety. However, more pervasive forms of social phobia may shade imperceptibly into AVPD, and the two disorders may coexist.

Although, in theory, OCD and OCPD are "discontinuous," there are cases in which the distinction is not clear. For example, you may see a perfectionistic, overly scrupulous individual whose frequent house cleaning is ego-syntonic until it begins to interfere with social and occupational functioning—at which time the features of OCD may be present (Rasmussen and Eisen 1992). OCPD may sometimes resemble schizoid personality disorder, because both types of patient may show constricted affect and value work over relationships; however, the patient with OCPD is less prone to (ego-syntonic) social isolation than is the schizoid individual (Vaillant and Perry 1985).

Passive-aggressive personality disorder is sometimes hard to distinguish from DPD; however, the features of resentment, obstructionism, and scorn for people in authority are more typical of PAPD. Vaillant and Perry (1985) point out that, in the past, women who would meet the criteria for PAPD have been labeled as "histrionic" or "borderline." However, "the passive-aggressive personality is more stable and less flamboyant, dramatic, affective, and openly aggressive than the histrionic and borderline personalities" (Vaillant and Perry 1985, p. 986).

Table 9–9. Differential diagnosis of Cluster C personality disorders

Personality disorder	Conditions in differential diagnosis
Avoidant	Schizoid personality disorder Social phobia Agoraphobia
Dependent	Agoraphobia Passive-aggressive personality disorder[a]
Obsessive-compulsive	Obsessive-compulsive disorder Schizoid personality disorder
Passive-aggressive[a]	Oppositional defiant disorder (preempts PAPD if patient is under 18 years of age) Dependent personality disorder Histrionic personality disorder Borderline personality disorder

[a]In DSM-IV, considered a "personality disorder not otherwise specified."

Adjunctive Testing

Neuroendocrine and Neuroimaging Techniques

A recent computerized search of the literature failed to turn up any studies in this area, which is consistent with the review by Siever and Davis (1991). Clearly, electroencephalographic, positron-emission tomography, magnetic resonance imaging, and neuroendocrine studies of the Cluster C disorders are sorely needed.

Neuropsychiatric Testing

The MMPI profiles of AVPD and DPD patients are similar in many ways, reflecting, perhaps, Meyer's view that "dependent personality disorders can be seen as successful avoidant personality disorders. They have achieved a style that elicits the desired relationships, though at the cost of any consistent self-expression" (Meyer 1983, p. 206). Thus, on the MMPI, both AVPD and DPD patients may show the 2-7/7-2 profile (2, depression; 7, psychasthenia). Meyer asserts that for both disorders, a low scale 5 (masculinity-femininity) score is common, reflecting "acceptance of the stereotypal feminine role." Scale 0 tends to be elevated in both conditions, owing to social withdrawal. With PAPD, the 3-4/4-3 pattern is common (3, hysteria; 4, psychopathic deviant), with scale 4 reflecting the aggressive component of the individual's temperament. In OCPD, MMPI scales tend to show a "low profile"; that is, scales are rarely elevated, owing to the patient's reticence. An exception may be scale 9 (hypomania), which may be elevated as a result of "how autocratic and dominant the individual is in personal relationships" (Meyer 1983, p. 209).

On the Rorschach, AVPD and DPD patients again show some responses in common (e.g., responses of passivity such as seeing animals being killed). The DPD patient often produces reponses in concert with the perceived expectations of the examiner. The OCPD patient tends to show many Dd responses, a high F+%, and relatively few color-based responses—reflecting (respectively) the OCPD patient's preoccupation with minor details, relatively high "ego-strength," and emotional constriction (Carr 1985). The PAPD patient shows responses on the Rorschach that reflect his or her pattern of relating (e.g., seeing "people arguing," or "animals sneaking around," etc.). PAPD patients may also show odd combinations of aggressive and passive responses, such as "children with guns" (Meyer 1983).

Treatment Directions and Goals

Somatic Approaches

Ellison and Adler (1990) have summarized the studies suggesting a role for medication in the Cluster C disorders; specifically, beta-blockers, MAOIs, and alprazolam may prove useful. This approach is based more on extrapolation from the treatment of social phobia than on direct, placebo-controlled studies of Cluster C patients. Thus, Liebowitz et al. (1986a) found phenelzine to be effective in the treatment of social phobia and imply that it could be useful in other "rejection-sensitive" states. Ellison and Adler related a case of a 37-year-old man with social anxiety but not a fear of "humiliation" in public; low self-esteem; and hypersensitivity to rejection. The authors believed that a diagnosis of AVPD was warranted. Alprazolam 0.5 mg tid proved effective, with the patient noting greater ease in joining group conversations and attending social activities.

There is little empirical evidence that medication per se is useful in the treatment of PAPD patients, and the risk of noncompliance, misuse, or overdose must be considered carefully (Perry 1989b). Roughly the same may be said of patients with DPD. Whereas the pharmacological treatment of OCD is now well established, the use of medication for OCPD has not yet been substantiated by empirical trials.

Psychosocial Approaches

Psychodynamic, interpersonal, and cognitive-behavioral approaches have all been applied to the Cluster C disorders, utilizing individual, group, and family formats (Frances and Widiger 1989; Perry 1989a, 1989b; Salzman 1989). For all this therapeutic activity, the course and prognosis of these disorders is largely unknown, or—in the case of PAPD—rather unencouraging (Vaillant and Perry 1985). Countertransference feelings—almost always "negative"—are a major problem in the treatment of these disorders. Thus, the patient with OCPD may invite protracted power struggles with the therapist; the patient with DPD may evoke the therapist's fear of being "sucked dry," etc. Much of the dynamic work with Cluster C patients entails the "corrective emotional experience" of sympathetic and empathic understanding. The direct encouragement of assertive behavior is also appropriate, "after establishing the patient's sense of security in the treatment relationship" (Frances and Widiger 1989, p. 2761). On the other hand, becoming overly directive runs the risk of setting up a pathological transference-countertransference relationship, in which the patient manipulates the "authoritarian" therapist into "running" his or her life (Perry 1989b).

Addressing the cognitive distortions common to Cluster C individuals may be helpful—for example, examining the assumption of an AVPD patient that "it would be horrible if I got rejected by someone." Occasionally, so-called paradoxical approaches may be useful— for example, encouraging an AVPD patient to "get yourself rejected" in a social relationship (Frances and Widiger 1989). However, in my experience, such paradoxical interventions may backfire if the patient has some "borderline" features (Greenberg and Pies 1983). Finally, despite our earlier call for "empathy," there is also a place for well-timed confrontation and limit setting with some Cluster C patients, particularly the hostile and demanding passive-aggressive patient (Hackett and Stern 1991).

Details of the psychotherapeutic treatment of Cluster C individuals may be found in the sources cited above.

Integrated Case History

Mr. Tempesta, a 24-year-old single male employed as a firefighter, was seen in the ER after making superficial lacerations on his wrists. He seemed despondent and tearful and was quickly referred to the psychiatric resident on call. The patient stated that he had gotten into an argument with his most recent girlfriend "because I think she's been fooling around on me." The patient had been drinking prior to the altercation and acknowledged episodic alcohol abuse. He had cut his wrists in the past, usually in the context of some social turmoil. The current self-injury occurred when, according to the patient, "my girl told me it was none of my damn business what she did after she left my apartment." He denied recent history of severe depression, appetite disturbance, change in weight, or sleep disturbance. However, the patient did acknowledge, "I can't even remember the last time I was really happy." He also gave a history of considerable affective instability that did not reach the level of frank mania or major depressive episodes.

The patient had never had a psychiatric hospitalization. However, because he continued to express suicidal ideation, as well as veiled threats to "even up the score" with his girlfriend, he was admitted to the inpatient psychiatric unit.

Developmental history obtained from the patient's mother was notable for head injury at age 3, with brief loss of consciousness. Although the mother initially attributed the injury to "an accident," close questioning revealed that the patient had been struck by his father, who "was pretty drunk at the time." The patient's mother had also been physically abused by her husband and had "taken off for a few months" throughout the course of her rather stormy marriage. During these absences, the patient had been left alone with his father, or else "shipped off" to a maternal aunt.

The patient had a poor school history, with many incidents of truancy, trouble with authority figures, and so forth. He had managed to graduate from high school with below-average grades, and supported himself with a variety of menial jobs. He had passed the civil service exam, however, and was able to secure a job with the local fire deparatment. Recently, he had had an altercation with his supervisor, resulting in suspension from work.

Mental status exam on the unit showed no evidence of frank cognitive impairment or psychosis. His affect was labile, with episodes of angry outbursts interspersed with tearfulness. On less structured interviewing, the patient related feeling "empty inside . . . like I got to have somebody around all the time just to feel whole." At times he felt "like I'm not really there . . . I got to cut myself sometimes just to make sure I'm real." He denied pertinent symptoms of a schizophrenic nature.

On psychological testing, the patient showed elevation of scales 3, 4, and 7 (hysteria, psychopathic deviance, psychasthenia, respectively). The Rorschach showed poor form level and many contaminations. The psychologist's comment on the Rorschach testing was, "This almost looks like a remitted schizophrenic."

Computed tomography scan with contrast was within normal limits. A sleep-deprived EEG showed no focal epileptiform activity, but did show some abnormalities described as "mild local suppression of alpha activity" in temporal regions, "suggestive of old head injury." Evoked potential testing revealed reduction in P300 amplitude.

The working diagnosis by the inpatient psychiatric resident was "Axis I: Episodic alcohol abuse. Axis II: Borderline personality disorder. Axis III. s/p head trauma with possible electroencephalographic abnormalities (? related to Axis II symptoms)."

In light of the patient's affective instability and somewhat abnormal EEG, a trial on valproate (Depakote) was begun, with plasma levels maintained at around 60 ng/ml. The patient was also engaged in a brief, supportive form of psychotherapy, focusing on managing stress, identifying precipitants of self-injurious behavior, and finding alternatives to alcohol abuse. After discharge from the unit, he participated in a group for patients with severe personality disturbance and also attended AA meetings. Follow-up 6 months after discharge found the patient affectively stable, with no more instances of wrist cutting. He still experienced feelings of inner "emptiness" and difficulty being alone. However, he was better able to deal with these feelings without recourse to self-injury or substance abuse.

Conclusion

The diagnosis and treatment of personality disorders is, to say the least, a therapeutic challenge. Aside from the ambiguities of presentation, there is the vexing problem of comorbidity—both with other personality disorders and with Axis I disorders. The comorbidity of personality disorder and substance abuse is a particularly difficult management problem (O'Malley et al. 1990). The ego-syntonic quality of the personality disorders makes them especially refractory to traditional "insight-oriented" psychotherapies; unfortunately, medications, too, have only a limited role. If all this sounds terribly pessimistic, you should take some encouragement from D. Adler (1990), who reminds us that "therapeutic nihilism often results from unrealistic goals. . . . we must counter our own rigidities with flexibility. The focus of treatment is on helping people, rather than pursuing theoretical therapeutic ideals" (p. 39).

References

Adler D: Personality disorders: theory and psychotherapy, in Treating Personality Disorders (New Dir Ment Health Serv 47). Edited by Adler D. San Francisco, CA, Jossey-Bass, 1990, pp 17–42

Adler G: The borderline-narcissistic personality disorder continuum. Am J Psychiatry 138:46–50, 1981

Adler G: Narcissistic personality disorder, in Treatments of Psychiatric Disorders, Vol 3. Washington, DC, American Psychiatric Association, 1989, pp 2736–2741

Akhtar S: Schizoid personality disorder: a synthesis of descriptive features. Am J Psychother 41:499–518, 1987

Akiskal HS: Borderline: an adjective still in search of a noun, in Handbook of Borderline Disorders. Edited by Silver D, Rosenbluth M. Madison, CT, International Universities Press, 1992, pp 155–176

American Psychiatric Association: Diagnostic and Statistical Manual of Mental Disorders [DSM-I]. Washington, DC, American Psychiatric Association, 1952

American Psychiatric Association: Diagnostic and Statistical Manual of Mental Disorders, 2nd Edition. Washington, DC, American Psychiatric Association, 1968

American Psychiatric Association: Diagnostic and Statistical Manual of Mental Disorders, 3rd Edition. Washington, DC, American Psychiatric Association, 1980

American Psychiatric Association: Diagnostic and Statistical Manual, 3rd Edition, Revised. Washington, DC, American Psychiatric Association, 1987

American Psychiatric Association: Diagnostic and Statistical Manual, 4th Edition. Washington, DC, American Psychiatric Association, 1994

Andrulonis PA, Glueck BC, Stroebel CR, et al: Organic brain dysfunction and the borderline syndrome. Psychiatr Clin North Am 4:47–66, 1981

Arieti S: Interpretation of Schizophrenia, 2nd Edition. New York, Basic Books, 1974

Bear DM, Fedio P: Quantitative analysis of interictal behavior in temporal lobe epilepsy. Arch Neurol 34:454–467, 1977

Bear D, Levin D, Blumer D, et al: Interictal behavior in hospitalized temporal lobe epileptics: relationship to idiopathic paychiatric syndromes. J Neurol Neurosurg Psychiatry 45:481–488, 1982

Beeber AR, Kline MD, Pies RW, et al: Hysteroid dysphoria in depressed inpatients. J Clin Psychiatry 45:164–166, 1984

Brinkley J, Eitman S, Freidel R, et al: Low-dose neuroleptic regimens in the treatment of borderline patients. Arch Gen Psychiatry 36:319–326, 1979

Cadoret RJ, O'Gorman TW, Troughton E, et al: Alcoholism and antisocial personality: interrelationships, genetic, and environmental factors. Arch Gen Psychiatry 42:161–167, 1985

Carr AC: Psychological testing of personality, in Comprehensve Textbook of Psychiatry/IV, 4th Edition, Vol 1. Edited by Kaplan HI, Sadock BJ. Baltimore, MD, Williams & Wilkins, 1985, pp 514–535

Chapin D, Wightman L, Lycaki H, et al: Difference in the reaction time between subjects with schizotypal and borderline personality disorder. Am J Psychiatry 144:948–950, 1987

Chodoff P: Histrionic personality Disorder, in Treatments of Psychiatric Disorders, Vol 3. Washington, DC, American Psychiatric Association, 1989, pp 2727–2736

Cleckley H: The Mask of Sanity, 4th Edition. St Louis, MO, CV Mosby, 1964

Coccaro EF, Siever LJ, Klor HM, et al: Serotonergic studies in patients with affective and personality disorders: correlates with suicidal and impulsive aggressive behavior. Arch Gen Psychiatry 46:587–599, 1989 [correction: 47:124, 1990]

Cornelius JR, Soloff PH, Perel JM, et al: A preliminary trial of fluoxetine in refractory borderline patients. J Clin Psychopharmacol 11:116–120, 1991

Cowdry RW: Psychopharmacology of borderline personality disorder: a review. J Clin Psychiatry 48 (No 8, Suppl):15–22, 1987

Cowdry RW: Psychobiology and psychopharmacology of borderline personality disorder, in Handbook of Borderline Disorders. Edited by Silver D, Rosenbluth M. Madison, CT, International Universities Press, 1992, pp 495–508

Cummings JL: Clinical Neuropsychiatry. Orlando, FL, Grune & Stratton, 1985

Ellison JM, Adler D: A strategy for the pharmacotherapy of personality disorders, in Treating Personality Disorders (New Dir Ment Health Serv 47). Edited by Adler D. San Francisco, CA, Jossey-Bass, 1990, pp 43–64

Frances AJ, Widiger T: Avoidant personality disorder, in Treatments of Psychiatric Disorders, Vol 3. Washington, DC, American Psychiatric Association, 1989, pp 2759–2761

Freedman AM, Kaplan HI, Sadock BJ: Modern Synopsis of Psychiatry. Baltimore, MD, Williams & Wilkins, 1972

Glueck S, Glueck E: Delinquents and Non-Delinquents in Perspective. Cambridge, MA, Harvard University Press, 1968

Goldberg SC, Schulz SC, Schulz PM, et al: Borderline and schizotypal personality disorders treated with low-dose thiothixine vs placebo. Arch Gen Psychiatry 43:680–690, 1986

Goldman RG, Bruder GE, Stewart JW, et al: Personality and perceptual asymmetry in depression, in New Research Program and Abstracts, 145th Annual Meeting of the American Psychiatric Association, Washington, DC, May 1992, NR90, p 69

Gorten G, Akhtar S: The literature on personality disorders, 1985–88: trends, issues, and controversies. Hosp Community Psychiatry 41:39–51, 1990

Grant I: Personality disorders, in Harrison's Principles of Internal Medicine, 12th Edition. Edited by Wilson JD, Braunwald E, Isselbacher KJ, et al. New York, McGraw-Hill, 1991, pp 2135–2139

Greenberg R, Pies R: Is paradoxical intention risk-free? A review and case report. J Clin Psychiatry 44:66–69, 1983

Gunderson JG: Borderline personality disorder, in Treatments of Psychiatric Disorders, Vol 3. Washington, DC, American Psychiatric Association, 1989, pp 2749–2759

Gunderson JG, Singer MT: Defining borderline patients: an overview. Am J Psychiatry 132:1–10, 1985

Gunderson JG, Zanarini MC: Current overview of the borderline diagnosis. J Clin Psychiatry 48 (No 8, Suppl):5–11, 1987

Gunderson JG, Kolb JE, Austin V: The Diagnostic Interview for Borderline Patients. Am J Psychiatry 138:896–903, 1981

Hackett TP, Stern TA: Suicide and other disruptive states, in Massachusetts General Hospital Handbook of General Hospital Psychiatry, 3rd Edition. Edited by Cassem NH. St Louis, MO, Mosby Year Book, 1991, pp 281–307

Herman JL, Perry JC, van der Kolk BA: Childhood trauma in borderline personality disorder. Am J Psychiatry 146:490–495, 1989

Kagan J, Moss H: The stability of passive and dependent behavior from childhood through adulthood. Child Dev 31:577–591, 1960

Kagan J, Reznick JS, Snidman N: The physiology and psychology of behavioral inhibition in young children. Child Dev 58:1459–1473, 1987

Kaplan HI, Sadock BJ: Synopsis of Psychiatry, 5th Edition. Baltimore, MD, Williams & Wilkins, 1988

Kernberg O: Borderline Conditions and Pathological Narcissism. New York, Jason Aronson, 1975

Kohut H: The Restoration of the Self. New York, International Universities Press, 1977

Kutcher SP, Blackwood DHR, St Clair D, et al: Auditory P300 in borderline personality disorder and schizophrenia. Arch Gen Psychiatry 44:645–650, 1987

Lasch C: The Culture of Narcissism. New York, Warner Books, 1979

Liebowitz MR: Somatic therapy, in Treatments of Psychiatric Disorders, Vol 3. Washington, DC, American Psychiatric Association, 1989, pp 2678–2688

Liebowitz MR, Klein DF: Inter-relationship of hysteroid dysphoria and borderline personality disorder. Psychiatr Clin North Am 4:67–87, 1981

Liebowitz MR, Fyer AJ, Gorman JM, et al: Phenelzine in social phobia. J Clin Psychopharmacol 6:93–98, 1986a

Liebowitz MR, Stone MH, Turkat ID: Treatment of personality disorders, in American Psychiatric Association Annual Review, Vol 5. Edited by Frances AJ, Hales RE. Washington, American Psychiatric Press, 1986b, pp 394–400

Linehan MM: Behavior therapy, dialectics, and the treatment of borderline personality disorder, in Handbook of Borderline Disorders. Edited by Silver D, Rosenbluth M. Madison, CT, International Universities Press, 1992, pp 415–434

Lishman WA: Organic Psychiatry, 2nd Edition. Oxford, UK, Blackwell Scientific, 1987

Lucas PB, Gardner DL, Wolkowitz OM, et al: Dysphoria associated with methylphenidate infusion in borderline personality disorder. Am J Psychiatry 144:1577–1579, 1987

MacKinnon RH, Michels R: The Psychiatric Interview in Clinical Practice. Philadelphia, PA, WB Saunders, 1971

Marmar CR: Personality disorders, in Review of General Psychiatry, 2nd Edition. Edited by Goldman HH. Norwolk, CT, Lange Medical Books, 1988, pp 401–424

Masterson JF: Psychotherapy of the Borderline Adult. New York, Brunner/Mazel, 1976

Meissner WW: Theories of personality and psychopathology: classical psychoanalysis, in Comprehensive Textbook of Psychiatry/IV, 4th Edition, Vol 1. Edited by Kaplan HI, Sadock BJ. Baltimore, MD, Williams & Wilkins, 1985, pp 337–418

Meissner WW: Paranoid personality disorder, in Treatments of Psychiatric Disorders, Vol 3. Washington, DC, American Psychiatric Association, 1989, pp 2705–2711

Meyer RG: The Clinician's Handbook. Boston, MA, Allyn & Bacon, 1983

Nemiah J: Obsessive-compulsive disorder, in Comprehensive Textbook of Psychiatry/IV, 4th Edition, Vol 1. Edited by Kaplan HI, Sadock BJ. Baltimore, MD, Williams & Wilkins, 1985, pp 904–917

Nigg JT, Silk KR, Westen D, et al: Object representations in the early memories of sexually abused borderline patients. Am J Psychiatry 148:864–869, 1991

O'Malley SS, Kosten TR, Renner JA: Dual diagnosis: substance abuse and personality disorder, in Treating Personality Disorders (New Dir Ment Health Serv 47). Edited by Adler D. San Francisco, CA, Jossey-Bass, 1990, pp 115–138

Perry JC: Dependent personality disorder, in Treatments of Psychiatric Disorders, Vol 3. Washington, DC, American Psychiatric Association, 1989a, pp 2762–2770

Perry JC: Passive-aggressive personality disorder, in Treatments of Psychiatric Disorders, Vol 3. Washington, DC, American Psychiatric Association, 1989b, pp 2783–2790

Pies R: Psychotherapy Today: A Consumer's Guide to Choosing the Right Therapist. St Louis, MO, Manning-Skidmore-Roth, 1991

Raine A: Sex differences in schizotypal personality in a nonclinical population. J Abnorm Psychol 101:361–364, 1992

Rasmussen SA, Eisen JL: Epidemiology and differential diagnosis of obsessive-compulsive disorder. J Clin Psychiatry 53 (No 4, Suppl):4–10, 1992

Reid WH, Burke WJ: Antisocial Personality Disorder, in Treatments of Psychiatric Disorders, Vol 3. Washington, DC, American Psychiatric Association, 1989, pp 2742–2748

Rizzuto A, Peterson RK, Reed M: The pathological sense of self in anorexia nervosa. Psychiatr Clin North Am 4:471–489, 1981

Robins LN: Deviant Children Grown Up: A Sociological and Psychiatric Study of Sociopathic Personality. Baltimore, MD, Williams & Wilkins, 1966

Rosenbaum JF, Biederman J, Gerten M, et al: Behavioral inhibition in children of parents wih panic disorder and agoraphobia. Arch Gen Psychiatry 45:463–470, 1988

Salzman L: Compulsive personality disorder, in Treatments of Psychiatric Disorders, Vol 3. Washington, DC, American Psychiatric Association, 1989, pp 2771–2782

Schulz SC, Cornlius J, Schulz PM, et al: The amphetamine challenge test in patients with borderline personality disorder. Am J Psychiatry 145:809–814, 1988

Siever LJ: The neurobiology of personality disorders: new developments and implications for treatment. Presentation at "New Frontiers in Neuropsychiatry: A Practical Update," CME, Inc, Montreal, August 9, 1992

Siever LJ, Davis KL: A psychobiological perspective on the personality disorders. Am J Psychiatry 148:1647–1658, 1991

Siever LJ, Klar H: A review of DSM-III criteria for the personality disorders, in American Psychiatric Association Annual Review, Vol 5. Edited by

Frances AJ, Hales RE. Washington, DC, American Psychiatric Press, 1986, pp 279–314

Sifneos PE: Two different kinds of psychotherapy of short duration, in Brief Therapies. Edited by Barten HH. New York, Behavioral Publications, 1971, pp 82–90

Silverstein SM, Raulin ML, Pristach EA, et al: Perceptual organization and schizotypy. J Abnorm Psychol 101:265–270, 1992

Soloff RH, George A, Nathan R, et al: Progress in pharmacotherapy of borderline disorders: a double-blind study of amitriptyline, haloperidol, and placebo. Arch Gen Psychiatry 43:691–697, 1986

Stone MH: Schizoid personality disorder, in Treatments of Psychiatric Disorders, Vol 3. Washington, DC, American Psychiatric Association, 1989a, pp 2712–2718

Stone MH: Schizotypal personality disorder, in Treatments of Psychiatric Disorders, Vol 3. Washington, DC, American Psychiatric Association, 1989b, pp 2719–2726

Stone MH: The borderline patient: diagnostic concepts and differential diagnosis, in Handbook of Borderline Disorders. Edited by Silver D, Rosenbluth M. Madison, CT, International Universities Press, 1992, pp 3–28

Stringer AY, Joseph NC: Methylphenidate in the treatment of aggression in two patients with antisocial personality disorder. Am J Psychiatry 140:1365–1366, 1983

Vaillant GE, Perry JC: Personality disorders, in Comprehensive Textbook of Psychiatry/III, 3rd Edition, Vol 2. Edited by Kaplan HI, Freedman AM, Sadock BJ. Baltimore, MD, Williams & Wilkins, 1980, pp 1562–1590

Vaillant GE, Perry JC: Personality disorders, in Comprehensive Textbook of Psychiatry/IV, 4th Edition, Vol 1. Edited by Kaplan HI, Sadock BJ. Baltimore, MD, Williams & Wilkins, 1985, pp 958–986

Welch LW, Bear D: Organic disorders of personality, in Treating Personality Disorders (New Dir Ment Health Serv 47). Edited by Adler D. San Francisco, CA, Jossey-Bass, 1990, pp 87–102

Whitman R, Trosman H, Koenig R: Clinical assessment of passive-aggressive personality. Archives of Neurology and Psychiatry 72:540–549, 1954

Widiger TA, Frances A, Spitzer RL, et al: The DSM-III-R personality disorders: an overview. Am J Psychiatry 145:786–795, 1988

Zimmerman M, Coryell W: DSM-III personality disorder diagnosis in a non-patient sample. Arch Gen Psychiatry 46:682–689, 1989

10

Alcoholism and Other Substance Use Disorders

> Drink has drained more blood . . . plunged more
> people into bankruptcy . . . slain more children . . .
> driven more to suicide . . . than any other poisoned
> scourge that ever swept the death-dealing waves
> across the world.
>
> Evangeline Cory Booth, Salvation Army
> Commander (quoted in biography
> by P. W. Wilson)

Consider that in the United States today, somewhere over 13 million people have some form of alcohol abuse or dependence. Consider further that alcoholism is associated with at least 50% of traffic fatalities, 50% of homicides, and 25% of suicides (Kaplan and Sadock 1988). If there were no other substances in this country to abuse, alcohol would create more than enough problems. Add to alcoholism the abuse of cocaine, amphetamines, opioids, and prescription sedative-hypnotics and you will appreciate the scope of the substance abuse problem.

In this chapter, we apply our biopsychosocial model to three broad groups of substance use disorders: those related to central nervous system (CNS) depressants, to CNS stimulants, and to hallucinogens. However, we will devote most of our discussion to the abuse of alcohol, opioids, barbiturates, and cocaine, because arguably the greatest harm to society (if not the individual) stems from these agents. Alcoholism will be given particular emphasis, as it is (after heart disease and cancer) the third largest health problem in the United States today.

Preliminary Definitions and Nosology

The "drug abuse" literature is rife with ambiguous terms, not all of which are used in the most recent editions of the DSM. For example, the term "alcoholism" was not officially sanctioned in DSM-III-R, and it is still not in DSM-IV. Instead, DSM-III-R and DSM-IV utilize the concepts of substance *dependence* and *abuse* (American Psychiatric Association 1987, 1994). The basic features of substance dependence are summarized in our first vignette.

Vignette

Mr. Lonahte, a 34-year-old married electrician, presented to his family physician with a complaint of insomnia ("I wake up real early and feel kinda wired"). He denied any other physical or emotional problems and became slightly irritated when his physician began to explore a number of other areas. Eventually, however—and after a meeting with the patient's wife—the physician was able to determine the following. Over the past 5 years, the patient had increasing difficulty "sticking with what he says" about his drinking. For example, at parties, Mr. Lonahte would tell his wife, "I'm just gonna have a couple of beers," then would proceed to have six or seven. He had attempted to "cut down" upon the urgings of his wife, but, as he put it, "Once that drink is in my hands, Doc, I just lose count."

The patient's wife had begun to "hide" beer and liquor in various parts of their house, but, invariably, the patient would locate the alcohol, sometimes spending several hours late at night "rummaging through the closets." Mr. Lonahate's drinking had begun to affect his ability to work. According to his wife, "Once, Joe actually showed up drunk on the job, and the boss sent him home. Another time, he showed up so shaky, the boss called me and said Joe had the DTs." The patient had begun to withdraw from his wife and spend more and more time with his "buddies," who also drank heavily. Despite warnings from both his wife and his boss, the patient had continued this pattern of alcohol use. He had also gradually increased the amount of alcohol he used, because, "I just don't get the kick I used to out of a couple of beers."

Mr. Lonahte's experience with alcohol is paradigmatic of psychoactive substance *dependence* in general, with a couple of exceptions. (For example, characteristic withdrawal symptoms may not be seen with cannabis, phencyclidine [PCP], or hallucinogens.) Note that in our vignette, the concepts of *tolerance* and *withdrawal* are introduced. Tolerance refers to the need for markedly increased amounts of the substance to produce the same physical or psychological effect. (Alternatively, tolerance denotes a progressively diminishing effect, given the same dose of the substance.) Tolerance that develops to one drug after exposure to another (usually related) drug is termed *cross-tolerance*. A related term, *cross-dependence,* denotes the ability of one drug to suppress the manifestations of physical dependence produced by another (Jaffe 1975). The term *withdrawal* (or abstinence syndrome) refers to the collection of signs and symptoms that follow the (usually sudden) discontinuation of a substance of dependence. Withdrawal differs fundamentally according to the stimulating or depressing nature of the substance.

In DSM-IV the term *substance abuse* is defined as a maladaptive pattern of substance use leading to significant psychosocial impairment or distress (American Psychiatric Association 1994). This pattern may be characterized by an inability to fulfill major role obligations at work or home; use of the substance in physically hazardous situations (e.g., driving); recurrent legal problems related to substance use; or continued substance use despite severe interpersonal problems related to use. Such a pattern is generally seen in the early stages of psychoactive substance use, particularly with drugs less likely to promote marked withdrawal symptoms.

DSM-IV further classifies *substance-related disorders* into 12 main syndromes for any given substance. Thus, under "Alcohol Use Disorders," we find the categories of dependence, abuse, intoxication, withdrawal, delirium, dementia, amnestic disorder, psychotic disorder, mood disorder, anxiety disorder, sexual dysfunction, and sleep disorder. This basic breakdown applies for most of the major classes or types of substance (e.g., amphetamines, cannabis, cocaine, opiates, and sedative-hypnotics).

Not all syndromes occur with every substance; for example, withdrawal from cannabis is not considered a bona fide syndrome, and dementia is associated primarily with alcohol and sedative-hypnotics.

The term *addiction*, although not used in DSM-IV, is still a useful construct in some instances. Addiction has been defined by the World Health Organization as a behavioral pattern of drug use characterized by overwhelming involvement with the use of a drug; compulsive drug-seeking behavior; and a high tendency to relapse after withdrawal from the agent. Addiction, in this sense, exists along a continuum of psychosocial dysfunction.

Overview of Psychoactive Substances of Abuse

Central Nervous System Depressants

The CNS depressants are a heterogeneous group, consisting of (among others) alcohol, opiates, and a variety of so-called sedative-hypnotic agents. The last category includes barbiturates, methaqualone-type agents, and the benzodiazepines. In general, CNS depressants produce varying degrees of drowsiness and impairment of motor coordination, judgment, and memory. The signs and symptoms of alcohol intoxication are almost too well known to require a summary: overconfidence, impaired performance, emotional outbursts, hyperactivity, slurred speech, and—in higher doses—stupor and coma. (In large doses, any of the CNS depressants can produce respiratory suppression, stupor, coma, and death.) Animal studies have demonstrated a high degree of cross-dependence among the CNS depressants; for example, most sedative-hypnotics will show some cross-dependence with one another, with alcohol, and with barbiturates. When the CNS depressants are suddenly withdrawn, a general pattern of *rebound hyperexcitablity* ensues; for example, the user becomes more irritable, restless, and tremulous. In a very gross sense, withdrawal of CNS depressants leads to a state of sympathetic nervous system overarousal.

Despite the similarities among the CNS depressants, there are important qualitative differences. The opioid compounds, in particular, seem to have important neurophysiological differences with respect to other depressants; indeed, some authorities would consider the opiates in a separate category altogether. Thus, as Jaffe and Martin (1975) note,

> high doses of barbiturates, or gross intoxication with alcohol produce significant analgesia, but only in association with sedation and impairment of motor coordination, intellectual acuity, emotional control, and judgment. For a given degree of analgesia, the mental clouding produced by therapeutic doses of morphine is considerably less pronounced and of a qualitatively different character; morphine and related drugs rarely produce the garrulous, silly, and emotionally labile behavior frequently seen in alcohol and barbiturate intoxication. (p. 248)

Central Nervous System Stimulants

The CNS stimulants represent a variety of sympathomimetic drugs, including cocaine, amphetamines, methylphenidate, pemoline, phenmetrazine, and diethylpropion. While all these agents tend to increase general arousal, their subjective effects depend to some extent on the user (Jaffe 1975). Thus, moderate doses of amphetamine given orally to normal subjects may produce a spectrum of mood states (e.g., mild euphoria, anxiety, irritability, or even transient drowsiness). In higher doses, the CNS stimulants tend to produce more stereotyped responses. Typically, the user is hyperactive, suspicious, and often frankly paranoid. Indeed, amphetamine psychosis has often been used as a "chemical model" for schizophrenia, although PCP-induced psychosis may be a closer fit. Some users attempt to antagonize the hyperstimulating effects of these drugs via simultaneous use of opioids—hence, the heroin and cocaine "speedball."

For many years, a "withdrawal" syndrome from sudden discontinuation of CNS stimulants was either discounted or minimized. To be sure, there is nothing so dramatic as the withdrawal that follows, say, sudden discontinuation of barbiturates. But there is a recognizable pattern of prolonged sleep, general fatigue, lassitude, and depression that may be quite profound. Because both amphetamines and cocaine suppress REM sleep, there is also a marked "REM rebound" phenomenon during withdrawal.

Hallucinogens

It may seem that the hallucinogens are merely relics of "the 60s," but there has been an upsurge of both clinical and theoretical interest in some of these agents. The hallucinogens are usually said to include lysergic acid diethylamide (LSD) and related compounds; PCP and related arylcyclohexylamines; dimethyltryptamine (DMT), mescaline, and other natural substances; and a few less common substances like MMDA (5-methoxy-3,4-methylenedioxyamphetamine).

Although marijuana (and its chief psychoactive ingredient, THC [delta-9-tetrahydrocannabinol]) is usually not included in this grouping, we shall do so for both didactic and clinical reasons. For example, at very high blood levels, marijuana *can* produce some of the same effects as LSD, including distorted perception of body parts, synesthesia, and, occasionally, true psychotic symptoms (Jaffe 1975).

Alcohol-Induced Mental Disorders

The Central Concept

We already described the features of alcohol dependence in our first vignette. Now consider the following case.

Vignette

Ms. Snemert was a 32-year-old chronic "alcoholic" whose typical pattern was a drinking binge of 2 weeks or so, followed by a month or two of relative sobriety. She presented to the psychiatric emergency room with the chief complaint that "the cops have planted bugs under my skin." She was disoriented to day and date and seemed quite tremulous and diaphoretic. Her pulse, blood pressure, and temperature were elevated, and her pupils were dilated and reactive. The patient reported the feeling that "bugs are crawling all over me," and she attributed this to "a police plot to get me." She also reported seeing "cockroaches" out of the corner of her eye. Laboratory studies showed a blood alcohol level of less than 0.10% and slightly elevated GGT (gamma-glutamyl transpeptidase); other liver function tests were within normal limits. The patient stated that she had not had anything to drink in the past 2 days, but that prior to that she had been drinking one quart of vodka per day. Toxic screen for other substances of abuse was negative.

You have probably recognized the classic symptoms of delirium tremens (DTs) in this case. The tip-off here is the elevated autonomic findings in a disoriented person with visual and tactile hallucinations. Auditory hallucinations may be reported (see discussion of alcohol hallucinosis in next subsection) and are usually of a threatening nature. Grand mal seizures are common in alcohol withdrawal states and often precede the onset of delirium. DTs represent the most serious of the alcohol withdrawal syndromes, associated with a mortality of between 5% and 20%, depending on treatment and the presence of intercurrent medical problems (Kaplan and Sadock 1988; Lishman 1987). If death occurs, it is usually due to cardiovascular collapse, infection, hyperthermia, or self-injury (Lishman 1987). DTs usually appear within 24 to 72 hours after cessation of or marked reduction in drinking; however, DTs may not appear until a week after the last drink, in some cases (Hackett et al. 1991).

A variety of other alcohol-related states are of concern to psychiatrists, but particularly alcohol idiosyncratic intoxication ("pathological intoxication"), alcohol hallucinosis, and alcohol amnestic disorder (Korsakoff's syndrome). The main features of these conditions (as well as DTs) are summarized in Table 10–1. We will say more about each condition when we discuss the biopsychosocial perspective. Finally, although the signs and symptoms of acute alcohol intoxication hardly need detailed description, you should be aware of the relatively rare state known as "alcoholic paranoia." Affected patients often harbor

Table 10–1.   Alcohol-related neuropsychiatric syndromes

Syndrome	Pathophysiology	Physical features	Psychiatric features
Delirium tremens	Alcohol withdrawal; ? reticular system dysfunction; limbic system hyperirritability; ? "kindling" over time; ? if REM rebound basis of vivid hallucinations.	Elevated pulse and blood pressure; sweating, tremor, fever seizures.	Disorientation; perceptual distortions (visual/tactile) paranoia, agitation.
Alcohol hallucinosis	Usually associated with ethanol withdrawal, but may occur while drinking; ? related to schizophrenia.	Tinnitus common; less psychomotor agitation than in DTs.	Orientation, sensorium WNL; often auditory (sometimes visual) hallucinations of command or derogatory type; paranoid delusions common.
Alcohol idiosyncratic intoxication	? Encephalitic or traumatic brain damage predisposes; some patients show temporal lobe spiking on EEG after small amount of alcohol.	Markedly increased psychomotor activation; rage, violence, followed by prolonged sleep.	Confusion, disorientation, transient delusions and/or hallucinations; amnesia for rage episode.
Alcohol amnestic disorder/ alcohol encephalopathy[a]	Thiamine deficiency; impaired absorption of thiamine from gut; lesions in thalamic nuclei and mamillary bodies.	Ataxia, ophthalmoplegia, nystagmus; may be cerebellar signs, peripheral neuropathy, and hypotension.	"Quiet global confusion," mild delirium; impaired short-term memory; confabulation, emotional lability.

Note. ? = hypothesized; WNL = within normal limits.
[a]Usually considered together as Wernicke-Korsakoff syndrome.
Source. Lishman 1987.

the belief that a spouse or lover has been unfaithful, and this belief is accompanied by the usual findings of slurred speech, ataxia, alcohol on the breath, and so forth (McNeil 1987).

Historical Development of the Disorders

The use and abuse of alcohol have ancient origins. Distillation was in evidence as early as the first century A.D., and one of the oldest "temperance tracts"—the Egyptian text "The Wisdom of Ani"—was written about 3,000 years ago! The "disease model" of alcoholism, however, is much more recent (Mello and Mendelson 1975). For centuries, alcoholism was considered a form of moral transgression or social deviance, to be dealt with solely through the criminal justice system. Gradually, the "addiction" concept began to be applied to alcohol abuse, evolving later into our present "biobehavioral" model (Mello and Mendelson 1975). This model does not posit a "linear physical causality" between alcohol use and "alcoholism"; rather, as Mello and Mendelson (1975) point out,

> the model assumes that expression of the disorder depends on an interaction between the individual, the agent of the disease (alcohol), and the environment in which the disease process develops. . . . even infectious disease is often more closely related to host-resistance factors and environmental variables than to the presence or even the virulence of any given infectious agent. (p. 376)

Although the term "alcoholism" is fraught with ambiguity, we will use it for the sake of convenience in various parts of our discussion. We may define alcoholism as "a disease marked by the chronic, excessive use of alcohol that produces psychological, interpersonal, and medical problems" (Kaplan and Sadock 1988, p. 221).

The Biopsychosocial Perspective

Biological Factors

Let's begin with the thing itself: ethanol. We still do not know the exact physiological mechanism of ethanol intoxication or withdrawal, though recent research has turned up some intriguing findings. Apparently, alcohol, barbiturates, and benzodiazepines share a common mechanism: they suppress brain function (at least in part) by activating the GABAergic system (Giannini and Miller 1991). You may recall that GABA (gamma-aminobutyric acid) is an inhibitory neurotransmitter that slows, relaxes, and eventually paralyzes cognitive and motor function. It may seem paradoxical, then, that in low doses, ethanol may have a "stimulating" effect on behavior. Although explanations for this effect differ, most data suggest that ethanol first acts on the reticular formation; impairment of reticular function leads to increased excitability of the cortex. Thought processes and motor coordination become jumbled or disrupted, giving the appearance of "stimulation." Later, there are direct toxic effects on cortical neurons (Lishman 1987). There is impairment of memory consolidation, perhaps underlying the anterograde amnesia seen with alcoholic "blackouts." In these episodes, the intoxicated individual may behave normally but have no recollection (when sober) of significant events during the drinking bout. Intriguingly, the person may recall these events when intoxicated again, suggesting some form of "state-dependent learning." Alcohol also seems to antagonize excitatory NMDA receptors (Paul 1992) and to interfere with neuronal membrane function.

A blood alcohol level of 150 to 250 mg/100 ml is usually correlated with obvious signs of intoxication. However, individual and racial variations are common; for example, many Asian individuals show increased flushing, vasodilation, and dizziness after ethanol consumption compared with Caucasians exposed to the same dose (Mello and Mendelson 1975). There is some evidence that "high risk" subjects are physiologically more sensitive than control subjects to the effects of ethanol. Pollock et al. (1983) examined the electroencephalogram (EEG) after alcohol administration in 134 high-risk (HR) sons of alcoholic males and 70 sons of nonalcoholic males, matched for age and social class. The HR subjects showed greater increases in slow alpha energy and greater reductions in fast alpha energy than did the control subjects after oral ethanol administration. Other studies (Schuckit 1987) suggest that sons of alcoholic individuals seem to have decreased reaction to modest doses of ethanol, and lower-amplitude P300 waves in response to cortical activation.

Family studies have shown a three- to fourfold increase in risk for alcoholism in the children of alcoholic individuals, without clear evidence of increased vulnerability to other primary psychiatric illnesses (Schuckit 1987). Some recent research has found an association between alcoholism and the gene that codes for the D_2 dopamine receptor (Blum et al. 1990), but many questions have arisen regarding the validity of this work.

The sex of parent and offspring may influence the genetic "transmission" of alcoholism (Pollock et al. 1987). Thus, both alcoholic males and females more frequently come from homes in which the father is alcoholic; also, whereas daughters of alcoholic mothers have higher rates of alcoholism than those in the general population, sons of alcoholic mothers do not. The precise genetic (or psychosocial?) implications of these findings are not yet clear, but the role of both biological and environmental factors in alcoholism seems indisputable. Indeed, Cloninger et al. (1981) have proposed that two types of familial alcoholism exist: type I, which occurs in both male and female children of alcoholic individuals and may be influenced in its severity by environmental factors; and type II, which is limited to males, associated with a history of criminality in the biological father, and less susceptible to environmental effects (Table 10–2). We will say more about sociopathy and alcohol abuse in discussion of the differential diagnosis.

What about biological factors in alcohol withdrawal and other alcohol-related brain syndromes? Ballenger and Post (1978) have

Table 10–2. Types of alcoholism

Type I	Type II
Later onset of drinking	Earlier onset
Loss of control over drinking	Spontaneous alcohol seeking
Strong gene-environment effect	Postnatal effects weak; criminal behavior in father
Transmitted to men and women	Transmitted mainly to men

Source. Extensively modified from Dinwiddie and Cloninger 1991.

proposed that the phenomenon of "kindling" could be applied to alcohol withdrawal syndromes. They have hypothesized that limbic system hyperirritability accompanies each alcohol withdrawal episode and that, over time, this local irritability "kindles" increasingly widespread subcortical structures. Such long-term changes in neuronal excitability may relate to the progression from tremor to seizures to delirium—and perhaps even to personality changes between episodes of withdrawal. On a more molecular level, there is evidence that withdrawal from drugs that affect GABA causes a rebound excess of norepinephrine, epinephrine, and dopamine, which are under GABAergic control (Giannini and Miller 1991). These increases may account for the increased alertness, hypertension, increased motor activity, and other "hypersympathetic" phenomena seen in withdrawal. Noradrenergic function may be especially related to the autonomic hyperactivity of alcohol withdrawal, because cerebrospinal fluid levels of MHPG (3-methoxy-4-hydroxyphenylglycol) appear to rise commensurately with autonomic disturbance (Fujimoto et al. 1983).

The pathophysiology of so-called pathological (alcohol idiosyncratic) intoxication remains quite mysterious. Although the classical description emphasizes ingestion of "small" amounts of alcohol as a precipitant, the experimental evidence for this is weak (Lishman 1987). Some patients who show this phenomenon also show changes in the EEG during alcohol infusion, but these changes do not correlate with the disturbed behavior (Maletsky 1976). Nevertheless, there is speculation that abnormal temporal lobe activity may underlie this disorder. There is also modest evidence showing that brain-damaged persons have a higher than expected susceptibility to pathological intoxication.

Wernicke-Korsakoff syndrome, although linked to thiamine deficiency and medial temporal lobe pathology, is undoubtedly more complicated. For example, some evidence points to frontal lobe dysfunction in the etiology of "confabulation." Some Korsakoff patients exhibit personality changes such as apathy, lack of insight, or self-neglect, which also suggest frontal lobe involvement (Lishman 1987).

Finally, there is considerable evidence of the direct, toxic effects of alcohol on the brain (Lishman 1987). Even in the absence of nutritional deficiencies (e.g., thiamine deficiency in Wernicke-Korsakoff syndrome), alcohol causes alterations in dendritic morphology in the hippocampus and inhibits the normal, reactive "sprouting" of dendrites in response to brain injury. These phenomena could account for the pervasive abnormalities seen in the computed tomography (CT) scans of alcoholic individuals, as we will discuss under adjunctive testing.

Psychological Factors

A common psychoanalytic aphorism is "The superego is soluble in alcohol." This view epitomizes the psychoanalytic understanding of alcoholic individuals—that is, as persons "with harsh superegos who are self-punitive [and who] turn to alcohol as a way of diminishing their unconscious stress" (Kaplan and Sadock 1988, p. 222). Traditional formulations posit that alcoholic individuals are "fixated at the oral stage of development" and that the "alcoholic personality" tends to be shy, isolated, impatient, irritable, anxious, hypersensitive, and sexually repressed (Kaplan and Sadock 1988). Zimberg (1989) has reviewed the evidence suggesting that in "primary" alcoholism (i.e., alcoholism without coexisting major psychiatric disorders), "conflict with dependent needs is a major psychological factor that contributes to alcoholism. This conflict may have developed because of childhood rejection by one or both parents, overprotection, or forcing premature responsibility on a child, particularly if a parent is alcoholic" (pp. 1094–1095). Furthermore, according to Zimberg (1989),

> the psychological conflict observed in alcoholics consists of low self-esteem along with feelings of worthlessness and inadequacy. These feelings are denied and repressed and lead to unconscious needs to be taken care of and accepted. Since these dependent needs cannot be met in reality, they lead to anxiety and compensatory needs for control, power, achievement, and elevated self-esteem. Alcohol tranquilizes the anxiety; more importantly, it creates pharmacologically induced feelings of power, omnipotence, and invulnerability in men and enhanced feelings of womanliness in women. (p. 1095)

Object-relations theorists have also hypothesized "psychostructural" deficits in alcoholic individuals (Donovan 1986). Balint (1969) described alcoholic individuals in the following way:

> Their object relationships, though usually fairly intense, are shaky and instable. . . . the first effect of intoxication is invariably the establishment of a feeling that everything is now well between them and their environment. . . . the yearning for this "feeling of harmony" is the most important cause of alcoholism, or for that matter, any form of addiction. (pp. 55–56)

Not all authorities agree with these dynamic formulations, and many would find them unhelpful in treatment (see subsection on treatment goals and directions). As Mello and Mendelson (1975) note,

> The psychiatric literature on alcoholism contains countless theories which attempt to conceptualize alcoholism in terms of a psychodynamic formulation, a psychosocial developmental model, or as the outgrowth of specific personality characteristics such as depression, dependence, immaturity, hostility, and social isolation . . . [but] the most plausible and ingenious theories concerning the psychological determinants of alcoholism have contributed little to the development of effective treatment and, for the most part, have been difficult to subject to rigorous experimental scrutiny. (p. 383)

We will delve a bit more into this controversy later. For now, suffice it to say that while some alcoholic individuals may show the dynamics posited by Zimberg, not all do so; moreover, it is often hard to tell which came first—the alcoholism or the "dynamics." For example, the mere act of repetitive intoxication, withdrawal, and disruption of the individual's personal and family life can generate abysmally low self-esteem and feelings of worthlessness.

Sociocultural Factors

It is hard to disentangle some of the supposed sociocultural factors in alcohol abuse/dependence from possible biogenetic factors. For example, Native Americans, black women (and perhaps ghetto-reared black males), and Eskimos are at higher risk than the general population for the development of alcoholism; however, the cultural and genetic components of this vulnerability are not precisely known

(Mello and Mendelson 1975). (The "flushing" response to alcohol seen in about two-thirds of Asian persons, however, is present at birth and could account for the relatively low rate of alcoholism in this group.) Jews and "conservative Protestants" apparently use alcohol less frequently than do "liberal Protestants" and Catholics (Kaplan and Sadock 1988).

"Heavy drinkers" (variously defined) are more likely than not to be male, single or divorced, living in urban areas, from lower socioeconomic classes, and poorly educated, when compared with "moderate" drinkers. Adult drinking problems also seem to be associated with early school problems, delinquency, other drug use, and broken homes—but again, it is hard to know what to infer from these facts. For example, do early school problems lead to later alcohol abuse, or do the school problems and the alcohol abuse both stem from some common biological diathesis?

You should not conclude from all this that well-educated, upper-middle-class whites are immune to alcoholism. In one study by Vaillant et al. (1975), physicians actually showed a higher incidence of drug or alcohol misuse than did control subjects (36% vs. 22%). A recent study of resident physicians showed that, in comparison with age-matched nonphysician control subjects, the residents had a higher rate of "past-month use" of alcohol and benzodiazepines; however, "heavy" alcohol or drug use was not seen in the resident group (P. H. Hughes et al. 1991). Certainly, the presence of severe stress combined with the ready availability of drugs places physicians at significant risk for substance abuse. Waiters, bartenders, longshoremen, musicians, authors, and reporters seem to have high cirrhosis (and presumptively, alcoholism) rates; accountants, mail carriers, and carpenters have relatively low rates. It is intriguing to note that of eight Americans who won the Nobel Prize for literature, four were clearly alcoholic and one was a heavy drinker (Goodwin 1985).

Finally, what is the role of the family in the etiology of alcoholism? Donovan (1986), in an excellent synthesis of biopsychosocial factors in this disorder, notes that "alcoholism can be seen as both the cause and the effect of family dysfunction" (p. 6). In particular, "by isolating and infantalizing the alcoholic, the family system can serve to maintain his or her drinking" (p. 6).

Pitfalls in the Differential Diagnosis

Organic Disorders

Intoxication due to virtually any sedative-hypnotic, anxiolytic, or other CNS depressant can resemble alcohol intoxication; moreover, as DSM-III-R noted, "the presence of alcohol on the breath does not exclude the possibility that another psychoactive substance is responsible for the intoxication" (p. 128). Alcohol intoxication may also share some signs and symptoms with neurological diseases such as cerebellar ataxia or multiple sclerosis (American Psychiatric Association 1987). Alcohol withdrawal resembles withdrawal from any CNS depressant, although auditory, visual, and tactile hallucinations are less common in withdrawal from narcotics or barbiturates (Dubovsky 1988). Alcohol idiosyncratic intoxication may sometimes be mistaken for the interictal disinhibition seen in temporal lobe epilepsy (American Psychiatric Association 1987); however, in temporal lobe epilepsy, the clinical history is usually positive for other features such as olfactory hallucinations, ictal stereotypies, and fuguelike episodes not associated with violence. Alcohol hallucinosis may be confused with various types of "organic hallucinosis." In theory, the hallucinogens (LSD, mescaline) are more likely to produce visual hallucinations than the auditory type experienced in alcohol hallucinosis; however, the distinction does not always hold, because some patients with alcohol hallucinosis do have hallucinations in the visual realm. The amnestic pattern seen in Wernicke-Korsakoff syndrome may be seen in any process that causes bilateral damage to medial temporal lobe structures (e.g., the mammillary bodies, fornix, and hippocampus). However, the presence of nystagmus, ataxia, and peripheral neuropathy helps distinguish Wernicke-Korsakoff syndrome from other organic causes of amnesia, such as head trauma, anoxia, or transient global amnesia (Cummings 1985).

Other Psychiatric Disorders

Alcohol intoxication, withdrawal, hallucinosis, and amnestic syndromes may resemble a number of "functional" psychiatric disorders. The overconfidence, emotional outbursts, ebullience, and hyperactivity of the intoxicated individual may, of course, suggest hypomania or mania. The clinical history will help distinguish the two, as will associated features of ethanol intoxication, such as slurred speech or ataxia. You should remember, however, that substance abuse is a common complication of mania and that some acutely manic patients may also be intoxicated.

The psychiatric manifestations of DTs and/or alcohol hallucinosis are sometimes mistaken for schizophrenia and related disorders. With classic DTs, the presence of disorientation and (typically) visual or tactile hallucinations should help you make the diagnosis; with alcohol hallucinosis, the distinction may be more subtle. The clinical history in this situation is critical: if a bout of heavy drinking has preceded (by 2 or 3 days) the presentation of auditory hallucinations and paranoid ideation, think seriously about alcohol hallucinosis. (Information from a family member may be essential in corroborating this.)

Vignette

A 27-year-old male with a history of a "psychotic episode" presented to the ER with the complaint of accusatory "voices" telling him, "You're gonna fry for your crimes," and the associated belief that the mayor's office "is out to get me." The patient was oriented to day and date. There was no formal thought process disorder. He denied alcohol consumption or street drug use in the past 2 days. Physical examination was essentially within normal limits, except for mild tachycardia and elevated blood pressure. However, the patient complained of intermittent "ringing" or "buzzing" in his ears. A diagnosis of "brief reactive psychosis" was made, and the patient was given 100 mg of chlorpromazine po, followed by 50 mg im. Two hours later, he suffered a grand mal seizure. A CT scan of the brain and the EEG were negative. On the evening of admission to the ER, the patient's brother appeared and related that the patient had been drinking heavily 3 days prior to assessment. The revised diagnosis was "alcohol hallucinosis, withdrawal seizure, possibly precipitated by chlorpromazine."

The red herring in this vignette was the patient's (legitimate) denial of alcohol use in the preceding 2 days; an important clue was

the presence of tinnitus. There is some evidence that alcohol hallucinosis is related to disturbance of the auditory pathways; interestingly,
when tinnitus is one-sided, the hallucinations usually seem to originate
only from that side (Hackett et al. 1991).

There is considerable overlap between alcohol abuse and mood
disorders, and a number of studies suggest that drinking behavior is
influenced by the presence of a depressive disorder (O'Sullivan et al.
1983). In some patients, the mood disorder predates the onset of
alcoholism; in others, the converse is true. The determination of
which disorder is "primary" is often difficult. One clue is the rapidity
with which active (primary) alcoholic individuals recover from their
apparent "depression"—often within a month or so of achieving
sobriety. Consider the following vignette.

Vignette

Mr. Dual, a 35-year-old unemployed electrician, was admitted to
the psychiatric unit with a diagnosis of "major depression." He
complained of insomnia, weight loss, decreased libido, and suicidal
ideation over the past 2 months, which he attributed to the recent
breakup of his marriage. On initial presentation, Mr. Dual appeared
lethargic, sad, and tearful. He scored 18 (severe) on the Beck
Depression Inventory (BDI), and a dexamethasone suppression test
(DST) came back elevated (8 A.M. cortisol = 9 µg/dl, normal < 5).
A careful history revealed that over the past 6 weeks, the patient had
been drinking "a half a bottle of whiskey" per day, and at times
substantially more than this. After 3 weeks on the psychiatric unit,
the patient appeared markedly less depressed. His BDI score had
dropped to 4 (mild depression), and his DST had normalized.

There is also considerable overlap between alcoholism and various
anxiety states, particularly agoraphobia, obsessive-compulsive disorder
(OCD), and social phobia (Kushner et al. 1990). Moreover, alcohol
withdrawal shares several signs and symptoms with panic disorder and
other anxiety states (e.g., tremulousness, tachycardia, sweating, palpitations, and subjective distress).

How might comorbidity between alcohol abuse and anxiety disorders arise? A common genetic predisposition is one possibility.

However, some patients, particularly those with agoraphobia, may control their anxiety with alcohol. Subsequent withdrawal may then set off panic attacks. (Strictly speaking, such an "organic factor" would vitiate the diagnosis of panic disorder; rather, the patient would receive the diagnois of organic anxiety syndrome.) The clue to panic disorder is the "spontaneous," rapidly escalating, and circumscribed quality of the attacks, and the often overwhelming fear of dying or of "going crazy." Alcohol withdrawal occurs more gradually and continues for a longer period of time than the attacks seen in panic disorder; moreover, the fear of dying or of going crazy is usually not pronounced in alcohol withdrawal, unless the person is responding to a frightening delusion or hallucination.

Although Wernicke-Korsakoff syndrome is usually unmistakable in its classic form, some patients with this syndrome may show features suggesting a manic psychosis. Such patients often show a "fantastic type" of confabulation "in which a sustained and grandiose theme is elaborated, usually describing far-fetched adventures and experiences which clearly could not have taken place at any time" (Lishman 1987, p. 29).

We alluded earlier to the overlap or comorbidity of alcoholism and sociopathy. You will recall that in the typology of Cloninger (1987; Cloninger et al. 1981), type II alcoholism is limited to males and is associated with criminality in the biological father. Furthermore, the typical type II alcoholic individual is posited to show a high propensity to use drugs, a high degree of "novelty seeking," and a low tendency to avoid harm. In a study that examined these personality traits in men whose fathers had severe alcohol-related problems (vs. subjects with no family history of alcoholism), Schuckit et al. (1990) were unable to confirm Cloninger's typology. Indeed, Schuckit et al. concluded that "it is likely that the prototype type 2 alcoholic actually has a separate disorder, antisocial personality disorder" (p. 482) and that excessive alcohol and drug use in such individuals is "secondary" to antisocial personality disorder. While this controversy is being worked out, keep in mind that both antisocial and borderline personality disorders are in the differential diagnosis of alcohol abuse and dependence. Finally, hyperactivity predisposes to sociopathy; both have a genetic component, and both are associated with later alcoholism (Tarter et al. 1977).

Adjunctive Testing

Imaging and Electroencephalographic Studies

Many studies of chronic alcoholism have demonstrated cerebral atrophy on CT scans, in perhaps 50% to 70% of cases (Lishman 1987). Cortical shrinkage and/or ventricular dilatation are common, especially affecting the frontal lobes. Such changes may be seen before clinical evidence of mental impairment and are apparently not related to progression of liver disease (Dano and Le Guyader 1988; Lishman 1987). CT changes are correlated to some degree with impairment of memory and intelligence (see discussion of neuropsychiatric testing), at least in advanced cases.

Pollock et al. (1983) have summarized the electroencephalographic findings in chronic alcoholic individuals. Many individuals show "poorly synchronized" EEGs characterized by deficient alpha activity. There is some evidence that persons with a genetic predisposition to alcoholism show such deficient alpha activity and that alcohol use actually serves as "self-medication" for this deficiency. Pollock et al. also found that, in comparison with control subjects, the biological sons of alcoholic individuals show greater increases of "slow alpha energy" and greater decreases of "fast alpha energy" after alcohol administration. We have already alluded to abnormal event-related potentials in alcoholic persons; specifically, the P300 component appears less developed in alcoholic individuals than in control subjects (Begleiter et al. 1980).

Neuroendocrine Studies

There is no consistent or "diagnostic" neuroendocrine abnormality in alcoholism. However, Schuckit (1991) notes the following common hormonal changes: increased serum cortisol levels, which can remain elevated during heavy drinking; decreased vasopressin secretion at rising blood alcohol concentrations, and the opposite with falling ethanol levels; a modest and reversible decrease in serum thyroxine (T_4); and a more marked decrease in serum triiodothyronine (T_3). You should also keep in mind a useful set of nonendocrine indicators of alcoholism: normal or slightly elevated MCV (mean corpuscular volume) and elevated GGT, uric acid, and tri-glycerides (Schuckit 1991).

Neuropsychiatric Testing

Lishman (1987) has reviewed the abundance of psychological test data pertaining to alcohol abuse. The first point to keep in mind is that cognitive testing should be deferred for as long as feasible after sobriety is attained, because substantial recovery of function occurs during the first few weeks of abstinence. Nevertheless, even after a year of total abstinence, deficits show up on tests of psychomotor speed, perceptual-motor function, visuospatial competence, and abstracting ability (Lishman 1987). Memory impairment of varying degrees can occur—including impaired acquisition of new material—even in the absence of frank Wernicke-Korsakoff syndrome. On the revised Wechsler Adult Intelligence Scale (WAIS-R), alcoholic individuals often show significantly lower scores on digit symbol, block design, object assembly, and picture arrangement, suggesting impaired visuomotor coordination (Meyer 1983).

The MacAndrew Alcoholism Scale (MAC) is a specialized Minnesota Multiphasic Personality Inventory (MMPI) scale used in the diagnosis of general "addiction proneness"; high scorers on the MAC tend to be impulsive, energetic, nonconforming, and superficial in their social relationships (Newmark 1985). Other common MMPI profiles in alcoholic individuals include the 4-2 pattern and the 1-2/2-1 pattern (Meyer 1983). (Note that scale 2 indicates severity of depressive features.) On the Rorschach, a high percentage of oral and anatomical responses is common, accompanied by a low F+% (Meyer 1983).

Treatment Directions and Goals

The 18 basic "ingredients" of treating the substance-abusing patient are nicely summarized by Dubovsky (1988) and are presented in condensed form in Table 10–3. These are general guidelines, but they clearly apply to the treatment of the alcoholic patient.

Before discussing the specific somatic and psychosocial interventions used in alcoholism, let's get a broad view of treatment, utilizing the following vignette.

Vignette

Mr. Daniels, a 40-year-old married father of two, was referred for psychiatric treatment by his primary physician, who was the first to confront the patient about his excessive use of alcohol. According to the patient's wife, "Jack has just gotten out of hand. It used to be a few too many beers now and then. But now it's gotten to the point where he's either sloshed or withdrawing so bad, he shakes. And

Table 10–3.   Basic approach to alcohol or other substance abuse

Detoxify the patient.

Confront the patient's denial gradually.

Change the patient's environment.

Establish a positive relationship.

Adopt a "disease model."

Treat associated problems (e.g., depression).

Insist on abstinence.

Assess motivation.

Involve the family.

Arrange periodic toxicology screens.

Avoid medications that promote dependence.

Help the patient recognize psychosocial precipitants of substance abuse.

Encourage exercise.

Refer the patient to self-help groups, such as AA.

Arrange residential treatment in some cases.

Consider mandated treatment in some cases.

Expect relapses.

"Leave the door open" to individuals who refuse treatment.

Source.   Extensively modified from Dubovsky 1988.

he's been violent, too—I don't trust him around me and the kids." The psychiatrist first interviewed Jack and found very strong denial of his drinking problem. Jack also seemed poorly motivated for treatment, offering only "to drop in at AA once and a while." The psychiatrist did not confront this denial aggressively at first, and asked the patient and his wife to come back in 2 weeks. He asked Jack to "see what you can do to cut down on drinking, and we will take it from there next time." Jack grudgingly agreed to this. Two weeks later, the patient and his wife returned. His wife confronted Jack in the presence of the psychiatrist, stating, "If anything, Jack has been even worse in the last 2 weeks." The psychiatrist told Jack that inpatient detoxification was necessary in order to get treatment started. After considerable pressure from his wife—including the threat of her leaving him—Jack agreed.

After a 10-day "detox," Jack was discharged with a contract to attend AA three times per week and to find a "sponsor" there. He continued to meet weekly with the psychiatrist, who gradually helped Jack understand alcoholism as a disease, not as a "moral weakness." The psychiatrist insisted on total abstinence, despite Jack's frequent claims that "I could just drink socially now and then, if you'd give me half a chance." Jack was also taught to recognize the stressors at home and at work that helped precipitate a drinking bout. Despite his apparent willingness to abstain, Jack was told that—from time to time—he might be asked to submit a blood sample to detect the presence of alcohol. Jack did well with this approach for 1 month but then had a brief relapse after "a big blowup with my boss." The psychiatrist explained that this was "par for the course," and treatment resumed with increased attendance at AA.

Somatic Approaches

The somatic treatment of alcohol intoxication has yet to be invented, although experimental drugs are being tested. Stimulants and caffeine do not hasten sobriety, and sedative-hypnotics are contraindicated during acute intoxication (Dubovsky 1988). Occasionally, haloperidol is used to control severe agitation or intoxication-related psychosis, but antipsychotics increase the risk of seizures. Thus, mechanical restraint is preferred for disinhibited behavior associated with severe intoxication.

The pharmacological treatment of choice in alcohol withdrawal states is a benzodiazepine. A typical regimen is chlordiazepoxide (Librium) 25–50 mg po every 2 to 4 hours. Although this agent is often given intramuscularly, it is not well absorbed by this route. In contrast, lorazepam in doses of 1 to 4 mg every 2 to 4 hours is well absorbed via intramuscular or oral administration. Keep in mind that the acute effects of a benzodiazepine are not related to its plasma half-life, but to its lipophilicity and its resultant distribution in various "body compartments" (Greenblatt 1991). Thus, a single dose of a highly lipophilic, "long half-life" agent such as diazepam may have a rapid onset of action, but it may also have a rapid diminution of clinical effects, because of its high lipophilicity; that is, it quickly penetrates, but then quickly exits, the lipid-rich CNS, later to be distributed in extra-CNS lipid stores. As a result of these properties, diazepam may have to be given several times per day during the initial stages of alcohol withdrawal. Over the ensuing few days, less lipophilic, long-acting metabolites accumulate, permitting less frequent dosing. Gradual tapering of the benzodiazepine may commence over 5 to 7 days. Because patients with alcoholism often have impaired hepatic function, you should consider the use of benzodiazepines that do not require oxidative metabolism (e.g., lorazepam or oxazepam). Dosage should be titrated so as to mitigate signs of sympathetic overarousal while avoiding oversedation. Thiamine, 100 mg im, then 100 mg po qd, should always be administered to the withdrawing alcoholic individual in order to avert possible Wernicke-Korsakoff syndrome. (Thiamine should be given prior to the patient's first meal in order to avoid depleting body stores of thiamine used for carbohydrate metabolism.) Electrolytes should be checked to rule out, for example, hypokalemia, hypomagnesemia, and hypophosphatemia (Ciraulo and Ciraulo 1988), which in some cases may require treatment.

The treatment of alcohol hallucinosis is a bit controversial, though many clinicians advocate benzodiazepines as the initial approach. If hallucinations and/or paranoia continue past the first 24 hours or so, some clinicians add (or substitute) a high-potency antipsychotic such as haloperidol (Ciraulo and Ciraulo 1988; Kaplan and Sadock 1988). Cases that continue beyond 30 days or so should be viewed with an eye toward rediagnosis—as the onset of a schizophreniform disorder, for example.

States of "pathological intoxication" are probably best treated with physical restraint and/or intramuscular lorazepam, although the latter has the potential for further disinhibiting the patient; unfortunately, there are few controlled studies offering guidance on this question. Antipsychotic agents are generally not recommended for pathological intoxication (Magliozzi and Schaffer 1988). Because there is some evidence linking this condition with seizure disorder, further workup and possible anticonvulsant therapy may be indicated.

The pharmacological treatment of alcoholism after detoxification has been reviewed by Ciraulo and Ciraulo (1988). Essentially, you may want to consider the use of antidepressants, lithium, or disulfiram (Antabuse). Each of these approaches has its pros and cons, and none has been established as being clearly effective in preventing alcoholic relapse. The use of benzodiazepines after "detox" is very controversial, though Ciraulo and Ciraulo (1988) conclude the following:

> There is an important but limited place for benzodiazepines in the treatment of alcoholics. When there is a diagnosable anxiety disorder that persists for 2–3 weeks after detoxification, benzodiazepines may be used. Chlordiazepoxide, oxazepam, and halazepam may have less potential for abuse than other drugs in this class. No greater than a 1-week supply of medication should be given at any one time. Pill counts, urine drug screens, and periodic benzodiazepine plasma levels should be obtained to ensure that dosage is not being escalated and that other drugs are not being taken surreptitiously. (p. 134)

Other authorities generally advise against the use of benzodiazepines in alcoholic patients, and would probably manage a primary anxiety disorder in such patients with a sedating tricyclic (such as doxepin 25 mg/day), buspirone, or a beta-blocker. Certainly, the rationale for use of benzodiazepines should be carefully documented in such cases and consultation obtained.

The use of tricyclics for nondepressed alcoholic patients in the "post-detox" stage may be of some short-term value but has no demonstrable advantage over placebo after about 3 weeks (Guttmacher 1988). Alcoholic patients with a clear-cut "primary" depressive disorder, on the other hand, merit the same pharmacological treatment as do nonalcoholic patients with major depression. The data thus far on the use of lithium have been conflicting, with some studies showing a benefit in maintaining abstinence (Fawcett et al. 1987).

Although the research literature on the efficacy of disulfiram is less than convincing, some specialists advocate its use in certain circumstances (Whitfield 1982). Disulfiram alone is not an appropriate treatment; rather, its use should be part of a comprehensive program including the elements summarized in Table 10–3. The usual dose of disulfiram is 125 to 500 mg/day. Its biochemical effect is to inhibit aldehyde dehydrogenase, the enzyme that breaks down ethanol; in the presence of alcohol, acetaldehyde accumulates, producing the characteristic reaction of flushing, tachycardia, tachypnea, headache, and nausea. Though rare, fatal alcohol-disulfiram reactions have been reported. Disulfiram also inhibits dopamine beta-hydroxylase, the enzyme that converts dopamine to norepinephrine; in theory, and occasionally in fact, this may lead to psychotic symptoms. Keep in mind that even the alcohol contained in aftershave lotion may precipitate an adverse reaction. Disulfiram may also cause hepatic changes, and LFTs should be monitored regularly. Patients should be fully informed of the above concerns and should also be warned that even within 2 weeks of stopping Antabuse (disulfiram), they can experience adverse effects from alcohol.

Psychosocial Approaches

The elements of psychosocial treatment are contained in Table 10–3. However, because the issue of individual psychotherapy often arises, we will look at this in greater detail. Whitfield (1982) has summarized what might be called the "conservative/nondynamic" view:

> If the patient is still drinking, most intensive psychotherapeutic techniques will be to no avail. The initial effort of the psychotherapist should be to work with the patient toward abstinence, and

eventually toward regular participation in group treatment. It is suggested that the psychotherapist utilize a combined confrontative, supportive, and directive approach. . . . individual supportive psychotherapy, which all physicians can provide, is useful to continue the patient's education about the disease . . . and the recovery process; monitor the patient's functioning in important life areas, such as family, job, and interpersonal relations; evaluate the patient's ego strength and psychopathology; and assist the patient in change and growth. (p. 451)

But how will you assist the patient in "change and growth"? Is a psychodynamically oriented approach helpful, or will it only "stir up trouble"? Frances et al. (1989), while acknowledging risks to the psychodynamic approach, still believe it useful for some alcoholic patients. The best candidates are those with "a firmly structured intrapsychic conflict at any psychosexual level that leads to a repeated negative pattern beyond an immediate crisis" (p. 1105–1106) Dynamic therapy is also best suited to patients with "a capacity for insight, intimacy, identification with the therapist, average or superior intelligence, time, money, and high motivation" (Frances et al. 1989, p. 1106). The dynamic approach actually begins with more general supportive maneuvers. But soon "other issues such as problems in self-care, self-esteem, and specific conflicts over assertiveness, problems handling aggression, alcohol's role in either allowing or distancing from a sexual life, and issues around control may become prominent" (Frances et al. 1989, p. 1107).

Insistence on abstinence is essential, and concomitant attendance at AA may be helpful. The therapist must constantly monitor the complex transference and countertransference problems that may develop in working with the alcoholic patient.

Steinglass (1989) has reviewed the indications for "family therapy" in the treatment of alcoholism, citing preliminary evidence of its efficacy. Family treatment may be indicated when "reorganization around the alcoholic symptom has occurred in the family" (p. 1112)—for example, when the family's daily routines, rituals, and problem-solving strategies have begun to revolve around the identified patient's alcoholism.

Emrick (1989) has reviewed the use of AA, concluding that the clinician "should become familiar with AA and its associated organizations [Al-Anon, Alateen] and strive to utilize these self-help resources whenever appropriate" (p. 1162). AA, of course, is a "leaderless group." More conventional group therapeutic approaches to alcoholism have also been used with some success (see Pattison and Brandsma 1989 for a review).

Finally, behavioral approaches to alcoholism have also been advocated (Litman 1989). In behavioral terms, "excessive drinking is seen as a learned response . . . shaped and maintained because of its rewarding consequences" (Litman 1989, p. 1125). Behavioral treatments include the use of "covert sensitization" and "contingency management." The former entails the use of "aversive verbal imagery" coupled with visualization of scenes involving alcohol. Contingency management involves identifying target behaviors to be controlled (e.g., walking past a favorite bar) and finding "effective reinforcers" to counteract these behaviors. (Disulfiram, although sometimes considered a form of "chemical aversion," has been discussed under somatic approaches.)

Opioid (Narcotic) Abuse and Dependence

The prototypic opiates morphine and codeine (3-methoxymorphine) are derived from the juice of the opium poppy, *Papaver somniferum*. The semisynthetic drugs produced from morphine include hydromorphone (Dilaudid), codeine, diacetylmorphine (heroin), and oxycodone. Purely synthetic opioids include meperidine (Demerol), propoxyphene (Darvon), and the "heroin substitute" methadone (Jaffe and Martin 1975). As Schuckit and Segal (1991) note, "Despite claims to the contrary, all of these substances (including almost all prescription analgesics) are capable of producing euphoria as well as psychological and physical dependence when taken in high enough doses over prolonged periods of time" (p. 2151).

Opiates bind to specific types of receptors in the CNS and elsewhere in the body; these receptors in turn mediate the well-known opiate effects of analgesia, respiratory depression, constipation, and euphoria. The classic opioids are mu-receptor agonists. The compounds nalorphine and pentazocine (Talwin) are mixed opiate agonists-antagonists; naloxone and naltrexone are pure antagonists (see discussion of treatment later in this section). Endogenous opiate peptides (enkephalins and endorphins) appear to be natural ligands for opioid receptors and probably play a role in analgesia, memory, learning, and stress tolerance (Daniels and Martin 1991).

The acute effects of opiates on the CNS include nausea, decreased pain perception, euphoria (probably via limbic system effects), and sedation. In larger doses, markedly decreased respirations; bradycardia; pupillary miosis; stupor; and coma may result. Withdrawal from opiates typically produces diarrhea, rhinorrhea, profuse sweating, muscle twitching, mild fever, increased respiration, piloerection ("goose bumps"), and diffuse body pain (Schuckit and Segal 1991). With short-acting opiates such as heroin, morphine, and oxycodone, withdrawal signs (lacrimation, yawning, rhinorrhea, sweating) may begin 8 to 12 hours after the last dose, peak at 48 to 72 hours, and subside over 7 to 10 days. With longer-acting opiates such as methadone, withdrawal usually begins 24 to 48 hours after the last dose, peaks at 3 days or so, and lasts up to several weeks (Ciraulo and Ciraulo 1988).

Epidemiology of Abuse

Epidemiological studies carried out between 1981 and 1983 showed that just under 1% of the population in the United States met DSM-III criteria for opioid abuse or dependence at some time in their lives (Kaplan and Sadock 1988). More than 50% of urban heroin-addicted individuals come from single-parent homes, and many addicted persons have disturbed family relationships (Jaffe and Kleber 1989). Roughly 70% of narcotic-addicted individuals have another psychiatric disorder, usually depression, anxiety, alcoholism, or personality disorder (Dubovsky 1988; Jaffe 1986). Schuckit and Segal (1991) distinguish two broad types of opiate-abusing individuals: the "medical" abuser and the "street" abuser. The medical abuser is often an individual with a chronic pain syndrome who misuses prescribed analgesics. Physicians, nurses, and pharmacists are also at high risk because of their easy access to narcotics. The street abuser is typically a high-functioning individual who began by "experimenting" with tobacco, alcohol, and marijuana; some such street abusers may meet the criteria for antisocial personality disorder. Opiate-abusing individuals have a death rate 2 to 20 times that of the general population; suicide, murder, anaphylactic reactions to intravenously injected impurities, and a high incidence of human immunodeficiency virus (HIV) infection all contribute to this figure (Dubovsky 1988).

Treatment of Clinical Syndromes

Opiate intoxication (e.g., due to overdose) is usually treated with the narcotic antagonist naloxone 0.01 mg/kg im or iv, repeated in 3 to 10 minutes if no response occurs (Schuckit and Segal 1991). It is important to support the patient's vital signs until the body detoxifies the opiate, and to monitor the patient for at least 24 hours after an opiate overdose (longer periods may be required if a long-acting opiate was used). Intravenous fluids and respiratory support may be necessary.

Opiate withdrawal is generally managed using methadone or clonidine (Ciraulo and Ciraulo 1988). The average methadone dose is 30 to 40 mg/day, with larger doses for some tolerant abusers who have been using very high doses of opiates. Although outpatient detoxification is possible, inpatient treatment permits closer monitoring and protection from further illicit drug use. Clonidine, an alpha$_2$ agonist, is used in doses of 0.3 to 0.5 mg/day, with monitoring for possible hypotension and dizziness.

Methadone maintenance is a widely used strategy in the management of opiate addiction. Although methadone may have mood-elevating effects in some addicted individuals, methadone maintenance leads nevertheless to reduced opioid (and nonopioid) drug use, reduced criminal behavior, and decreased depressive symptoms (Jaffe and Kleber 1989). Depending on the nature of the program, maintenance doses can range from 20 to 120 mg/day. The compound L-alpha-acetylmethadol (LAAM) is a long-acting synthetic narcotic substitute that may be given only three times per week; however, some patients experience nervousness and stimulation not commonly seen with methadone.

The partial mu-receptor agonist buprenorphine, when given chronically, blocks the subjective effects of morphine or heroin. In outpatient settings, buprenorphine appears to be as effective as low-dose methadone, but systematic studies are lacking (Jaffe and Kleber 1989). Finally, the narcotic antagonist naltrexone (Trexan) is used in a manner analogous to that of disulfiram (Dubovsky 1988). An oral dose of 150 mg/day will precipitate an abstinence syndrome when the patient uses a narcotic, perhaps leading to a high rate of attrition from treatment. The underlying theory behind the use of narcotic antagonists, however, is that the blocking of opiate effects discourages drug-seeking behavior and thus "deconditions" the addicted individual (Kaplan and Sadock 1988).

Barbiturate Abuse and Dependence

Prior to the advent of benzodiazepines, barbiturates were widely used as sedative-hypnotic agents. Pentobarbital (Nembutal), secobarbital (Seconal), and amobarbital (Amytal) are now under the same federal controls as morphine and have been largely supplanted as sedative-hypnotics by the benzodiazepines. Secobarbital ("reds," "downers"), pentobarbital ("yellow jackets," "nembies"), and combinations of secobarbital and amobarbital ("reds and blues") are common on the black market (Kaplan and Sadock 1988). Intoxication with barbiturates (and other sedative-hypnotics) generally resembles alcohol intoxication: the individual achieves a state of "disinhibition euphoria," characterized by elevated mood, increased energy, and reduced anxiety (Smith et al. 1989). Unsteady gait, slurred speech, memory impairment, and nystagmus may also be seen. Barbiturates are unique among CNS depressants in that as tolerance develops, there is not a concomitant increase in the lethal dose level—as occurs, for example, in opiate addiction. Thus, as the barbiturate-addicted individual uses higher and higher doses to achieve intoxication, he or she comes progressively closer to the lethal dose. The upshot of this is a high rate of accidental fatal barbiturate overdose (Renner and Gastfriend 1991). Withdrawal from barbiturates is not only uncomfortable but also dangerous; abstinence phenomena may include seizures, delirium, and fatal hyperthermia (Ciraulo and Ciraulo 1988).

Epidemiology of Abuse

As Grinspoon and Bakalar (1980) have noted, the availability of barbiturates "on the street" is only part of the problem; many patients are maintained in their habit by well-intentioned physicians. Indeed, chronic intoxication usually occurs in a 30- to 50-year-old person who obtains the barbiturate from a physician rather than from an illegal source. Often, such individuals are of the middle or upper class, and began taking a barbiturate as a prescribed "sleeper." Episodic intoxication, on the other hand, is usually seen in teenagers or young adults who ingest barbiturates to "get high" (Grinspoon and Bakalar 1980). Finally, intravenous barbiturate users are mainly young adults heavily involved in the illegal drug culture and are often identifiable by their large, visible skin abscesses. (Alcoholic individuals may also use barbiturates to relieve the "shakes" during withdrawal.)

Treatment of Clinical Syndromes

Acute barbiturate intoxication is usually evident when serum concentrations of long-acting barbiturates exceed 4 mg/dl (Lovejoy and Linden 1991). Pupils are usually constricted, and hypothermia is common. Initial management involves repetitive administration of activated charcoal; hemodynamic and respiratory support; correction of temperature and electrolyte derangement; and monitoring for pulmonary complications such as pulmonary edema. In severe cases, hemodialysis may be necessary.

Early signs of barbiturate withdrawal include apprehension, muscular weakness, tremor, orthostatic hypotension, anorexia, and myoclonic jerks; by the second or third day, grand mal seizures or delirium may occur. Treatment usually begins by establishing the severity of the patient's tolerance by means of a "test dose" of pentobarbital 200 mg po on an empty stomach. Depending on the degree of intoxication produced—ranging from somnolence to no sign of intoxication at all in extremely tolerant patients—the patient's daily pentobarbital requirement is estimated (see Ciraulo and Ciraulo 1988 for details). A typical daily dose of pentobarbital for moderate tolerance after test dose is 700 mg/day. Some clinicians recommend the longer-acting phenobarbital for stabilization and withdrawal; doses are one-third those suggested for pentobarbital. The total barbiturate requirement is given in divided doses every 6 hours until the patient is stable for 2 to 3 days, and then the dose is reduced by 10% every 1 to 2 days (Dubovsky 1988).

Cocaine and Other Stimulant Abuse

Cocaine Abuse

The National Institute on Drug Abuse has estimated that each day 5,000 people try cocaine for the first time and that over 1,000,000 Americans now abuse cocaine regularly (Albukeirat and Mackler 1992). In 1985, there were over 550 cocaine-related deaths, mainly from myocardial infarctions in relatively healthy individuals (Kaplan and Sadock 1988). Cocaine has taken a sort of downward spiral since the Incas dubbed it a "gift from the Sun God"; but then the Incas chewed wads of coca leaves in a manner that produced stimulation but little euphoria (Kleber 1988). This is a far cry, however, from the effects of "crack" cocaine in our own culture. (Incidentally, yes, Coca-Cola actually did contain cocaine until 1903, when caffeine was substituted as the principal stimulant [Kleber 1988].)

Cocaine ("snow," "coke") is an alkyloid derived from the shrub *Erythroxylon coca,* which is indigenous to Bolivia and Peru. Cocaine and other abused stimulants have multiple actions on multiple neurotransmitters (Volpe 1992). All of these drugs affect dopamine, norepinephrine, serotonin, and acetylcholine. The autonomic arousal produced by cocaine is probably due to its inhibitory effect on norepinephrine reuptake. Cocaine's euphoriant effect is usually attributed to its blockade of dopamine reuptake and to the subsequent effect of dopamine on the mesolimbic and mesocortical "reward pathways" (Volpe 1992). Using animal "self-administration" models, it has been shown that cocaine is a potent reinforcer in rats, cats, dogs, baboons, and virtually every other species tested (Fischman 1988). Cocaine also impairs tryptophan and serotonin metabolism, possibly accounting for its disruptive effects on sleep (Volpe 1992).

In humans, cocaine produces consistent self-reported psychological changes (e.g., increased "vigor and arousal," self-confidence, friendliness, talkativeness, and sense of well-being). Such benign effects pass quickly into cocaine intoxication, characterized by extreme agitation, irritability, impaired judgment, aggressiveness, impulsive sexual behavior, and manic excitement. Drug-induced paranoid psychosis is not uncommon. Tachycardia, hypertension, and mydriasis are accompanying features (Kaplan and Sadock 1988). Cocaine intoxication is usually short-lived—on average, full recovery occurs within 48 hours, assuming no cardiovascular or neurological complications. Unfortunately, fatal cardiac events, rupture of preexisting atrioventricular malformations, seizures, transient neurological deficits, and intracranial hemorrhage have all been observed in connection with cocaine abuse (Albukeirat and Mackler 1992).

The most common route of cocaine administration is intranasal— that is, "snorting" the drug in the form of a white powder. Peak plasma levels are achieved in this way within about 30 minutes; most users are "ready" for another dose about 50 minutes after first inhaling the drug (Fischman 1988). Intravenous cocaine use is popular among "serious" abusers; this route causes an intense "rush" within a minute or two. (Bear in mind the risk of HIV infection in this subgroup.) In recent years, two heat-stable, smokable forms of cocaine have been produced. "Freebase" cocaine requires elaborate equipment to produce and flammable solvents such as ether; in contrast, "crack" is easily and cheaply made by mixing cocaine with baking soda and water. In either case, the cocaine is absorbed efficiently through the lungs and goes very rapidly to the brain. Blood levels peak almost immediately, which produces a rapid, intense "rush." Withdrawal, craving, reintoxication, and withdrawal occur in rapid cycles that can propel the "crack" user for many days.

Even if recovery from intoxication is routine, the abusing individual faces the discomfort of cocaine abstinence. This first ("crash") phase of abstinence may mimic major depression with melancholia and may be more akin to the alcoholic individual's "hangover" than to true withdrawal (Gawin 1988). The second phase—true withdrawal—begins 12 hours to 1 week after the last use of cocaine and is characterized by a constellation of symptoms: anhedonia, anergia, hypersomnia, lethargy, craving for cocaine, anxiety, and irritability (Gawin 1988). Suicidal ideation may also be present. (Some of these effects may relate to depletion of dopamine stores in individuals who chronically abuse cocaine.) Over the course of the ensuing 1 to 10 weeks, these depressive symptoms usually "clear up," unless, of course, there is an underlying major depression that the abusing individual was "treating" with cocaine. A full discussion of comorbidity and "dual diagnosis" would take us far afield, but you should know that in four systematic studies using DSM-III criteria (American Psychiatric Association 1980), chronic affective disorders were present in nearly 50% of stimulant-abusing individuals seeking treatment (Gawin 1988). Stimulant abuse is also quite common among schizophrenic patients, and one can speculate on the role these dopaminergic agents play in the "self-medication" of negative features in schizophrenia (Lehman et al. 1989). Finally, we should note that many cocaine-abusing individuals also abuse alcohol and that the combination of these drugs produces a potent and highly addictive euphoriant compound called cocaethylene (Randall 1992). Other addicted individuals combine cocaine with heroin in the so-called speedball—often a deadly combination, as the death of actor John Belushi demonstrated.

Epidemiology of Abuse

There are indications that cocaine use in general has "leveled off" or even declined in recent years, but use of "crack" may not be following this pattern (Kleber 1988; Pope et al. 1990). Although weekly cocaine use among college seniors apparently declined from 30% to 20% between 1978 and 1989, this is still a substantial number of users. There seems to be a correlation—if not a causal link—between marijuana use and subsequent cocaine use. Kleber (1988) hypothesizes that "once a person breaks a certain psychological barrier with marijuana, the likelihood of trying an even 'better' drug increases" (p. 5). During the 1970s and 1980s, cocaine use "spread from the jet set to the business community to the sports world and finally to lower socioeconomic groups and to adolescents of all socioeconomic groups" (Kleber 1988, p. 4).

Treatment of Clinical Syndromes

Cocaine intoxication, if uncomplicated by delirium, extreme paranoia, or urgent medical problems, does not require active treatment beyond observation over 24 hours or so (Gawin and Ellinwood 1989). On the other extreme, treatment of cocaine overdose is a medical emergency, calling for control of ventricular arrythmias, hypertension, tachycardia, tonic-clonic seizures, and so forth (Mendelson and Mello 1991). "Middle cases" may come to the attention of psychiatrists because intoxicated patients may appear hypomanic, manic, or transiently delusional. Anderson and Tesar (1991) recommend the use of a small amount of a high-potency antipsychotic in such cases (e.g., haloperidol 2 to 5 mg im), but keep in mind the risk of lowering the seizure threshold with neuroleptics. Lorazepam 1 to 2 mg im might be a reasonable alternative.

Cocaine abstinence and withdrawal, although distinctly unpleasant, generally remit spontaneously. However, preliminary evidence suggests that two classes of medication—dopamine agonists and tricyclics—may reduce cocaine craving in the short-term (Gawin 1988). Amantadine and bromocriptine have been the most commonly used dopamine agonists, but there are few well-controlled studies demonstrating long-term efficacy. Methylphenidate may be of use in cocaine-abusing individuals with residual or preexisting attention-deficit/hyperactivity disorder (ADHD) (Khantzian 1983). Of the tricyclics, desipramine has been most studied, though trazodone and imipramine have also been used. While desipramine does seem to reduce cocaine craving and use, conclusive trials are still pending (Gawin 1988). Although, in theory, monoamine oxidase inhibitors could be useful, cocaine relapse would present a grave risk of hypertensive encephalopathy. It is still too early to know whether the selective serotonin reuptake inhibitors will prove useful in treating cocaine abstinence, but preliminary data are not impressive.

Pharmacotherapy should be only one component in the overall

approach to cocaine abuse (Millman 1988). Initial evaluation requires a thorough assessment for concurrent use of alcohol, opiates, and other drugs of abuse; medical complications (e.g., excoriated ulcers due to picking at "cocaine bugs"); and premorbid psychopathology. In addition to educating the patient about cocaine itself, the clinician must help the patient to end drug-related associations and activities and to form a carefully selected support network. The basic components of treatment are summarized in Table 10–4, following Millman (1988).

Continued participation in 12-step–type groups is also important, although such groups sometimes take an "antipsychiatric" stance, which may interfere with treatment of comorbid mood disorders or other psychopathology. Cognitive-behavioral, supportive-expressive, and interpersonal psychotherapies have all been used with some success (Millman 1988). However, in my own experience, failure to treat the cocaine abuse as a "primary problem" is a sure prescription for relapse. Whatever the patient's comorbid or premorbid psychopathology (cf. Khantzian 1985), the actual use of cocaine must be brought under control before psychotherapy (or pharmacotherapy, for that

Table 10–4. Preventing cocaine relapse: initial treatment

Help the patient recognize warning signs of relapse.

Help the patient combat "euphoric recall" (i.e., the tendency to remember only positive aspects of cocaine use).

Help the patient avoid the temptation to "master" use of cocaine (e.g., using it "once in a while").

Reinforce negative aspects of cocaine use (e.g., "crashing," getting in trouble with the police or family, etc.).

Help the patient avoid powerful conditioned stimuli for cocaine use (e.g., cocaine pipes, white powder, old "drug contacts," etc.).

Insulate "slips" so that they do not become full-blown relapses.

Teach the patient adaptive ways of coping with depression and other feelings that used to elicit drug craving.

Help the patient develop rewarding alternatives to drugs.

Source. Extensively modified from Millman 1988.

matter) can succeed. Gawin and Ellinwood (1989) recommend the use of hospitalization and/or pharmacotherapy (discussed earlier in this section) if abstinence does not closely follow initiation of outpatient treatment.

Amphetamine Abuse

Although we have focused on cocaine, amphetamine abuse may be making a comeback, after a decade of decreased use (Gawin and Ellinwood 1989). Amphetamines are usually taken orally but can be injected or snorted (Kaplan and Sadock 1990). Recently, a smokable form of methamphetamine—"crystal methamphetamine" (or "crystal")—has appeared as a frequent cause of toxic psychosis; in Hawaii, "crystal" seems to have replaced "crack" as the drug of choice (Jackson 1989).

The signs and symptoms of acute amphetamine abuse are similar to those of cocaine intoxication, and, as with cocaine, a "let-down" or "crash" occurs with sudden abstinence. A cycle of "runs" (i.e., heavy use for several days) and crashes is seen with amphetamine abuse, much as with the use of "crack," though the time interval between uses is generally longer with amphetamines. (The half-life of amphetamines, at more than 4 hours, is longer than that of cocaine, which has a half-life of about an hour.) In the general hospital setting, the most common type of amphetamine abuse involves the patient who began using amphetamines to control obesity and who later became a chronic abuser (Renner and Gastfriend 1991). The other classic syndrome is a paranoid psychosis in the absence of delirium; this psychosis is often confused with an acute schizophreniform psychosis but is usually brief and self-limited. (An exception to this may be psychosis due to "crystal" abuse, which may present as a paranoid psychosis with auditory hallucinations lasting several days or even weeks.) Acidification of the urine using ammonium chloride may speed elimination of amphetamine, and a brief course of antipsychotic medication may be helpful in diminishing paranoia. Lorazepam or clonazepam may be useful in controlling hyperactivity and agitation, and antihypertensives may be necessary. Postamphetamine depression often extends for several months and may respond to antidepressants;

however, well-controlled studies are lacking (Renner and Gastfriend 1991). Finally, amphetamine-like reactions have also been reported with abuse of phenylpropanolamine (Dietz 1981).

Integrated Case History

Mr. Snow was 34-year-old single businessman who had been referred to the outpatient psychiatry service by his family practitioner. The diagnosis was "cocaine abuse," but the patient minimized this by stating, "My family doc worries too much." The patient acknowledged cocaine use "now and then" via the nasal route. He denied any history of intravenous drug use. According to Mr. Snow and confirmatory school history, the patient had a long history of disturbed behavior. In elementary school, he had been "hard to manage," with a history of mild conduct disturbance and disciplinary actions. The term "hyperactive" had been used in one report by the school psychologist. The patient was thought of as "bright," however, and had done fairly well in junior high and high school, despite disciplinary problems related to marijuana use. He obtained a business degree from a 2-year college and had functioned quite successfully, running his own florist business. In his mid-20s, the patient began to experience what he called "feeling in the pits for weeks on end." During these episodes, the patient exprienced anhedonia, insomnia, poor appetite, and fleeting suicidal ideation. He stated that he first began using cocaine "to get myself out of the blues." However, after "getting in with a bunch of guys who like to do dope," the patient's cocaine use became more frequent. (According to his family practitioner, the patient would snort cocaine four to five times per week.) The psychiatrist—concerned with the patient's minimizing and the "social circles" fostering his habit—advised a brief inpatient "detox" on a dual-diagnosis unit. The patient reluctantly agreed to this. On the inpatient unit, the treatment team concluded that Mr. Snow suffered from adult ADHD, with superimposed recurrent major depression. Although Mr. Snow's cocaine habit had evolved into an autonomous "disorder," the team felt that a trial on methylphenidate (20 mg/day) would be worthwhile. After 3 weeks, the patient reported feeling "calmer than I can remember feeling in years . . . and not as down." He attended groups on the unit aimed at teaching cocaine users to recognize the warning signs of relapse, to avoid "cocaine cues" (e.g., old social contacts), and to cope with depression in adaptive ways. He was referred to a 12-step program but was maintained on methylphenidate.

Marijuana (THC)

The brevity of our discussion of marijuana should not persuade you that marijuana is a "benign," "harmless," or merely "recreational" drug. To be sure, the damage done by marijuana pales before that of alcohol or cocaine. And it is probably true that infrequent use of marijuana—say, three or four times a year—poses few problems for the majority of users. Nevertheless, marijuana and its chief active ingredient, delta-9-tetrahydrocannabinol (THC), can produce subtle psychological problems in some individuals and severe reactions in a few. Mild intoxication usually produces a subjective sense of relaxation and mild euphoria, accompanied by some impairment in thinking, concentration, and visuomotor function (Mendelson and Mello 1991). These effects are heavily colored by the user's expectations and environment. High doses tend to produce behavioral effects similar to those in severe alcohol intoxication, and may precipitate severe emotional reactions in persons with premorbid neurotic or psychotic disorders (e.g., panic attacks, paranoia, or visual hallucinations). Inexperienced users partaking of "strong" marijuana preparations may be especially prone to such adverse reactions. According to Anderson and Tesar (1991),"rest and reassurance is generally all that is required, with recovery in a few hours" (p. 461). Earlier reports of a specific "amotivational syndrome" and cannabis-induced brain atrophy have not been confirmed; nonetheless, "chronic marijuana abusers may lose interest in common socially desirable goals and devote progressively more time to drug acquisition and use" (Mendelson and Mellow 1991, p. 2156). Mild withdrawal effects can also occur with chronic use, with severity related to dosage and duration of use. Recently, a case report suggested that fluoxetine-marijuana interaction may precipitate mania, perhaps via a serotonergic mechanism (Stoll et al. 1991).

Phencyclidine

Phencyclidine (PCP, "angel dust") is actually a dissociative anesthetic used in veterinary medicine; that is, it dissociates pain perception from conscious awareness. Perhaps this accounts, in part, for anecdotal reports of PCP users breaking handcuffs and fracturing the bones of their wrists, and yet experiencing no pain! Recent surveys suggest an increase in phencyclidine use, whether taken by mouth, by cigarette, or by injection; it is also used as an adulterant in THC, LSD, amphetamine, and cocaine (Mendelson and Mello 1991). PCP intoxication may mimic an "acute schizophrenic reaction," and there is considerable theoretical interest in a "phencyclidine model" of schizophrenia. (Phencyclidine interacts with NMDA receptors, which respond to the excitatory amino acid neurotransmitter glutamate; it has been suggested that the psychotomimetic effects of PCP are related to effects on the NMDA receptor [Javitt and Zukin 1990].) PCP can produce a highly variable clinical picture, ranging from stupor to violent agitation; Anderson and Tesar (1991) note that "a quiet patient [on PCP] is not necessarily reassuring" (p. 461). Multidirectional nystagmus, hypertension, tachycardia, and elevated CPK (perhaps reflecting muscle damage during struggling) are common associated findings. The components of management include physical restraint in severe cases, acidification of the urine, and symptomatic use of high-potency antipsychotics, benzodiazepines, or beta-blockers. (Note that if CPK is very high, acidification of the urine should be deferred because of the risk of precipitating myoglobin in the renal tubules.) Phenothiazines should be avoided in the early stages of toxicity because their (central) anticholinergic side effects may add to those of phencyclidine and thus worsen the psychosis.

Other Drugs of Abuse

We have certainly not provided "exhaustive coverage" of the many possible drugs of abuse. Thus, we have noted LSD only in passing, despite the occasional appearance of the patient who has "dropped some acid." We have said virtually nothing about nicotine, despite the following appropriate caveat from J. R. Hughes et al. (1992): "In reality, smoking causes three times the number of deaths as all other forms of drug abuse combined, can be as intractable as other severe dependencies, and is linked to several psychiatric disorders" (p. 1118). It is hoped that the references provided will encourage you to pursue the topic of substance abuse in more detail.

Conclusion

A particularly vexing problem for the psychiatrist today is the so-called dual-diagnosis patient—a problem we have only adumbrated here. As Osher and Kofoed (1989) note, dually diagnosed patients, compared with either psychiatrically ill or chemically dependent patients, show increased rates of hospitalization, homelessness, criminal acts, and suicidal behavior. Dual-diagnosis patients also show poor medication compliance and poor response to traditional substance abuse treatment. We need vastly improved methods of both diagnosing and treating these patients. Certainly any psychiatric evaluation is deficient if it does not include a detailed inquiry regarding alcohol and other drugs of abuse. And because patients frequently conceal or minimize their illicit drug use, you should strongly consider obtaining blood and urine "screens" for illicit drugs when evaluating suspicious cases. Ongoing attention to both the psychiatric and the substance-related disorder is critical. We might profitably close with this observation by Osher and Kofoed (1989): "Abstinence is not the end of substance abuse treatment for the dually diagnosed patient. . . . maintenance requires an ongoing connection between the patient and trusted health care providers" (p. 1027).

References

American Psychiatric Association: Diagnostic and Statistical Manual of Mental Disorders, 3rd Edition. Washington, DC, American Psychiatric Association, 1980
American Psychiatric Association: Diagnostic and Statistical Manual of Mental Disorders, 3rd Edition, Revised. Washington, DC, American Psychiatric Association, 1987

American Psychiatric Association: Diagnostic and Statistical Manual of Mental Disorders, 4th Edition. Washington, DC, American Psychiatric Association, 1994

Anderson WH, Tesar G: The emergency room, in Massachusetts General Hospital Handbook of General Hospital Psychiatry, 3rd Edition. Edited by Cassem NH. St Louis, MO, Mosby Year Book, 1991, pp 445–464

Albukeirat FA, Mackler SA: The epidemic of cocaine-related neurologic catastrophies. Resident and Staff Physician 38:33–40, 1992

Balint M: The Basic Fault. London, Tavistock, 1969

Ballenger JC, Post RM: Kindling as a model for alcohol withdrawal syndromes. Br J Psychiatry 133:1–14, 1978

Begleiter H, Porjesz B, Tenner M: Neuroradiological and neurophysiological evidence of brain deficits in chronic alcoholics. Acta Psychiatr Scand Suppl 286(Vol 62):3–13, 1980

Blum K, Noble EP, Sheridan PJ, et al: Allelic association of human dopamine D_2 receptor gene in alcoholism. JAMA 263:2055–2060, 1990

Ciraulo DA, Ciraulo AM: Substance abuse, in Handbook of Clinical Psychopharmacology. Edited by Tupin JP, Shader RI, Harnett DS. Northvale, NJ, Jason Aronson, 1988, pp 121–158

Cloninger CR: Neuogenetic adaptive mechanisms in alcoholism. Science 236:410–416, 1987

Cloninger CR, Bohman M, Sigvardsonn S: Inheritance of alcohol abuse: cross fostering analysis of adopted men. Arch Gen Psychiatry 38:861–868, 1981

Cummings JL: Clinical Neuropsychiatry. Orlando, FL, Grune & Stratton, 1985

Daniels GH, Martin JB: Neuroendocrine regulation and diseases of the anterior pituitary and hypothalamus, in Harrison's Principles of Internal Medicine, 12th Edition. Edited by Wilson JD, Braunwald E, Isselbacher KJ, et al. New York, McGraw-Hill, 1991, pp 1655–1678

Dano P, Le Guyader J: Cerebral atropy and chronic alcoholism. Rev Neurol (Paris) 144:202–208, 1988

Dietz AJ: Amphetamine-like reactions to phenylpropanol amine. JAMA 245:601–602, 1981

Dinwiddie SH, Cloninger CR: Family and adoption studies in alcoholism and drug addiction. Psychiatric Annals 21:206–213, 1991

Donovan JM: An etiologic model of alcoholism. Am J Psychiatry 143:1–11, 1986

Dubovsky SL: Concise Guide to Clinical Psychiatry. Washington DC, American Psychiatric Press, 1988

Emrick CD: Alcoholics Anonymous, in Treatments of Psychiatric Disorders, Vol 2. Washington, DC, American Psychiatric Association, 1989, pp 1151–1162

Fawcett J, Clark DC, Aagesen CA, et al: A double-blind placebo-controlled trial of lithium carbonate therapy for alcoholism. Arch Gen Psychiatry 44:248–256, 1987

Fischman MW: Behavioral pharmacology of cocaine. J Clin Psychiatry 49 (No 2, Suppl):7–10, 1988

Frances RJ, Khantzian EJ, Tamerin JS: Psychodynamic psychotherapy, in Treatments of Psychiatric Disorders, Vol 2. Washington, DC, American Psychiatric Association, 1989, pp 1103–1110

Fujimoto A, Nagao T, Ebara T, et al: Cerebrospinal fluid monamine metabolites during alcohol withdrawal syndome and recovered state. Biol Psychiatry 18:1141–1152, 1983

Gawin FH: Chronic neuropharmacology of cocaine: progress in pharmacotherapy. J Clin Psychiatry 49 (No 2, Suppl):11–16, 1988

Gawin FH, Ellinwood EH: Stimulants, in Treatments of Psychiatric Disorders, Vol 2. Washington, DC, American Psychiatric Association, 1989, pp 1218–1240

Giannini AJ, Miller NS: Biopsychiatric approach to drug abuse. Resident and Staff Physician 37:47–52, 1991

Goodwin DW: Alcoholism and alcoholic psychosis, in Comprehensive Textbook of Psychiatry/IV, 4th Edition, Vol 1. Edited by Kaplan HI, Sadock BJ. Baltimore, MD, Williams & Wilkins, 1985, pp 1016–1025

Greenblatt DJ: Benzodiazepine hypnotics: sorting the pharmacokinetic facts. J Clin Psychiatry 52 (No 2, Suppl):4–10, 1991

Grinspoon LG, Bakalar JB: Drug dependence: nonnarcotic agents, in Comprehensive Textbook of Psychiatry/III, 3rd Edition, Vol 2. Edited by Kaplan HI, Freedman AM, Sadock BJ. Baltimore, MD, Williams & Wilkins 1980, pp 1614–1628

Guttmacher LB: Somatic Therapies in Psychiatry. Washington, DC, American Psychiatric Press, 1988

Hackett TP, Gastfriend DR, Renner JA: Alcoholism: acute and chronic states, in The Massachusetts General Hospital Handbook of General Hospital Psychiatry, Littleton, MA, Mosby Year Book, 1991, pp 9–22

Hughes JR, Bickel WK, Higgins ST: Alcohol and addictions (letter). Am J Psychiatry 149:1118, 1992

Hughes PH, Conard SE, Baldwin DC, et al: Resident physician substance use in the United States. JAMA 265:2069–2073, 1991

Jackson JG: Hazards of smokable methamphetamine. N Engl J Med 321:907, 1989

Jaffe JH: Drug addiction and drug abuse, in The Pharmacological Basis of Therapeutics, 5th Edition. Edited by Goodman LS, Gilman A. New York, Macmillan, 1975, pp 284–324

Jaffe JH: Opioids, in Psychiatry Update: The American Psychiatric Press Annual Review, Vol 5. Edited by Frances AJ, Hales RE. Washington,

DC, American Psychiatric Press, 1986, pp 137–159

Jaffe JH, Kleber HD: Opioids: general issues and detoxification, in Treatments of Psychiatric Disorders, Vol 2. Washington, DC, American Psychiatric Association, 1989, pp 1309–1331

Jaffe JH, Martin WR; Narcotic analgesics and antagonists, in The Pharmacological Basis of Therapeutics, 5th Edition. Edited by Goodman LS, Gilman A. New York, Macmillan, 1975, pp 245–283

Javitt DC, Zukin SR: The role of excitatory amino acids in neuropsychiatric illness. J Neuropsychiatry Clin Neurosci 2:44–52, 1990

Kaplan HI, Sadock BJ: Synopsis of Psychiatry, 5th Edition. Baltimore, MD, Williams & Wilkins, 1988

Khantzian EJ: Cocaine dependence: an extreme case and marked improvement with methylphenidate treatment. Am J Psychiatry 140:784–785, 1983

Khantzian EJ: The self-medication hypothesis of addictive disorders: focus on heroine and cocaine dependence. Am J Psychiatry 142:1259–1264, 1985

Kleber HD: Cocaine abuse: historical, epidemiological, and psychological perspectives. J Clin Psychiatry 49 (No 2, Suppl):3–6, 1988

Kushner MG, Sher KJ, Beitman BD: The relation between alcohol problems and the anxiety disorders. Am J Psychiatry 147:685–695, 1990

Lehman AF, Myers CP, Corty E: Assessment and classification of patients with psychiatric and substance abuse syndromes. Hosp Community Psychiatry 40:1019–1025, 1989

Lishman WA: Organic Psychiatry, 2nd Edition. Oxford, UK, Blackwell Scientific, 1987

Litman G: Behavior therapy, in Treatments of Psychiatric Disorders, Vol 2. Washington, DC, American Psychiatric Association, 1989, pp 1125–1131

Lovejoy FH, Linden CH: Acute poison and drug overdosage, in Harrison's Principles of Internal Medicine, 12th Edition. Edited by Wilson JD, Braunwald E, Isselbacher KJ, et al. New York, McGraw-Hill, 1991, pp 2163–2182

Magliozzi Jr, Schaffer CB: Psychosis, in Handbook of Clinical Psychopharmacology. Edited by Tupin JP, Shader RI, Harnett DS. Northvale, NJ, Jason Aronson, 1988, pp 1–48

Maletsky BM: The diagnosis of pathological intoxication. J Stud Alcohol 37:1215–1228, 1976

McNeil GN: Anxiety, in Handbook of Psychiatric Differential Diagnosis. Edited by Soreff SM, McNeil GN. Littleton, MA, PSG Publishing, 1987, pp 1–56

Mello NK, Mendelson JH: Alcoholism: a biobehavioral disorder, in American Handbook of Psychiatry, 2nd Edition, Vol 4. Edited by Arieti S. New York, Basic Books, 1975, pp 371–403

Mendelson JH, Mello NK: Commonly abused drugs, in Harrison's Principles of Internal Medicine, 12th Edition. Edited by Wilson JD, Braunwald E, Isselbacher KJ, et al. New York, McGraw-Hill, 1991, pp 2155–2157

Meyer RG. The Clinician's Handbook of Psychopathology of Adulthood and Late Adolescence. Boston, MA, Allyn & Bacon, 1983

Millman RB: Evaluation and clinical management of cocaine abusers. J Clin Psychiatry 49 (No 2, Suppl):27–33, 1988

Newmark CS: Major Psychological Assessment Instruments. Boston, MA, Allyn & Bacon, 1985

Osher RC, Kofoed LL: Treatment of patients with psychiataric and psychoactive substance abuse disorders. Hosp Community Psychiatry 40:1025–1030, 1989

O'Sullivan K, Whillans P, Daly M, et al: A comparison of alcoholics with and without co-existing affective disorder. Br J Psychiatry 143:133–138, 1983

Pattison EM, Brandsma JM: Group therapy, in Treatments of Psychiatric Disorders, Vol 2. Washington, DC, American Psychiatric Association, 1989, pp 1117–1124

Paul SM: Drugs, receptors, and brain messenger systems. Presentation at "New Frontiers in Neuropsychiatry: A Practical Update," CME, Inc, Montreal, August 7, 1992

Pollock VE, Volavka J, Goodwin DW, et al: The EEG after alcohol administration in men at risk for alcoholism. Arch Gen Psychiatry 40:857–861, 1983

Pollock VE, Schneider LS, Gabrielli WF, et al: Sex of parent and offspring in the transmission of alcoholism: a meta-analysis. J Nerv Ment Dis 175:668–673, 1987

Pope HG Jr, Ionescu-Pioggia M, Aizley HG, et al: Drug use and lifestyle among college undergraduates in 1989: a comparison with 1969 and 1978. Am J Psychiatry 147:998–1001, 1990

Randall T: Cocaine, alcohol mix in body to form even longer lasting, more lethal drug. JAMA 267:1043–1044, 1992

Renner JA, Gastfriend DR: Drug addiction, in Massachusetts General Hospital Handbook of General Hospital Psychiatry, 3rd Edition. St Louis, MO, Mosby Year Book, 1991, pp 23–38

Schuckit MA: Biological vulnerability to alcoholism. J Consult Clin Psychol 55:301–309, 1987

Schuckit MA: Alcohol and alcoholism, in Harrison's Principles of Internal Medicine, 12th Edition. Edited by Wilson JD, Braunwald E, Isselbacher KJ, et al. New York, McGraw-Hill, 1991, pp 2146–2150

Schuckit MA, Segal DS: Opioid drug use, in Harrison's Principles of Internal Medicine, 12th Edition. Edited by Wilson JD, Braunwald E, Isselbacher KJ, et al. New York, McGraw-Hill, 1991, pp 2151–2154

Schuckit MA, Irwin M, Mahler HIM: Tridimensional personality questionnaire scores of sons of alcoholic and non-alcoholic fathers. Am J Psychiatry 147:481–487, 1990

Smith DE, Landry MJ, Wesson DR: Barbiturate, sedative, hypnotic agents, in Treatments of Psychiatric Disorders, Vol 2. Washington, DC, American Psychiatric Association, 1989, pp 1294–1308

Steinglass P: Family therapy, in Treatments of Psychiatric Disorders, Vol 2. Washington, DC, American Psychiatric Association, 1989, pp 1111–1117

Stoll AL, Cole JO, Likas SE: A case of mania as a result of fluoxetine-marijuana interaction. J Clin Psychiatry 52:280–281, 1991

Tarter RE, McBride H, Buonpane N, et al: Differentiation of alcoholics. Arch Gen Psychiatry 34:761–768, 1977

Vaillant GE, Bovowale NC, McArthur C: Some psychologic vulnerabilities of physicians. N Engl J Med 287:372–375, 1975

Volpe JJ: Effect of cocaine use on the fetus. N Engl J Med 327:399–404, 1992

Whitfield CL: Outpatient management of the alcoholic patient. Psychiatric Annals 12:447–458, 1982

Zimberg S: Individual management and psychotherapy, in Treatments of Psychiatric Disorders, Vol 2. Washington, DC, American Psychiatric Association, 1989, pp 1093–1102

Conclusion

Long textbooks often conclude with high-minded gener-
alities; these, of course, are rarely read. Let us instead
conclude our examination of psychiatric diagnosis and treatment with
a case that brings forward a wealth of specifics—and, I hope, ties
together many aspects of the biopsychosocial approach we have labored over at length.

Vignette

The patient was a 23-year-old female referred by the inpatient
psychiatric service for psychopharmacological consultation. Her admission to the inpatient unit was precipitated by suicidal ideation
related to the imminent death of her grandmother. The patient had
made statements to the effect that "maybe I should beat my grandmother to the punch." The patient had a nearly lifelong history of
psychiatric disturbance, beginning as early as the third grade, at
which time the she was "hearing my name being called." There was
evidence of significant physical and sexual abuse during childhood,
and the patient carried diagnoses of posttraumatic stress disorder
(PTSD) and recurrent major depression with psychotic features.
There was also a strong suggestion of complex partial seizures,
though several electroencephalograms (EEGs) had failed to show
evidence of a clear seizure focus. There was, however, a history of
head trauma, including head banging. There was no history of
significant substance abuse.

I would like to thank James Uhl, M.D., and Richard I. Shader, M.D., for their
helpful comments on the case presented in this chapter.

The patient's typical symptom complex included visual and tactile hallucinations, as well as auditory distortions or hallucinations such as "hearing bees in the wall." She described episodic sensations of "rats crawling on my skin." Occasionally, she would hear "a million voices"; at other times, she would hear a specific "voice" of a derogatory nature ("telling me why people hate me"). The patient could not identify this voice. She also experienced episodes in which her visual field would constrict in a tunnel-like manner, during which, as she described it, "words get stuck in my brain." Typically, the patient would be unable to carry on a conversation with others during these episodes but could hear what others were saying. At other times, the patient experienced what she herself described as "dissociative episodes," during which she would reexperience traumata from childhood (principally sexual abuse by family members). She would have these "flashbacks" as often as once a day, sometimes precipitated by trauma-related stimuli, sometimes spontaneously. There was no history clearly suggestive of fugue states or alternate identities.

The patient related a history of compulsive and/or self-injurious behavior, principally "scrubbing my body clean until my skin is raw." She related this behavior to the sense of "feeling dirty . . . not literally, but in a shameful sense." This "scrubbing" would bring some transient psychic relief, but the behavior would usually resume within a few hours.

On mental status examination, the patient was alert and cooperative. She admitted occasional suicidal ideation. Her affect was surprisingly cheerful in relation to her mood. There was no formal thought process disorder, loose associations, and so forth. She was oriented to day and date, and recalled three of three items at 2 and 5 minutes. Serial sevens were within normal limits, and her drawing of a clock face reading "ten past two" was also normal.

Laboratory data and physical examination were unremarkable.

The patient's current pharmacological regimen included clozapine, trazodone, valproate, and sertraline. Past trials had included carbamazepine, lithium, phenelzine, fluoxetine, and nortriptyline; none had been especially effective except phenelzine, which "worked pretty well" for the patient's depressive symptoms.

What can we say about such a polymorphous presentation? How would you diagnose and treat such a patient? My first inclination is generally to presume that visual and tactile hallucinations are "organic" in origin, until proved otherwise. We would certainly wonder if a seizure focus in the temporal or occipital region might be provoking some of this patient's experiences, despite the "negative" electroencephalographic results. On the other hand, many peculiar visual, tactile, and auditory perceptions might be expected as posttraumatic dissociative phenomena.

But what about the patient's experience of a voice "telling me why people hate me"? Isn't this the sort of Schneiderian auditory hallucination characteristic of schizophrenia? Or could it be consistent with a psychotic depression? On the other hand, could the bizarre, multimodal nature of the patient's internal perceptions point to a malingered illness? Or is the experience of "tunnel vision" more consistent with conversion disorder?

And what do we make of the patient's ritualized "scrubbing"? Is this part of an obsessive-compulsive disorder? Or does the connection to "feeling dirty" mark this as a symptom of major depression with psychotic features, or schizoaffective disorder? Can the entire clinical picture be explained most parsimoniously by a diagnosis of borderline personality disorder (BPD)? Is the patient "pathologically fused" to her ailing grandmother, such that the death of this "parenting" figure is tantamount to the death of the self?

I believe that the first thing a clinician should do in a case like this is admit confusion; this serves as an excellent antidote to premature closure or simplistic recommendations to the patient and referring physician. The next step is to seek consultation with an experienced colleague. After so doing, I was in a position to present my conclusions and recommendations to the referring psychiatrist.

I felt that the most parsimonious explanation of the patient's symptoms was a twofold diagnosis on Axis I: PTSD with dissociative features, and recurrent major depression with compulsive and psychotic features. On Axis II, I strongly suspected BPD. Despite the normal electroencephalograms, I listed complex partial seizures as a "rule out" on Axis III. (I could have listed the DSM-III-R designation "organic hallucinosis due to complex partial seizures" as a "r/o" on Axis I.)

I felt that extended psychotherapy was the most important intervention in this case. Treatment would follow the approaches we outlined in our discussion of PTSD (see Chapter 6) and BPD (see Chapter 9). As we noted in these earlier sections, neither PTSD nor BPD responds spectacularly well to pharmacological approaches. Indeed, both patients and therapists can develop inappropriate, "magical" expectations as to what medication can accomplish in such cases. Nevertheless, I felt that a trial on one or more serotonergic agents (e.g, paroxetine or fluvoxamine) would be worthwhile, aiming at the depressive, compulsive, and self-injurious dimensions of the patient's picture. (Serotonergic agents also show promise in PTSD.) Because an earlier trial on phenelzine had proved helpful, I suggested this as another option, noting that a trial on a monoamine oxidase inhibitor was incompatible with use of a selective serotonin reuptake inhibitor. Because clozapine had not proved especially helpful in this case—and carries with it a 1% incidence of agranulocytosis—I suggested that this could be replaced with a standard antipsychotic if clear signs of psychosis were present. I further advised obtaining a BEAM (brain electrical activity mapping) scan and neurological consultation to assess the role of temporal lobe pathology; if temporal lobe epilepsy emerged as a significant factor, trial on carbamazepine might be considered.

We have seen how this patient's clinical picture straddles several diagnostic categories: mood, anxiety, dissociative, somatoform, and personality disorders, and perhaps medical conditions as well. It should be clear by now that no simple model of psychopathology can completely explain this patient's symptoms, nor can a single treatment modality resolve them. The use of a complex biopsychosocial approach is our best hope in such a case—and this, after all, is the principal lesson we have been inculcating these many pages. All the rest is commentary.

Index

*Page numbers printed in **boldface** type refer to tables or figures.*